Progress in Child Health

Progress in Child Health
VOLUME ONE

EDITED BY

J A Macfarlane MB BChir MRCP
Consultant Paediatrician with special interest
in Child Health; Clinical Lecturer in Paediatrics,
University of Oxford

CHURCHILL LIVINGSTONE
EDINBURGH LONDON MELBOURNE AND NEW YORK 1984

CHURCHILL LIVINGSTONE
Medical Division of Longman Group Limited

Distributed in the United States of America by
Churchill Livingstone Inc., 1560 Broadway, New York,
N.Y. 10036, and by associated companies, branches and
representatives throughout the world.

First published 1984

ISBN 0 443 02791 9

British Library Cataloguing in Publication Data
Progress in child health.—Vol. 1
    1. Children—Care and hygiene—Periodicals
    613'.0432'05   RJ101

Printed in Singapore
by Richard Clay Pte Ltd

Preface

Progress in Child Health is a new venture to cover a rapidly expanding and very controversial field of interest not normally dealt with in this kind of publication. In spite of the very large number of people involved in the field of child health, including health visitors, general practitioners, clinical medical officers, school nurses and paediatricians, there has been a notable lack of up-to-date and authoritative texts on the subject. Much has been written concerning paediatrics and paediatric research but interest is now turning to the many other areas of research including psychology, epidemiology, and sociology involving child health.

I hope therefore that this yearly publication will ensure that professionals working in the field will have available to them the most recent ideas and research findings in a concise and readable form.

I would also like to take this opportunity of thanking all the contributors who were outstanding both because of the extraordinary high standard of their manuscripts and also because of the promptness with which they submitted them. Further I would like to thank Jill Howse for all her hard work in typing correspondence and re-typing manuscripts.

Oxford, 1984   J. A. Macfarlane

Contributors

Michael J Absolon MB, BChir, FRCS
Consultant Opthalmologist, Southampton Eye Hospital

P. A. Aspinall BSc, MSc, PhD
Honorary Research Fellow, Princess Alexandria Eye Pavilion, Edinburgh

Martin Bax MB, BCh, LMSSA, MRCP
Research Community Paediatrician, Community Paediatric Research Unit, St Mary's Hospital
Medical School, London

John C Catford MSc, MB, BChir, MRCP, MFCM, DCH
Specialist in Community Medicine, Wessex Regional Health Authority

Janet de Z Chaplais MA, BM, BCh, MRCP
Senior Registrar in Community Paediatrics, Community Health Offices, Radcliffe Infirmary,
Oxford

Jean Golding MA, PhD
Wellcome Trust, Senior Lecturer, Departments of Obstetrics and Child Health, University of
Bristol

Hilary Graham MA, PhD
Lecturer in Social Policy, University of Bradford

A. R. Hill BSc, PhD, FBCO
Principal Opthalmic Optician, Oxford Eye Hospital, and Honorary Research Fellow, Nuffield
Laboratory of Ophthalmology, University of Oxford

Judith M. Hockaday MD, MRCP
Consultant Paediatric Neurologist, John Radcliffe Hospital, Oxford

Susan Jenkins MBBS, MRCP, MRCS, LRCP, DCH
Senior Clinical Medical Officer, Paddington and North Kensington District; Honorary Lecturer, Community Paediatric Research Unit, St. Mary's Hospital Medical School, London

David P. H. Jones MB, ChB, MRC Psych, DCH, D(Obst), RCOG
Senior Registrar in Child Psychiatry, Park Hospital for Children, Oxford

Lennart Kohler MD
Professor, Director, The Nordic School of Public Health, Göteborg, Sweden

Anne Millo
Senior Orthoptist, Southampton Eye Hospital

Leon Polnay BSc, MBBS, MRCP, D Obst RCOG, DCH
Senior Lecturer in Child Health, The University of Nottingham, Queen's Medical Centre,
Nottingham

E. M. E. Poskitt MA, MB, BChir, FRCP
Senior Lecturer in Child Health, University of Liverpool; Honorary Consultant Paediatrician, Royal Liverpool and Alder Hey Children's Hospitals

M. P. M. Richards MA, PhD
Head of Child Care and Development Group, University of Cambridge; University Lecturer in Social Psychology, Cambridge

Euan M. Ross MD, FRCP, DCH
Senior Lecturer in Child Health and Community Medicine, The Central Middlesex Medical School, London

N. J. Spencer M Phil, MRCP, DCH
Consultant Paediatrician, Northern General Hospital, Sheffield

Margaret Stacey B Sc (Econ)
Professor, Department of Sociology, University of Warwick

Kingsley Whitmore MRCS, LRCP, DCH
Research Paediatrician, Thomas Coram Research Unit, London

Michael W. Yogman MD, MSc
Department of Pediatrics, Harvard Medical School and Division of Child Development, Department of Medicine, The Children's Hospital, Boston, Massachusetts, U.S.A.

Contents

The late walking child

INTRODUCTION

Delayed walking, whether accompanied by other developmental abnormalities or not, is often a worry for parents and a diagnostic problem for physicians. It affects some 3% of the British population of 18-month-old children (Neligan & Prudham, 1969). Late walkers are a heterogeneous group, including both normal children showing temporary gross motor delay only, with no clinical explanation for late walking, and children with a variety of clinical and neuropathological conditions responsible for late walking. While many of these conditions present and are diagnosed at less than 18 months of age (Table 1.1) the late walking population will contain a small proportion of children not previously recognised as being mildly physically or mentally handicapped. For example, in Oxfordshire there was a 5.9% incidence of neurological abnormality, previously unsuspected, in a series of 257 children

Table 1.1 Conditions associated with late walking in children assessed by paediatricians before 18 months of age and living in Oxfordshire at 18 months of age between 1978 and 1982

Condition	No of cases*
Cerebral palsy (all forms) (C.P)	40
Neurologically abnormal–? C.P	3
ESN (M)	11
ESN (S)	5
Congenital syndromes or diseases (with or without M.R)	19
Congenital C.N.S abnormality	10
Arrested hydrocephalus	3
Congenital orthopaedic abnormality	8
Down's syndrome	9
Acquired disease–spinal tumour	1
–chronic renal failure	1
Muscular dystrophy–Duchennes	1
–Congenital	1
Total	112

* These cases were identified from all possible sources but will inevitably be a slight underestimate.

† M.R. = mental retardation

referred because of late walking between 1978 and 1982 (Chaplais & Macfar-lane, unpublished data). Since it can be extremely hard to discriminate the normal late walker from the abnormal on clinical grounds at this age, those working in the community have to steer a course between under and over referral. In order to pick up, for example, cases of mild cerebral palsy or Duchenne's muscular dystrophy, a certain number of normal late walkers will need to be kept under surveillance or referred to specialists. If we are to keep this number to a minimum in order to avoid generating unnecessary parental anxiety, we need to have diagnostic guidelines. Since most general practitioners and health visitors are likely to come across only one or two late walkers per year, it would be helpful to refer to the results of surveys of late walkers carried out at specialist centres (Robson, Lundberg, 1979) or in the community (Hardie and Macfarlane 1980).

Late walkers in the population

The median age for the milestone of walking is found to vary between coun-tries and locally within countries, ranging from, for example 12.1 months in Denver, U.S.A. (Frankenburg & Dodds, 1967) to 13.6 months in Zurich (Handley, 1968). The proportion of non-walkers in the 18-month-old population will therefore be likely to show a corresponding variation. Neligan & Prudham (1969a) in their survey of Newcastle children looked for the poss-ible modifying effects of parameters such as sex, birth rank and social class, upon age of walking. They found that only social class was a significant influence in favour of children from social classes III and IV walking earlier than those from social classes I, II and V. The Oxford Late Walkers' Survey (Hardie & Macfarlane, 1980) did not show this social class effect, but there was a significantly increased incidence of children with either single parents or unemployed fathers among the late walker group as compared with a control group of 18-month-olds.

Ideally, according to Robson (1978) standards for milestones such as walking should be compiled from the local population. He compiled percen-tiles for motor milestones of children with different normal locomotor variants and children with mild motor disorders. Figure 1.1 shows the considerable overlap between these norms. The mean age for walking for hemiplegic children in Robson's South London sample was 15 months, and that for diplegic children was 24 months, hence the normal late walking child population falls between these two means.

Bryant et al (1979) also set out to cater for a local population when they standardised the Denver Developmental Screening Test (D.D.S.T) for Cardiff children. The D.D.S.T is now extensively used by health visitors and community physicians as an aid to screening for neurodevelopmental problems. Although Bryant did find differences between the milestones of Denver and Cardiff children, these are not thought to be important in terms

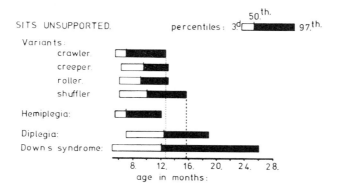

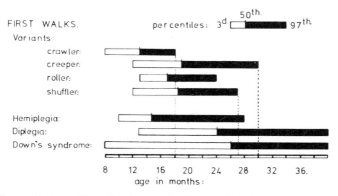

Fig. 1.1 Motor milestones. Normal variants and mild motor disorders
(Reproduced by kind permission of P. Robson)

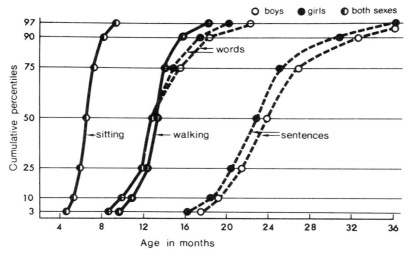

Fig. 1.2 Cumulative percentile curves for four standard developmental milestones
(Reproduced by kind permission of G. Neligan & B. Prudham)

of significantly affecting the numbers of children scored as having 'abnormal' or 'questionable' development.

As with some other developmental norms, the distribution curve for age of first walking is not normal but skewed towards the upper limit. The age of first walking for normal children has a modal value in the 12 to 14 month range, but the overall range of the distribution is from about 7 to 36 months. Hence, the age difference between the 97th percentile and the 50th percentile is about double that between the 3rd and 50th percentiles. Neligan & Prudham (1969b) found cumulative percentile curves a useful way of expressing data on first walking (Fig 1.2). The 97th percentile for this milestone fell at 18.4 months for Newcastle children. The Oxford Survey found that, of those children not walking by 18 months, 50% were walking by $19\frac{1}{2}$ months, 75% by 21 months and 97% by 24 months.

ASSESSMENT OF THE LATE WALKING CHILD

Clinical presentation of the normal late walkers

When assessing a late walking child it is essential to have a knowledge of normal locomotor development and its normal variants. Common to all surveys on late walking children is the observation that a deviant mode of locomotion before walking or a deviant sequence of early locomotor development is found in at least half of all late walkers. The incidence of bottom-shuffling in the normal population is between 8% and 9% (Lundberg, 1979) as compared with 48% in the Oxford late walking population for example. In that survey a further 3.5% of late walkers were 'creepers', 3.5% 'got up and walked' without any early form of locomotion and the remaining 45% were crawlers. The clinical characteristics and sequences of locomotor development found in these different groups of late walkers have been described by Robson (1970) and by Lundberg (1979). Although there appears to be considerable overlap in clinical presentation between the various deviant types, Lundberg has defined one group which stands out as a syndrome, which she has named The Idiopathic Late Walking Syndrome (I.L.W.S.) (1979). She carried out a prospective study on 65 children selected for dissociated gross motor delay (D.G.M.D), defined as marked gross motor delay without any abnormal neurological signs and contrasting with a normal fine motor-adaptive performance. Children entered the study at ages ranging from 7 to 23 months, and all had gross motor delay of unknown origin at 17 months, this age representing the 97th centile for first walking in Sweden. These late walkers were characterised by features which included shuffling (51%), an atypical or late pattern of learning to sit (79%), heredity for shuffling (30%) and heredity for late walking (19%). Muscular hypotonia (71%) more pronounced in the lower trunk, legs and feet was associated with hyperflexibility of joints, hyperextended knees and planovalgus feet. The muscle bulk in the lower legs was poorly developed and the feet were small and babyish. The children were reluctant to bear weight, having a preference for the 'sitting on air' posture when suspended under the arms, also known as a positive Foerster sign. Haidvogl (1979) described a similar syndrome of delayed motor development with dissociation of maturation among a series of children selected for 'sitting on air posture' from referrals for developmental delay or suspected cerebral palsy. Out of Lundberg's original 65 children presenting with D.G.M.D at 17 months, 35 (54%) were still normal at follow-up, and these were named 'idiopathic' late walkers. However 30 (46%) had developed a variety of clinical conditions accounting for late walking, and these were named the 'symptomatic' group. It was not possible to predict, on the basis of clinical signs and history at 17 months, which of these two groups a child with D.G.M.D would fall into, although a number of signs were found to favour a normal outcome. Hence it can be seen that the triad of shuffling, hypotonia and late sitting is no guarantee of normality. However, in a community-based sample of late walkers such as the Oxford series, the proportion of idiopathic late walkers is likely to be very much higher, so that the clinical picture described above would be a much more reassuring finding at 17 months. For example, in the Oxford sample of 257 18-month-old late walkers, from which the symptomatic late walkers with serious clinical conditions (see Table 1.1) had for the most part been removed by earlier referral and diagnosis, 116 (48%) of the 242 idiopathic late walkers were shufflers with mild to moderate selective hypotonia of the lower limbs and only one child in the neurologically abnormal group of 15 was a shuffler. This child had a mild spastic paraplegia.

The genetics of late walking are not straightforward. While Lundberg found a predominance of girls (69%) among her idiopathic late walkers, the sex incidence in the Oxford late walking sample was exactly equal. Heredity for shuffling in Robson's sample (1970) was strong enough to suggest a dominant mode of inheritance for this trait. However, there was no significant incidence of heredity for late walking in Robson's study, in contrast to Lundberg's (1979) incidence of 19% and Hardie & Macfarlane's (1980) incidence of 50% for heredity of late walking. The latter figure compares with an incidence of 16% for family history of late walking among a group of 48 Oxford-born children who walked before 18 months of age and who were seen as controls for another survey. Presumably the more 'normal' the population, the greater the likelihood of finding a family history of late walking. Interestingly in the Oxford survey, heredity for late walking was as strong for crawlers (50%) as for the collective group with deviant locomotion (50%). An earlier survey (Hardie & Macfarlane, 1980) of the first of 160 late walkers seen had suggested positive correlations between the shuffling trait, heredity for late walking and superior developmental assessment scores, but these findings were not confirmed in the larger sample of 243 children.

Abnormal late walkers

The Oxford Late Walking Childrens Survey

Other than large national child development surveys, this was the first survey to seek and assess late walking children in the community when in 90% of cases there had been no previous suspicion of abnormality and no apparent reason for referral to specialists. It was originally undertaken as part of the Oxford Cerebral Palsy Study, in an attempt to shed light upon our knowledge of the aetiology and incidence of this condition. 257 children in the Oxford area born between 1976 and 1981 and not taking six steps unaided at 18 months were referred by health visitors for developmental assessment and neurological examination at home by a paediatrician. An estimated 84% of all late walkers were referred in this way, the remainder having apparently evaded routine developmental surveillance at 18 months. Children subsequently suspected of being abnormal on the basis of a home visit were referred to a hospital paediatrician for diagnosis. 129 children who were already known to paediatricians either with known causes for late walking (112) (see Table 1.1) or normal (17) were not included in the survey. A further 18 were not seen because of objections from the primary health care team (10) or delayed referral (8).

The 257 late walkers assessed at home included eight cases of cerebral palsy (3.1%) and seven cases of minor neurological abnormality (2.8%), making a total of 5.9% previously unsuspected neurological abnormality. The eight cerebral palsy cases were all mild and included five cases of spastic paraplegia, one case of diplegia, one hemiplegia and one monoplegia. In 6 out of 8 cases (75%) there were abnormal perinatal events, severe in three cases (37.5%) whereas of the 242 normal late walkers only 15.4% had abnormal births, including 5.4% with severe complications.

Differential diagnosis of the abnormal late walkers

Can developmental assessment and examination at 18 months establish normality, or help to predict future abnormality in a late walker?

Cerebral palsy Although all severe and moderate cases of cerebral palsy will have presented at less than 18 months of age, the late walking population includes, as the Oxford Survey has shown, children in the so called 'grey area' of cerebral palsy, whose neurological signs when first seen may be subtle and still evolving. Lundberg (1979) stresses that mild cases of diplegia and simple ataxia may be impossible to diagnose from neurological signs before the age of 3. Robson (1971) has described the unpredictable and sometimes fluctuating neuropathological process followed by children with mild spastic diplegia, during which the initial phase of hypotonia in infancy progresses, via a phase of intermittent extensor activity, to overt spasticity by 18–24 months. In the case of three late walkers referred for the Oxford Survey, the gradual evolution of signs of spasticity did not allow a definite diagnosis to be made until the children were between 2 and $3\frac{1}{2}$ years of age. Robson (1971) has postulated that when the shuffling trait is inherited by a child destined to have spastic diplegia, the onset of hypotonia and hence the diagnosis of cerebral palsy may be delayed. The average age of diagnosis of cerebral palsy for shufflers in his series was 32 months, as compared with 17.2 months for non-shufflers. Since 1 in 8 children with spastic diplegia is a shuffler (Robson, 1970) it is easy to see how the diagnosis can be delayed. Two children in Lundberg's prospective series (1979) developed spastic hemiplegia and spastic diplegia respectively; neither of which was detectable at 17 months of age. To confuse the issue still further, apparent regression of neurological signs in cerebral palsy is being increasingly recognised, and makes it difficult to define mild cerebral palsy at this age. One late walker in the Oxford series, confidently diagnosed as ataxic cerebral palsy, showed subsequent regression of neurological signs and had to be reclassified at $2\frac{3}{4}$ years of age as having 'minor motor disorders'.

Do any guidelines emerge to help community workers sort out the 'confusing clinical picture' described by Robson? It is clearly not possible for health visitors, for example, to attempt to elicit subtle neurological signs, nor is it desirable for all 3% of the normal 18-month-old population to be referred to specialists. Granted that there is considerable overlap in clinical signs and developmental patterns between 'idiopathic' and 'symptomatic' cases at 18 months, a number of factors appear to favour a normal outcome. These include a normal pre-, peri-, and postnatal history, shuffling with heredity for shuffling, and an abnormal or late pattern of learning to sit (Lundberg, 1979). To this could be added a family history of late walking in either a parent or a sibling, which might enable reassurance to be given to parents of half of neurologically normal crawlers seen in the community. The task of diagnosing cerebral palsy in a hypotonic shuffler is clearly the job of a physician, since it depends upon eliciting such signs as brisk tendon reflexes and persistent ankle clonus (Robson, 1971). As regards cerebral palsy in its usual hypertonic form, one useful discriminating sign which was present among 6 out of 7 children with mild spastic paraplegia in the Oxford series was increased resistance to passive dorsiflexion at the ankle, together with a tendency to stand or walk round the furniture on the toes. In some cases hamstring shortening made sitting with legs outstretched uncomfortable for these children. These findings contrasted with the relative extreme ease of ankle dorsiflexion to well past the neutral position, together with the planovalgus foot posture found in practically all normal late walkers. Possibly health visitors and community physicians could be trained and encouraged to look for these features.

Mental retardation The 18-month-old late walking population is likely to include a proportion of mildly mentally retarded children (IQ 50–70). Though most will already be under surveillance for developmental delay, some may not be detectable by developmental assessment at 18 months. In many areas the health visitor has become responsible for routine developmental surveillance of 18 month olds. Her important role as part of a basic programme of health care surveillance offered by the primary health care team was endorsed by The Court Report (1976). The D.D.S.T offers a useful, quick aid for developmental assessment. More sophisticated and comprehensive screening tests have been devised for local use, for example, by Barber (1982) for screening of pre-school children in Glasgow and Drillien in Dundee. However the D.D.S.T has been recommended by Bryant (1980) as eminently suitable for use by health visitors and community workers. She warns against its use as anything other than a screening test, 'intended to alert the examiners to the presence of a developmental problem which needs fuller investigation'.

A number of factors, however, conspire to make 18 months a difficult age for assessment. Lundberg (1969) cast doubts upon the validity of the D.D.S.T at ages of below 30 months, even with the revised norms (Frankenburg et al, 1971). In her series, 20% of the children with mild mental subnormality were not scored as abnormal at initial assessment, but only at follow-up. There may, however be difficulties in identifying mild mental subnormality in children below 2 years by any method, and most psychologists would prefer to base a diagnosis upon a child's rate of progress over several assessments, rather than one single assessment. Frankenburg et al (1971) found that over-referral was more likely to occur than under-referral in the case of the non-ambulatory child. To reduce the number of over-referrals, they suggested re-screening all subjects scored as abnormal, and only referring after a second abnormal score.

From the point of view of the social class effect on development, 20 months appears to mark the 'watershed', before which children from lower social classes (III to V) are more advanced with gross motor skills, and after which children from social classes I and II begin to advance more rapidly with language and fine motor development. The late walking child can never be considered in isolation from his/her family and social background. Their typically placid and undemanding nature, together with their parents' frequent under-estimation of their potential, as compared with more precocious elder siblings, may interact to produce temporary delays in social, fine motor adaptive and language areas. Depending upon the home background, a late walker can be either over-protected, literally spoon fed and encouraged to remain dependent or, in a more disadvantaged home, under-stimulated and left to his/her own devices. Although he/she may appear at 18 months to be a mildly globally retarded child, when walking is finally achieved there is often a noticeable acceleration of development in all areas.

The results of an isolated D.D.S.T performed at 18 months must therefore be interpreted with caution. Bryant (1980) recommends the immediate referral of all children with an abnormal performance, or with a questionable performance due to more than two delayed items in one field of development. Children with a questionable performance, other than this, are kept under surveillance with repeat testing and referred if development does not normalise. According to Frankenburg et al (1971), two-thirds of all children scored as questionable on the D.D.S.T will be found to have IQ's over 80, therefore these borderline ESN(M) children should be rescreened.

The late walkers assessed at home for the Oxford survey between 18 and 21 months included 27 normal children who had previously been seen by paediatricians for reasons including developmental delay. They were found, not surprisingly, to include a significantly higher proportion (37.4%) of abnormal or questionable D.D.S.T scores than the sample as a whole (13.6%). Considering the D.D.S.T scores of the 215 children not previously referred to paediatricians, 192 (89.3%) had normal development in sectors other than gross motor. (Those who had started walking by the time of assessment had, of course, normal gross motor development as well). The remaining 23 (10.7%) had delays in social, fine motor or language sectors, which would, together with a persistently abnormal gross motor performance, qualify them for referral, according to Bryant's (1980) criteria. This group included four children (1.9%) with abnormal or questionable scores in two sectors other than gross motor, who would therefore qualify for immediate referral, regardless of gross motor normalisation. Were gross motor delay in the 10.7% of late walkers with D.D.S.T delays to normalise, then 11 (5.1%) would still remain in the questionable category and therefore qualify for follow-up. Bearing in mind the various difficulties in assessing the general development of late walkers, and the lack of clear predictive factors as regards outcome of IQ, a practical policy might be to retest all 18-month-old late walkers with abnormal or questionable tests at 21 months and again at 24 months and consider referral at 24 months if development had not normalised. Meanwhile the health visitor would be well placed with her easy access to the home to monitor the child's progress and advise parents as to suitable ways of encouraging general development.

Muscular dystrophy The frequency of Duchenne's muscular dystrophy (D.M.D) is 1:3000 to 1:5000 male births (Morton & Chung, (1959). Hence in a region the size of Oxfordshire, where there are 7000 deliveries per year, about one new case would be expected every year. The mean age of walking of D.M.D boys in Crisp et al's series (1982) was 17.2 months; hence, the late walking population includes nearly half of boys destined to develop D.M.D. Although clinical signs of the disease, including gait abnormalities, are rarely observed as early as 18 months, half the cases have symptoms before $2\frac{1}{2}$ years (Gardner–Medwin, 1979). Since the mean age of diagnosis nationally is as late as 5.6 years, there must in many cases be a delay on the part of clinicians in recognising this disease in its early stages. In some cases parents may be falsely reassured by the temporary functional improvement due to maturation of the nervous system which may occur in young D.M.D patients soon after starting to walk and before the inevitable deterioration sets in. Tragic case histories where diagnosis of D.M.D in an older sibling has not been made until after the birth of younger affected male siblings have prompted some to urge that serum creatine phosphokinase (CPK) estima-

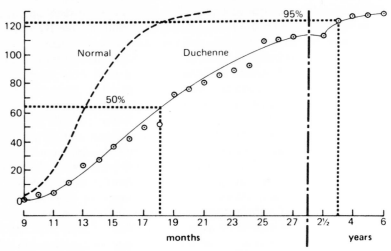

Fig. 1.3 Ages at which 130 Newcastle patients with D.M.D. began independent walking, compared with the normal range. Reproduced by kind permission of Gardner-Medwin et al

tions be carried out on all male late walkers. Gardner–Medwin et al (1978) have predicted an approximate relationship of one affected younger sibling birth prevented to 10 cases of D.M.D diagnosed by performing CPKs on 18-month-old late walkers. For example, in the Oxford region where one D.M.D case could be diagnosed at 18 months every 2 years by CPK testing, it would take 20 years for one recurrence to be prevented. There would be additional benefits in terms of identifying other relatives likely to be affected and offering genetic counselling to female carriers detected, and also as regards making provision for the D.M.D patient diagnosed and his parents at an early stage of the disease. However the effect of routine CPK testing on the normal male late walkers and their families, making up 1.5% of the population, should be taken into account. Prevention of recurrence of D.M.D on a nationwide scale may be better served by awaiting development of a reliable technique for female carrier detection.

Unfortunately there are no firm documented predictors for future development of D.M.D among late walkers as regards clinical characteristics or early developmental patterns which might enable selective CPK testing of male late walkers. Shuffling is apparently rare among D.M.D boys (Gardner-Medwin, personal observation), a family history of late walking would not be expected, and language delay is quite frequent (Dubowitz, 1965). However all these features are known to occur in normal late walkers, 25% of whom are crawlers with no family history.

Predictive value of assessment of late walkers

The significance of early delays in motor development is not fully understood. Neligan & Prudham (1969) assessed early walkers (<10 months) and late walkers (>17 months) for language and fine motor status at school entry age. A significant difference in performance was found among boys, but not among girls. Silva (1979) carried out a 3-year assessment of 1037 children in Dunedin, New Zealand, prospectively followed up from birth. The early motor-delayed group were 5–6 times more likely to be represented among those with very low language and fine motor performance at 3-year follow-up, compared with the normal range of children. However, between one-half and one-third of children with early motor delay scored within the average or better than average range on later testing. (It is not clear whether this survey includes any children with neuropathological or other reasons for late walking). Drillien (1983) in her Dundee child population survey investigated the predictive value of neurological assessment of the pre-school child. A highly significant excess of clumsiness, as observed and graded by teachers at school entry age was recorded for children who had previously been assessed at pre-school examinations (at 2 years and 3 years) as neurologically doubtful or abnormal. These groups also showed a greater degree of clumsiness than did clumsy children who had been neurologically normal on pre-school testing. It would appear therefore, that the late walking population may include a proportion of children at risk of having persisting neuro-developmental problems.

CONCLUSION

The late walking population is a heterogeneous group of children, some of whom are genetically destined to show an isolated gross motor delay, some with more generalised or global delay of unknown origin, some whose development has been temporarily delayed by adverse perinatal events, and some with known clinical or neuropathological causes for late walking. The effects of social deprivation and under-stimulation interacting with the above are important, though difficult to quantify.

A knowledge of the normal variants of locomotor development, together with an awareness of the range of conditions likely to be encountered may be helpful for those responsible for assessing 18 month olds. However it has not proved possible to divide late walkers into clearly defined clinical subtypes, not surprisingly, perhaps, in view of the interaction of social, environmental and genetic factors. The long-term significance of minor neurological problems at this age must await further follow-up studies.

REFERENCES

Barber J H 1982 Pre school Developmental screening—the results of a four year period. Health Bulletin 4014: 170–178

Bryant G M 1980 Use of the Denver Developmental Screening Test by health visitors. Health Visitor 53: 2–5

Bryant G M, Davies K J, Newcombe R G 1979 Standardisation of the Denver Developmental Screening Test for Cardiff children. Developmental Medicine and Child Neurology 21: 353-364

Crisp D E, Ziter F A, Bray P F 1982 Diagnostic delay in Duchenne's muscular dystrophy. Journal of the American Medical Association 247: 478–480

Court S D M (Chairman) 1976 Fit for the future. Report of The Committee on the Child Health Services. Command 66 London HSMO Vol 2.

Dubowitz V 1965. Intellectual impairment in muscular dystrophy. Archives of Disease in Childhood 40: 296–301

Frankenburg W K, Dodds J B 1967. The Denver Developmental Screening Test. Journal of Paediatrics 71: 181–191

Frankenburg W K, Goldstein A D, Comp B W 1971. The revised Denver Developmental Screening Test: its accuracy as a screening instrument. Journal of Paediatrics 79: 988–995

Gardner–Medwin D 1979 Controversies about Duchenne muscular dystrophy. (1) Neonatal screening. Developmental Medicine and Child Neurology. 21: 390–393

Gardner–Medwin D Bundly S Green S 1978 Early diagnosis of Duchenne muscular dystrophy. Lancet i: 1102

Haidvogl M 1979 Dissociation of Maturation: a distinct syndrome of delayed motor development. Developmental Medicine and Child Neurology 21: 52–57

Hardie J de Z, Macfarlane A 1980 Late Walking Children: a review of 160 late walkers in the Oxford area. Health Visitor 53: 466–468

Hindley C B 1968. Growing up in five countries. Developmental Medicine and Child Neurology 10: 715–724

Lundberg A 1979a Dissociated Motor development. Neuropaediatrie 10: 161–182

Lundberg A 1979b Gross and Fine Motor Performance in healthy Swedish children aged fifteen and eighteen months. Neuropaediatrie. 10: 35–50

Morton W E, Chung C S, 1959 Formal genetics of muscular dystrophy. American Journal of Human Genetics 11: 360–379

Neligan G, Prudham D 1969a Norms for four standard developmental milestones by sex, social class and place in family. Developmental Medicine and Child Neurology 11: 413–422

Neligan G, Prudham D 1969b Potential Value of four early developmental milestones in screening children for increased risk of later retardation. Developmental Medicine and Child Neurology 11: 423–431

Robson P 1970 Shuffling, hitching, scooting or sliding: some observations in 30 otherwise normal children. Developmental Medicine and Child Neurology 12: 608–617

Robson P 1978 Screening for children. Royal Society of Health Journal 98: 231–237.

Robson P, MacKeith R C 1971 Shufflers with spastic diplegic cerebral palsy: a confusing clinical picture. Developmental Medicine and Child Neurology 13: 651–659

Silva P A 1979 The significance of early delays in motor development. New Zealand Journal of Health, Physical Education and Recreation 12: 78–83

The diagnosis of migraine in childhood

INTRODUCTION

Migraine is defined by the World Federation of Neurology (1969) as a 'familial disorder characterized by recurrent attacks of headache widely variable in intensity, frequency, and duration. Attacks are commonly unilateral and are usually associated with anorexia, nausea and vomiting. In some cases they are preceded by, or associated with, neurological and mood disturbances. All the above characteristics are not necessarily present in each attack or in each patient'. While it is difficult to fault this widely accepted definition, it does not offer any objective or measurable diagnostic criterion, and there is in fact no test for migraine. It is a clinical diagnosis, based largely on the history, and as Pearce (1975) has pointed out, is under- or over-diagnosed according to which, and how many, of its characteristic features are regarded as prerequisite. For many reasons diagnosis can be more difficult, and less certain, in children.

Migraine is a common, usually minor disorder, and except in rare instances is without morbidity. In childhood its main importance lies in the fact that it is only one of many causes of headache, from the earliest years of life. While many of these are trivial, and benign, a few are serious, with grave morbidity if unrecognised. The need to distinguish the benign forms, of which migraine is a prominent example, from the rarer but sinister forms such as the headache of raised intracranial pressure, underlies much of the clinical attention to the subject. However, in addition, migraine needs to be distinguished from other 'non-organic' or benign headaches, to allow appropriate management, both in prescription, and management at home and at school. A comment such as 'It's just a headache, its nothing to worry about' may be intended as reassuring, but is usually puzzling, and at the least unhelpful, to those responsible for appraising school absence, or undone homework.

CRITERIA FOR DIAGNOSIS

Usually, migraine is diagnosed by identifying recurrent headaches, which are unilateral, associated with nausea (with or without vomiting) and preceded by an aura of focal neurological disturbance. In children this approach can be difficult, because the symptoms are often overshadowed by associated abdominal discomfort or may not be accurately reported; also, because of understandable concern, referral in childhood is likely to be made before the recurring pattern is clear. A further difficulty is that many cases will certainly fail to be diagnosed if the three criteria mentioned above are regarded as necessary. There is disagreement on this, and about the other so-called characterising features referred to in different studies. Over many years different authors have used various methods of case ascertainment. A widely accepted approach has been that of Vahlquist (1955) and Bille (1962) who made a diagnosis of migraine when headaches were paroxysmal (had a clear start and finish) and separated by free intervals and were associated with at least two of the following four features: one sided pain; nausea; visual aura; family heredity (parents or siblings). Friedman et al (1954) used seven criteria and recently Prensky & Sommer (1979) in the USA discussed their wide experience of cases diagnosed on the basis of three of six features: abdominal pain, nausea or vomiting; headache confined to one side; a throbbing or pulsatile quality of the pain; complete relief after a brief period of rest; an aura either visual, sensory or motor; a history of migraine headaches in one or more members of the immediate family.

This variation in approach explains the uncertainities of epidemiological study and the wide differences in reported prevalence (Table 2.1) In this country Congdon & Forsythe (1979) ascertained their large and well-studied childhood series on the basis of any three of the following four features: an aura; nausea; vomiting; a family history. They observed that had they used

Table 2.1 The incidence of headache and migraine in children aged 7 years and upwards

	No.	Age (years)		Frequent non-migraine	'Migraine'*
Vahlquist (1955)	1236	10–12		13.3%	4.5%
Dalsgaard-Nielsen et al (1969)	1075 boys	7–18			6.8%
	952 girls	7–18			7.5%
			Any Headache		
Bille (1962)	2304 boys	7–10	51%	4.2%	2.9%
	2136 boys	11–15	66%	7.6%	3.7%
	2288 girls	7–10	50%	4.2%	2.6%
	2265 girls	11–15	69%	11.2%	6.2%
			Headache in previous year		
Waters (1974) (b)	367 boys	10–16	85%		9.0%
(a)	390 girls	11–15	93%		10.5%
(b)	410 girls	10–16	93%		12.0%
Sparks (1978)	12543 boys	10–18			3.4%
	3242 girls	10–18			2.5%

* Ascertained on differing criteria.

Table 2.2 Characteristic features of migraine in 122 children with headache (data from Hockaday, 1979)

No. of features	No. of children
Three:	
Hemicrania, nausea/vomiting, aura.	20
Two:	
Hemicrania, nausea/vomiting	26
Hemicrania, aura	6
Nausea/vomiting, aura.	22
	54
One:	
Hemicrania	5
Nausea/vomiting	24
Aura	11
	40
None of above	8

Table 2.3 Characteristics of migrainous and tension headaches in 2000 cases (modified from Fig. 1, Friedman et al, 1954)

	Migraine (%)	Tension (%)
Family history of headache	65	40
Onset under age 20 years	55	30
Onset over age 20 years	45	70
Prodroma	60	10
Frequency constant or daily	3	50
Frequency less than once a week	60	15
Type throbbing	80	30
Location unilateral	80	10
Associated vomiting	50	10

the (stricter) criteria of Bille (1962) some of their cases would have been excluded from diagnosis for some years. Thus while for epidemological purposes such methods of case ascertainment are necessary, for clinical use they are less satisfactory. Ultimately, the only essential for the diagnosis of migraine is recurring headache.

It is simpler and for clinical purposes safer, to accept as migraine recurrent headaches that are clearly paroxysmal provided that there is return to full normal health (both mental and physical) between attacks and *that other causes of headache have been excluded*. In one study where cases were identified on this basis (Hockaday, 1979) it was found that one or more of the three chief features of migraine was actually present in almost every case, and that the headaches appeared similar whether or not these were present (Table 2.2). It is obviously possible that some headaches of muscle-tension origin will be misinterpreted as migraine; the two conditions have many common characteristics (Table 2.3). Often, both co-exist. However, the main purpose of the approach is the exclusion of other causes of headache and to this end the condition that there should be return to normal health between headache attacks is an important safeguard. So also is the period of observation which is necessary to establish that there is a recurring pattern with symptom-free intervals.

The presence or absence of a family history of migraine is not actually very helpful in clinical diagnosis. This is because it is likely to be unreliable: the diagnosis is even more difficult to establish on hearsay through relatives than by direct questioning of a patient. Moreover migraine (defined carefully on the basis of association with all three main characterising features) is not rare in the families of non-migraine subjects, and not much commoner in the families of migraine patients (Waters, 1971).

PREVALENCE

There have been a number of studies of the incidence of headache, and of migraine in school children aged 7 years and upwards (Table 2.1); the incidence in younger children is not known. The variation in findings must partly relate to the different methods of case collection (some by self-administered questionnaire) and selection. In the biggest recent study conducted by the Medical Officers of Schools Association (Sparks 1978) 3.4% of boys, and 2.5% of girls were regarded as migraine subjects. Of these over half had consulted their doctor about the symptoms. Even in Waters' study (1974) where the incidence of headaches was so high that by inference the great majority must have been trivial, 14% of all the children with headaches had consulted their doctor. That migraine must be common in children is clear from the observation that about 50% of adults describe onset of attacks before age 20 years, and over one-fifth before age 10 years (Selby & Lance 1960). Congdon & Forsythe (1979) found onset was before 5 years in one-third of cases presenting in childhood. The incidence is greater in boys than girls up to the age of puberty. Despite common hearsay, there is no evidence that subjects with migraine are more intelligent or of higher social class that either those without headache or those with non-migraine headache (Waters, 1971); it is possible they consult their doctor more readily. A link with allergy has not been established.

CAUSE

The process of events during an attack of migraine is fairly well established: in the first stage, when symptoms of the aura (indicating localised neurological dysfunction) occur, cerebral blood flow is reduced; the second, headache phase of the attack is accompanied by extracranial, and cerebral, vasodilatation (Marshall, 1978). However, what exactly causes this sequence of events is unknown, and the actual mechanism of the headache is not clear.

Certain amines and other chemicals which act on blood vessels causing vasoconstriction and reduced blood flow, are known to precipitate migraine. The response in migraine is, however, not simply one reflecting cerebral anoxia—the prodomal symptoms differ from those in ordinary vasovagal syncopal attacks. Abnormalities of platelet function have been observed in relation to the migraine attack, including increased aggregability, reduced enzyme activity, and release of the vasoactive amine 5-hydroxyptamine, as consistent findings. It is possible that these are merely late or secondary effects of whatever unknown factor is causing the migraine attacks. Various hypotheses suggest that migraine is primarily a disorder of platelets (Hannington, 1978) or of the blood brain barrier (Harper et al, 1977) or due to reactive hyperaemia in response to hypoxia (Burnstock, 1981). Whatever mechanisms are responsible must account for the enormous variation in clinical presentation both in, and between patients, and the well-known variability of action of certain agents or precipitating factors so that, although noxious on one occasion they may be harmless on another.

The evidence favouring a hereditary factor in migraine is relatively strong, but the mode is not clear. There is no biological marker, or test, for the predisposition to migraine, which must be what is inherited. Twin studies suggest an interplay of genetic and environmental factors. While a high incidence of migraine in near family members is often reported, this is difficult to establish epidemiologically. Most studies reach the tentative conclusion that there is autosomal dominant inheritance with incomplete penetrance, and that environmental factors are also important Raskin & Appenzeller, 1980). In these circumstances, the presence or absence of a family history is not a reliable diagnostic criterion.

While the original cause of migraine is not known, many immediate precipitants of attacks are recognised. Mental stress due to conflict at home or at school, difficulties in school work especially in relation to examinations, a hot and stuffy atmosphere as in the cinema or theatre, bright sunlight, TV flicker or grid patterns, late nights, fatigue, and hunger are all common factors. Physical stress as in athletics, or gymnastics may produce attacks. Bille (1962) observed a link with menstruation in nearly one-half of post-pubertal girls, but Sparks (1978) found only 21% of girls related attacks to menstruation, although many dated the onset of attacks from puberty. Congdon & Forsythe (1979) noted a relationship with travelling and cold. Dietary factors are often referred to, but the evidence is scanty. Double blind studies have failed to establish chocolate as a precipitant (Moffatt et al, 1974), and tyramine (thought to be the vasoactive substance in chocolate, cheese and alcohol) has been shown not to be a provoking factor in children (Forsythe & Redmond, 1974). An interesting precipitant is mild head trauma as in footballer's migraine (Matthews, 1972). Other instances of mild non-concussive head injury may be followed by severe migraine attacks, with profound neurological symptoms, e.g. blindness, or hemiplegia, alarming until their nature and transience is recognised (Haas et al, 1975).

FEATURES OF THE ATTACK

In between one-third and one-half of childhood cases migraine is of the *classical* type, that is, the headache is preceded or accompanied by an aura. The symptoms depend on which part of the brain is affected by this initial vasoconstrictor phase of the attack. In children, and probably also in adults (Lance & Anthony, 1966; Hockaday, 1979) the circulation to the posterior part of the brain and brainstem appears to be most often affected, causing the features of so-called basilar artery migraine. In this, the neurological deficit is usually mild, but is occasionally severe and alarming, especially in younger children. Symptoms include bilateral distortion or loss of vision; unsteadiness of gait with falling; sensory loss, sometimes bilateral; diplopia, vertigo, confusion, drowsiness, loss of consciousness. In other patients with classical migraine the aura is more restricted, affecting only one side, causing unilateral sensory or motor loss, or visual change, but this is less common in children, perhaps to some extent because of difficulties in history taking. There are other rare forms, well recognised in childhood, e.g. familial hemiplegic migraine (Glista et al, 1975), and ophthalmoplegic migraine (Raymond et al, 1977). In all types the kind of aura experienced can be very stereotyped, but in most patients it varies from attack to attack, and is indeed often missing.

In all forms of migraine in children, whether *classical* or *common* (without aura) there is almost always nausea and anorexia; sometimes there is severe prostration, and vomiting. When there is also abdominal discomfort, or pain, diagnosis can be difficult. Migraine can start at any time of day, often on rising. It rarely begins at night, and headache which wakes a child during the night should arouse suspicion of raised intracranial pressure. Most attacks last only a few hours or even less than one hour, and are terminated by a period of sleep; Congdon & Forsythe (1979) reported 61% lasting up to 5 hours, only 20% exceeding 10 hours. Attacks most often recur approximately once a month. A frequency as high as two to three attacks per week is sometimes observed (Congdon & Forsythe, 1979), but should arouse suspicion of other diagnosis.

Much is written about the distribution and quality of the headache in migraine. However, especially in children, details such as whether or not the headache is unilateral rather then bilateral, or throbbing rather than continuous, are not helpful in diagnosis—nor indeed are they always available in younger children. Some regard migraine as less likely if the headache is mild, but many patients both children and adults, maintain that their headache is not severe, and that the other features of the attack are more disturbing: the aura itself or the lethargy, malaise and nausea, are often the real reasons for disability. Generally fewer than 50% of children experience severe headaches.

It is difficult to evaluate the amount of disability and interference with schooling experienced by children with migraine. Actual absence from school is not common. Bille (1962) found that only 57 out of 756 children aged 10–15 years with migraine missed any school in a 5-month term. A study current in Oxford has so far shown only 20 absences due to headache out of a total of 836 absences recorded in 510 children. However these observations do not take account of the children whose attacks start during the school day. The MOSA study (Sparks, 1978) in 31 schools approximately half of which were boarding, observed a much higher absence rate (50%) amongst children with migraine: this could have been because in the boarding schools, sickness absence was easier to achieve. From clinical experience, it is probable that migraine quite often interferes with optimum school progress. It is certainly linked with school failure, but sometimes the primary problem is learning difficulty, with headache, albeit often genuine migraine, provoked or exacerbated by the difficulty, and offered as a more respectable presentation. The relationships are complex and each case needs close evaluation. Many headaches linked with school failure are not migraine, but are of muscle tension type, or purely psychogenic; their distinction from migraine may not be easy, and of course, both may occur in the same subject.

OTHER DISORDERS

It has been suggested that some of the other recurrent disorders of childhood where headache may be a feature represent forms of migraine. This is possible with some rare syndromes, such as alternating hemiplegia (Krageloh & Aicardi, 1980), transient global amnesia (Jensen, 1980), and benign paroxysmal torticollis (Deonna & Martin, 1981). It appears less likely that there is a link with paroxysmal abdominal pain (Christensen & Mortensen, 1975); this is a common disorder, but even so, the relationship although often suggested has never been proved. Vomiting and abdominal pain are of course common during attacks of migraine, and can sometimes obscure the headache. But the reported incidence of recurrent bouts of abdominal pain preceding the first onset of migraine was only 3.3% in one large childhood study (Congdon & Forsythe, 1979). Cyclical vomiting is another disorder sometimes regarded as a form of migraine; it is now uncommon. Headache has been noted at follow-up of children presenting in infancy with recurrent vomiting, but only as one of a variety of disorders suggesting psychopathology (Hammond, 1974; Reinhart et al, 1977). In retrospective studies migraine subjects claim a higher incidence of childhood bilious attacks (Waters 1972), but there has been no prospective study.

It is also difficult to be certain about the significance of the often discussed relationship between migraine and epilepsy: their occurence in the same patient could be due to the chance coincidence of two common disorders. Loss of consciousness occurring during the course of an attack of migraine is often merely postural syncope. However, loss of consciousness, which is not postural, and which is associated with convulsive movements or other epileptic features, can also occur during the course of a migraine attack. This is rare, but such features should be fully investigated, because occasionally they indicate an underlying organic lesion, such as cerebral angioma. Finally, some patients experience attacks in which it is impossible to make the distinction between migraine and epilepsy, either clinically, or on investigation; the mechanism is not clear (Swaiman & Frank, 1978).

It is sometimes suggested that benign paroxysmal vertigo is a form of migraine. Vertigo is a common symptom during the aura phase of migraine, suggesting brainstem or temporal lobe involvement, but the syndrome described by Basser (1964) is clinically, and on natural history, very different, and it is in most cases associated with vestibular nerve abnormality (Koenigsberger et al, 1970).

DIAGNOSIS

Diagnosis which is based on clinical history, and exclusion of underlying pathology, carries special difficulties in children. Important historical details of, for example, previous episodes of headache, head injury or associated symptoms such as nausea or vertigo, are often lacking, forgotten by the child, and not known to the parents. Change in nature of headache, such as the increasing severity of attacks in raised intracranial pressure, may not be recognised, and a child and his parents, accustomed to attacks of migraine, may be slow to appreciate the significance of slightly different symptoms due perhaps to meningitis. Routine investigation aimed at excluding important causes is not possible: the cases are too numerous and repeated hospital visits and investigations, some invasive and needing premedication, are undesirable in children. Plain X-ray of skull is not on its own a sufficient screening test (Honig & Charney, 1982) for cerebral tumour. However, the findings in a large series of children with headache thought to be migraine, and followed for at least 4 years, show that accuracy in diagnosis can be achieved by close attention to history (Congdon & Forsythe, 1979). Serious intracranial cause emerged in only two of 300 children, heralded in one by alteration of symptoms 6 years after onset, and in the other by the appearance of different symptoms after a 4-year remission.

In many instances, particularly in younger children, headache is merely one of a number of symptoms and signs which constitute a clear clinical picture of, for example, acute sinusitis or an acute exanthem; or it may result from fever of any cause. It is also a most important early symptom of intracranial infection and when accompanied by irritability, photophobia, vomiting, or drowsiness, it must be seriously and urgently investigated. Headache may be the only complaint in a child who has suffered a head injury. These and other aspects of differential diagnosis of acute headache arisising in a previously healthy child are discussed elsewhere (Hockaday, 1982).

More difficulty arises in considering recurrent, or chronic, headaches, where the cause is not immediately apparent. The great majority of these remain 'unexplained' (migraine, muscle-tension, psychogenic) or are found to be due to minor lesions (chronic sinusitis, malocclusion). A few are the result of serious neurological disease. The distinction demands close attention, and 'generally much more care has to be taken in children and clinical investigations should be done more often and sooner than in adults' (Heyck, 1968). The important distinctions are the differentiation of headaches resulting from raised intracranial pressure or distortion of intracranial pain sensitive structures, and of headaches arising from chronic scalp and cervical muscle tension.

Headache due to raised intracranial pressure

The quality or nature of a headache is not a very clear guide to its cause. There is no clear-cut line dividing the headache of migraine from that of raised intracranial pressure due to brain tumour. Brain tumour headaches often occur in the morning, or cause awakening from night sleep, they are often intense, prolonged and incapacitating, and they may become even more so as time passes (Honig & Charney, 1982). They are, however, sometimes mild, they are often intermittent and can remit for long periods, and they may be throbbing (suggesting a vascular cause) rather than constant.

The circumstances in which the headache occurs are more useful guides to diagnosis: thus headache due to raised intracranial pressure may be provoked, or made worse by manoeuvres which alter this pressure, such as coughing, sneezing, straining, exercise, recumbency and sleep. Sometimes trivial head trauma will alter the balance of cerebrospinal fluid circulation sufficiently to provoke headache, vomiting and drowsiness in a child with previously unsuspected brain tumour, or with so-called arrested congenital hydrocephalus. A large head circumference is an important clue to this latter possibility, which may not present until late childhood, or even adolescence.

The most important guide to the possibility of intracranial tumour in childhood (or other causes of raised intracranial pressure) is the associated psychic change, which is present often from an early stage, and almost always by the time of diagnosis. Concentration is impaired, cerebration slowed and learning interfered with; there is often personality change with apathy, depression or mood swings. There may only be slowing of intellectual development rather than regression. Slowing of growth, and other endocrine changes, for example diabetes insipidus leading to bed wetting, may occur. Some form of behaviour change, or interference with ordinary school progress, is so common that appraisal of these should be routine in every child presenting with headache, and on every occasion of follow-up.

A recent study (Honig & Charney, 1982) found that in the majority (85%) of children with headache due to brain tumour abnormal neurological signs developed within two months of the onset of thier headaches, and that these, or other features such as delayed growth, polydipsia, or behavioural change were present in virtually all cases within 4 months. Thus children with unexplained headaches should be carefully watched until this period of time had elapsed. Thereafter, the longer the follow-up with preservation of mental and physical health, the less likely is organic disease to emerge.

Headache due to scalp and cervical muscle tension

Headache due to cervical and scalp muscle tension resulting from anxiety is rare in very young children. It is common in older children, and can occur from the age of 5 or 6 years. It may be difficult to distinguish from migraine, and often both occur in the same child. Tension headache is usually non-paroxysmal and generalised or described as a tight band or feeling of heaviness; it recurs frequently and sometimes shows prolonged fluctuations. Children with tension headache appear pale, and they are generally anorexic, but rarely sick. There is often surprisingly little interference with ordinary activities. Mild analgesics are often not helpful. It is obviously less important to distinguish tension headache from migraine than to distinguish both from other more serious causes of headache. However, although management of the two conditions is similar with the emphasis on relieving the provoking stress factors in both, full treatment depends on proper understanding of the mechanisms involved, and every effort should be made to do this. Again, the history is all important.

INVESTIGATION

When no cause for headache is found at first presentation then the child should continue under intermittent observation until some satisfactory explanation is reached. Any headache which interferes with ordinary activity should be regarded as potentially serious until sufficient time has passed to show that it is not, or until investigation has excluded serious cause.

Investigation should be done if:

1. there are abnormal physical signs, including *inter alia* cranial bruit, head circumference exceeding the 90th centile, or head growth centile considerably greater than height centile;

2. accompanying symptoms are focal, or stereotyped, or included altered conscious level, or prominent vomiting.

3. the headache is related to straining, exercise or posture, or awakens from sleep;

4. the headache is not relieved by analgesics, or alters in quality, frequency, or severity;

5. there is any change in behaviour, personality, or physical and mental performance;

6. the child fails to grow at the normal rate, or shows slowing (or regression) of physical or mental development;

7. the child is under 5 years old.

It is beyond the scope of this chapter to discuss specific therapy but most children with migraine respond well to appropriate management. If a child with headache thought to be migraine fails to respond, the diagnosis should be reconsidered.

CONCLUSION

Migraine is common in childhood occurring in approximately 3% of boys and girls, from an early age. The disorder is usually mild. It may lead to disability because of frequent or severe attacks, or (rarely) because of permanent sequelae. Diagnosis can be difficult and depends more on the circumstances and temporal pattern of attacks, and continuing physical and mental well-being between attacks, than on the actual characteristics of the headache itself. The main clinical importance of migraine in children lies in the need to distinguish it from more serious causes of headache.

REFERENCES

Basser L S 1964 Benign paroxysmal vertigo of childhood. Brain 87: 141–152
Bille B 1962 Migraine in school children. Acta Paediatrica 51: Suppl 136, 13–151
Burnstock G 1981 Pathophysiology of migraine: a new hypothesis. Lancet i: 1397–1398
Christensen M F, Mortensen O 1975 Long term prognosis in children with recurrent
    abdominal pain. Archives of Disease in Childhood 50: 110–114.
Congdon P J, Forsythe W I 1979 Migraine in childhood. Developmental Medicine and Child
    Neurology 21: 209–216
Dalsgaard-Nielson T, Engberg-Pedersen H, Holm H E 1969 Danish Medical Bulletin
    17: 138–148
Deonna T, Martin D 1981 Benign paroxysmal torticollis in infancy. Archives of Disease in
    Childhood 56: 956–959
Forsythe W I, Redmond A 1974 Two controlled trials of tyramine in children with migraine.
    Developmental Medicine and Child Neurology 16: 794–799
Friedman A P, von Storch T J C, Merritt H H 1954 Migraine and tension headaches.
    Neurology 4: 773–788
Glista G G, Mellinger J F, Rooke E D 1975 Familial hemiplegic migraine. Mayo Clinic
    Proceedings 50: 307–311
Haas D C, Pineda G S, Lourie H 1975 Juvenile head trauma syndromes and their
    relationship to migraine. Archives of Neurology 32: 727–730
Hammond J 1974 The late sequelae of recurrent vomiting of childhood. Developmental
    Medicine and Child Neurology 16: 15–22
Hannington E 1978 Migraine: a blood disorder? Lancet ii: 501–502
Harper A M, MacKenzie E T, McCulloch J, Pickard J D 1977 Migraine and the blood-brain
    barrier. Lancet 2: 1034–1036
Heyck H 1968 Examination and differential diagnosis of headache. In: Vinken P J, Bruyn
    G W Handbook of Clinical Neurology, Vol 5, ch 3, p. 32. North Holland Publishers, New
    York
Hockaday J M 1979 Basilar migraine in childhood. Developmental Medicine and Child
    Neurology 21: 455–463
Hockaday J M 1982 Headache in children. British Journal of Hospital Medicine 27: 383–391
Honig P J, Charney E B 1982 Children with brain tumour headaches. American Journal of
    Diseases of Children 136: 121–124
Jensen T S 1980 Transient global amnesia in childhood. Developmental Medicine and Child
    Neurology 22: 654–667
Koenigsberger M R, Chutorian A M, Gold A P, Schrey M S 1970 Benign Paroxysmal
    Vertigo of Childhood. Neurology 20: 1108–1113
Krägeloh I, Aicardi J 1980 Alternating hemiplegia of infancy. Developmental Medicine and
    child Neurology 22: 784–791
Lance J W, Anthony M 1966 Some clinical aspects of migraine. Archives of Neurology
    15: 356–361
Marshall J 1978 Cerebral blood flow in migraine. In: Green R (ed) Current Concepts in
    Migraine Research, p. 131. Raven Press, New York

Matthews W B 1972 Footballer's Migraine. British Medical Journal i: 326–327
Moffatt A M, Swash M, Scott D F 1974 Effect of chocolate on migraine. Journal of
    Neurology, Neurosurgery and Psychiatry 37: 445–448
Pearce J 1975 Introduction. In: Modern Topics in Migraine, pp 1–7. William Heinemann
    Medical Books, London
Prensky A L, Sommer D 1979 Diagnosis and treatment of migraine in children. Neurology
    29: 506–510
Raskin N H, Appenzeller O 1980 Headache. Major Problems in Internal Medicine, Vol XIX
    W B Saunders Company, London
Raymond L A, Tew J, Fogelson M H 1977 Ophthalmoplegic migraine of early onset. Journal
    of Pediatrics 90: 1035–1036
Reinhart J B, Evans S L, McFadden D L 1977 Cyclic vomiting in children. Pediatrics
    59: 371–377.
Selby G, Lance J W 1960 Observations on 500 cases of migraine and allied vascular
    headache. Journal of Neurology Neurosurgery and Psychiatry 23: 23–32
Sparks J P 1978 The incidence of migraine in school children. The Practitioner 221: 407–411
Swaiman K F, Frank Y 1978 Seizure headaches in children. Developmental Medicine and
    Child Neurology 20: 580–585
Vahlquist B 1955 Migraine in Children. International Archives of Allergy 7: 348–355
Waters W E 1971 Migraine: intelligence, social class and familial prevalence. British Medical
    Journal i: 77–81
Waters W E 1972 Migraine and symptoms in childhood: bilious attacks, travel sickness and
    eczema. Headache 12: 55–61
Waters W E 1974 The Epidemiology of Migraine. Boehringer Ingelheim, Berkshire
World Federation of Neurology's Research Group on Migraine and Headache 1969
    Hemicrania 1: 3

Fetal alcohol syndrome and fetal alcohol effects

INTRODUCTION

Alcohol has been described as the most frequently known teratogenic cause of mental handicap in the Western world (Clarren & Smith, 1978) and damage to the fetus by alcohol as the largest known health hazard by a noxious agent that is preventable (Olegard et al, 1979). These are dramatic statements which raise the question why it took so long for the condition resulting from maternal alcoholism—fetal alcohol syndrome (FAS)—to be described (Jones et al, 1973). The answer to this may be that the features of FAS are not the only manifestations of the effects of alcohol on the fetus. Lesser degrees of damage produce a less clear-cut pattern of signs and such affected children can be considered as showing fetal alcohol effects but not FAS.

The prevalance of FAS varies from country to country and even between areas and ethnic groups within the same country. Nevertheless an extensive literature commenting on the consequences of maternal alcoholism for the fetus stretching over thousands of years shows that alcohol is, and always has been, a fairly frequent teratogen (Warner & Rosett, 1975). Yet drinking habits vary and maternal and fetal metabolism both affect the fetal response to alcohol. Damage to the fetus can vary from none at all to intra-uterine death or malformation with severe growth and mental retardation. Thus a confusing variety of fetal damage probably hindered the clinical definition of FAS since the full syndrome is only an extreme example in a vast range of abnormalities resulting from the effects of alcohol on the fetus.

CLINICAL FEATURES OF FAS

Table 3.1 lists some of the clinical features described in FAS. The variety of skeletal, cardiac, and other abnormalities associated with heavy maternal alcohol ingestion is too great to list every reported abnormality (Clarren & Smith, 1978; Iosub et al, 1981; Sandor et al, 1981; Cremin & Jaffer, 1981; Friedman, 1982; Pratt, 1982). None of the features listed in Table 3.1 is pathognomonic for FAS. It is consequently difficult to confirm a diagnosis

Table 3.1 Clinical features of FAS

Facial	Short palpebral fissures
	Anteverted nostrils
	Epicanthic folds
	Flat upper lip with hypoplastic philtrum
	Narrow vermilion border to upper lip
	Micrognathia
	Hypoplastic dental enamel
Cerebral	Microcephaly
	Mild to severe mental retardation
	Learning and behavioural difficulties
	Speech problems
	Hyperactivity
	Neonatal withdrawal symptoms
Growth	Prenatal growth retardation
	Postnatal growth retardation
Skeletal	Cleft palate
	Syndactyly
	Polydactyly
	Tetraectrodactyly
	Short metacarpals
	Epiphyseal fusion
	Vertebral anomalies
	Delayed bone age
Other	Cardiac abnormalities
	Renal abnormalities
	Obstructive jaundice and hepatic fibrosis
	Immunodeficiency
	Hypoplastic nails

Table 3.2 Complete FAS

Prenatal and/or Postnatal growth retardation	Weight, height and/or head circumference < tenth centile for gestational age
CNS involvement	Neurological abnormality, developmental delay, or intellectual impairment
Characteristic facial dysmorphology	At least two of the following: Microcephaly: head circumference < third centile Microphthalmia and/or short palpebral fissures Poorly developed philtrum, Thin upper lip and/or flattening of maxillary area

of FAS. Obviously not every presentation of the clinical features listed can be attributed to maternal alcohol consumption, particularly when this has been slight. The facial features of FAS are said to be as characteristic as those of Down's syndrome. We feel the facies is recognisable in the older child, but not as easily as that of Down's syndrome. The facies of the newborn with FAS may be uncharacteristic.

The Fetal Alcohol Study Group of the American Research Society on

Alcoholism has recommended that the term FAS be confined to children showing the features listed in Table 3.2. Children showing some, but not all, of these features together with other significant abnormalities in skeletal, cardiac or nervous system should be considered as showing the 'partial' or 'expanded' syndrome or simply fetal alcohol effects (Shaywitz et al, 1978; Rosett et al, 1981). The mothers of children with complete FAS are almost invariably chronic alcoholics. The mothers of children showing the partial syndrome have usually drunk less consistently in pregnancy, but have always consumed significant amounts of alcohol.

FAS IN THE NEONATE AND INFANT

Neurological problems

Mental handicap is the most important consequence of FAS. Brain damage is not always obvious in the neonatal period but may present as feeding problems and delayed milestones at a few months of age. Thus abnormal behaviour in the neonate may be the first sign to suggest a diagnosis of FAS or fetal alcohol effects.

Infants born to women who drink heavily until shortly before delivery may also develop true withdrawal symptoms (Nichols, 1967): these infants are restless, agitated, tremulous and hypertonic with increased respiratory rate and abdominal distension. Occasionally they have opisthotonos and convulsions. The half-life of alcohol in the fetus is short. The time of onset of withdrawal symptoms is therefore largely determined by the duration of maternal abstinence prior to delivery but is usually a matter of minutes or a few hours after delivery. This is in contrast to the symptoms of withdrawal from anticonvulsants or opiates which sometimes develop days after delivery. This acute alcoholic withdrawal resolves over the first few days of life, though it may impair feeding. The abnormalities of behaviour such as restlessness may make the child difficult to respond to with consequent effects on what may be an already disadvantaged situation in having an alcoholic mother.

Jitteriness, hyperexcitability, hypertonia and feeding difficulties persist beyond the neonatal period in some infants. Presumably these protracted symptoms relate to structural abnormalities in the central nervous system rather than to metabolic dependence on alcohol, since they do not finally disappear until 4 to 5 months of age. It seems likely that the gradual disappearance of these symptoms is due to myelinisation and maturation of the nervous system masking or suppressing this aspect of abnormal neurological function. Prolonged excitability and restlessness in early infancy may affect learning through abnormal mother-child interaction and therefore be partly responsible for the developmental retardation, emotional deprivation and behavioural abnormalities of later childhood.

Sleep studies on 3-day-old infants with FAS show a negative correlation between the time an infant spends sleeping and the amount of alcohol the mother consumed in the first trimester of pregnancy. The more the mother drank, the less the infant sleeps. The pattern of sleep in these infants is also different from that of infants whose mothers did not drink during pregnancy. Infants with FAS have more interruptions during periods of quiet sleep than the infants of non-drinking mothers. When awake, they also show an increased incidence of restlessness and major movements compared with control infants (Rosett et al, 1979).

Electroencephalographic (EEG) studies on neonates with FAS are abnormal. In one study abnormalities were demonstrable in all infants born to women who drank heavily throughout pregnancy and in two out of three infants born to women who abstained from alcohol after the first trimester but drank heavily until then. Abnormalities in somatosensory evoked responses were more consistently abnormal than either visual or 'photic driving' responses, although these responses were frequently abnormal too. Side differences in evoked responses were common (Havlicek & Childaeva, 1976; Olegård et al 1979).

Histopathology of the CNS abnormalities

Brain weights in infants and children with FAS are usually low. Reports of the histopathological abnormalities in these children are few but, when reported, the findings are often bizarre. Abnormal neuronal and glial cell migration leads to abnormal sheets of cells forming massive plaques of cells spreading over the brain surface and sometimes across the midline. These findings are not unique to FAS but are unusual in other conditions. Agenesis of the corpus callosum and cerebellar hypoplasia are other occasional findings (Jones & Smith 1975; Clarren et al, 1978). Spina bifida, meningomyelocoele and hydrocephalus do occur but are not particularly common features of FAS (Friedman, 1982). The lack of epidemiological studies which include histopathology of the brains of children born to alcoholic women makes it virtually impossible to know whether these abnormalities are more frequent in FAS than in other handicapping conditions.

Growth

Pre- and postnatal growth retardation is one of the diagnostic features of FAS, as growth seems to be one of the most sensitive indicators of the effects of alcohol on the fetus. This may be because alcohol can affect growth at any stage in pregnancy, whereas it has to be present in sufficient quantity at fairly precise times to cause many of the other congenital abnormalities associated with FAS. Birth weight is low in FAS, but birth length is proportionately more severely affected. Skull circumference is also low, but correlates less well with maternal alcohol consumption than weight or length (Streissguth et al, 1978). It is obviously not possible to know the full effect of alcohol in pregnancy on fetal growth since many infants, whose birth weights are within the normal range, might have had even higher birth weights had their mothers abstained throughout pregnancy.

One study of the birth weights of infants born to alcoholic women who did not change their drinking habits during pregnancy found the infants weighed, on average, 493 g less than the infants of women who were abstinent during pregnancy and drank little before that. Alcoholic women who managed to reduce their intake before pregnancy bore infants with a mean birth weight 258 g less than the non-drinking controls (Little et al, 1980). This suggests that some of the effects of alcoholism on birth weight persist even after the prospective mother stops drinking since the groups in this study were matched for race, education and smoking habits. Little (1977), however, found that women who drank the equivalent of 30 g of absolute alcohol, or more, per day in early pregnancy had infants with a birth weight on average 90.8 g less than non-alcohol drinking matched controls. When the women drank an equivalent amount of alcohol in the last trimester the infants weighed on average 160 g less at birth. The weight reductions in this study may seem slight but the amounts of alcohol consumed by these women were small and were at a level where FAS would not normally be expected.

Cardiac abnormalities

Congenital heart disease affects between 29% and 50% of children with FAS. Some studies report ostium secundum atrial septal defects as the commonest lesions but other studies suggest that simple or complex ventricular septal defects are as frequent as atrial septal defects. Naturally occurring population differences in the prevalence of types of congenital heart disease may determine the most likely teratogenic effect of alcohol on the fetus and thus account for some of the discrepancies between reports (Sandor et al, 1981).

Orthopaedic abnormalities

Congenital abnormalities involving the skeletal system are common in FAS and in fetal alcohol effects (Spiegel et al, 1979). Many different abnormalities are described and often consist of minor abnormalities of the digits. Abnormalities of one or more vertebrae are also common. Arthrogryposis may occur (Hermann et al, 1980; Jaffer et al, 1981; Cremin & Jaffer, 1981; Poskitt et al, 1982). Radiology frequently reveals orthopaedic abnormalities undetected at routine clinical examination. Epiphyseal fusion and the development of pseudo-epiphyses are common particularly in the hand and wrist. Synostoses, often involving the radius and ulna, are other common abnormalities diagnosed on skeletal survey. Bony fusions and bony abnormalities generally seem more common in the upper limbs than in the lower limbs, possibly because development of the upper limb occurs at a stage when the embryo is particularly vulnerable to alcoholic insult (Cremin & Jaffer, 1981; Jaffer et al, 1981). Alternatively upper limb development may occur before the time when a mother usually deliberately or spontaneously reduces her alcoholic intake because she is pregnant (Little et al, 1976). Many of the radiological abnormalities only become obvious as the infant grows, since the affected bones are not all ossified at birth.

FAS IN THE OLDER CHILD

Neurological function

Several studies of children with FAS or fetal alcohol effects estimate a mean IQ of 65 for affected children (Clarren & Smith, 1978; Iosub et al, 1981), although the range of IQ found is enormous and includes some children so severely retarded that their IQ cannot be estimated and other children with apparently normal intelligence. In general, the more severe the clinical manifestations of the effects of alcohol, the more severe the intellectual retardation, although this is not invariably so (Streissguth et al, 1978).

Children without significant mental retardation may nevertheless show signs of other brain dysfunction. Streissguth (1976) has described tremulousness, weak and primitive grasp, poor finger articulation and delay in establishing hand dominance in affected children. Poor attention and poor problem solving skills are other associated features. Shaywitz et al (1978) felt the full syndrome complex of FAS should include hyperactivity, attention deficiencies and school learning problems. Seventy-five per cent of older children with full or partial FAS show some behavioural problems and hyperactivity is a major handicap in 50%. Interestingly the children who are hyperactive are likely to become alcoholic themselves in later life (Goodwin et al, 1975). Over 80% of children have difficulties with speech even though their oropalatal mechanisms for speech are functioning normally, and happily these last difficulties seem to respond to speech therapy (Iosub et al, 1981).

It is not entirely clear how much the cerebral dysfunction of FAS can be blamed on irreversible intra-uterine damage and how much should be attributed to a postnatal environment of inappropriate rearing and deprivation in emotion and experience. Excellent fostering from birth does not overcome the mental retardation seen in the worst cases of FAS but it may alleviate some of the behaviour problems. A good home environment is likely to facilitate optimum mental development and thus minimise the effects of prenatal brain damage on ultimate ability. An alcoholic mother is unlikely to provide such an environment.

The EEG of older children with FAS shows excessive slowing with poor organisation in background rhythm, rhythmical slow delta waves and sharp activity arising particularly from the posterior part of the head (Root et al, 1975; Havlicek & Childaeva, 1976). In spite of the EEG appearance, epilepsy is not a particularly common accompaniment of FAS.

Growth

Although length is usually more affected than weight in the newborn with FAS, the reverse applies postnatally. Children with FAS are short but often very thin with weight further below the normal centiles than height (Clarren & Smith, 1978), which may reflect early feeding difficulties. Too few children have been followed into adult life to comment on pubertal development and final adult stature in FAS. Bone age is retarded although not usually as retarded as height age so these children probably become short adults. Investigation of the hypothalamo-pituitary axis has not demonstrated any abnormality which could account for the poor growth (Root et al, 1975; Tze et al, 1976).

Immunity

Postnatally some, if not all, children with FAS have altered immunity and an increased risk of infection. Johnson et al (1981) reviewed thirteen children with FAS and found an increased incidence of life threatening bacterial infections as well as a propensity to minor infections. Lymphopenia in FAS was similar to that in infants who were light for gestational age for other reasons. However, defective E rosette formation and mitogen stimulation, as well as low immunoglobulin levels, were assocaited with intrauterine exposure to alcohol and not with other causes of low weight for gestational age. More than one-third of children with FAS had immunoglobulin G (IgG) levels more than one standard deviation below that for normal controls although none had IgG below the level at which IgG replacement would normally be considered.

Recently Ammann et al (1982) described four cases of diGeorge syndrome where the mothers consumed substantial quantities of alcohol in early pregnancy. DiGeorge syndrome is a congenital disorder involving immunologic deficiencies and is of indeterminate aetiology. It is possible that it results from teratogenic insults such as alcohol, since the immunological abnormalities of diGeorge syndrome overlap with those described for complete FAS.

OTHER RISKS FOR FETUS AND CHILD

Women who drink large quantities of alcohol in pregnancy have an increased risk of spontaneous abortion in the second trimester (Harlap & Shiono, 1980). Kline et al (1980) compared the drinking habits of 616 women who had spontaneous abortions with those of 632 women who delivered infants of at least 28 weeks' gestation. Seventeen per cent of the women who had abortions, compared with only 8.1% of the women who carried to 28 weeks, drank alcohol at least twice a week during pregnancy. The authors estimated that more than one-quarter of pregnant women who drink alcohol at least twice a week will have spontaneous abortions compared with only 14% of women who drink less frequently. This increased risk is largely confined to the second trimester. The equivalent of more than 30 g of absolute alcohol drunk at any one time is associated with an increased risk of spontaneous abortion. Higher levels of ingestion do not carry a proportionately higher spontaneous abortion rate. Thus alcohol may act as a fetotoxin with a critical level above which the chances of fetal poisoning are greatly increased.

Small quantities of alcohol have noticeable effects on fetal breathing. In the third trimester a single drink of vodka produces significant suppression of respiratory movement. This occurs in the absence of changes in uterine activity and at blood alcohol levels well below those that cause acidosis or blood gas changes in the mother (Fox et al, 1978; Lewis & Boylan, 1979). Central nervous system depression, together with the problems of congenital abnormality and intra-uterine growth retardation probably contribute to the high perinatal mortality of FAS.

As already suggested unlike many insults that act on the child *in utero*, the damaging effects of maternal alcoholism do not necessarily cease at birth. These children are at risk of further damage from their chaotic family life. They are at risk of emotional deprivation, battering and neglect. Many end up in care or, perhaps worse, have intermittent spells in care. Many become alcoholic themselves in later life. Thus a diagnosis of FAS should alert those involved to the probability of continuing problems within the home and the likely need for constant supervision of the whole family.

HOW DOES ALCOHOL AFFECT THE FETUS?

There are many possible ways in which alcohol could damage the embryo and fetus. Unfortunately we can only speculate on which of these possibilities is most likely.

The epidemiology of FAS suggests that fetal as well as maternal factors affect the likelihood of fetal damage. Different congenital abnormalities in dizygotic twins with FAS indicate that there are genetic determinants of fetal susceptibility to alcohol (Christoffel & Salafsky, 1975). Monozygotic twins with FAS do not always have identical abnormalities (Palmer et al, 1974) but some of the differences between monozygotic twins could be explained by deformations due to intrauterine compression. Perhaps it is unreasonable to expect post-conception insults to produce identical effects with identical twin fetuses since teratogenic damage to singletons is not necessarily symmetrical.

It is not clear whether maternal nutrition, liver damage, the effect of other drugs or the level and duration of alcohol and its metabolites in the maternal blood is the main determinant of FAS. Not all chronic alcoholic women have infants with FAS. Presumably the individuality of maternal, as well as fetal, metabolism is relevant to the development of FAS.

Many alcoholic women are poorly nourished. They may be deficient in protein and energy stores or they may have specific nutrient deficiencies. Is there evidence to link poor maternal nutrition with the features of FAS?

Infants born to women who were in the first trimester of pregnancy at the height of the Dutch Famine Winter of 1944–45 showed an increased incidence of central nervous system abnormalities, although the numbers of infants born was so small that the significance of this finding is uncertain (Smith, 1947). Birth weights of infants born to mothers who were in the last trimester of pregnancy at the height of the famine were, on average, 9% below the weights of infants born before or after the famine. At age 19 these infants were of normal height, weight and intelligence. Thus the features of severe maternal malnutrition have little in common with the abnormalities and persisting growth retardation common in FAS (Stein & Susser, 1976).

Folic acid is one of the nutrients which may be below average levels in women who later deliver infants with spina bifida (Smithells et al, 1976) but, as we have already stated, spina bifida is not a particularly common accompaniment of FAS. The features of Fetal Anticonvulsant Syndrome and FAS are very similar and alcohol, phenytoin and phenobarbitone can all induce folic acid deficiency through malabsorption of folate and potentiation of liver metabolism of folate. All these drugs, however, have other effects in common which could be responsible for their similar teratogenic effects (Hill, 1976). Since there is a correlation, although not always a close one, between the amount a woman drinks and the severity of the features of FAS in her offspring (Ouellette et al, 1977), it seems possible that alcohol or its metabolites act directly on the fetus to produce the features of FAS. In early pregnancy alcohol acts as a fetotoxin and produces abortion but in order to exert a teratogenic effect it must damage the fetus without killing it. The wide variety of abnormalities produced by alcohol suggests that alcohol has a fairly non-specific effect on the fetus and can cause damage to many tissues at many stages in pregnancy.

What evidence is there that alcohol is directly responsible for the abnormalities of FAS? Work in animals has demonstrated repeatedly that abnormalities similar to those of FAS can result from exposure of embryonic and fetal animals to alcohol (Krous, 1981). Often, however, these studies use doses of alcohol that achieve blood levels in excess of those likely to be achieved by pregnant women. Nevertheless, infant rats born to mothers fed alcohol in insufficient quantities to affect birth weights show delayed neuronal maturation with reduced dendritic extensions and branching within the brain (Hammer & Schiebel, 1981). Since the development of dendritic connections is important both for maturation of brain function and for growth and development of other neurones, this sort of abnormality, if it occurs in FAS, could have profound effects on brain size and function.

It is possible that acetabldehyde, the first metabolite of alcohol, rather than alcohol itself is the teratogen for FAS. Disulfiram, which inhibits acetaldehyde metabolism, causes severe fetal damage when given to pregnant women (Nora et al, 1977). Individual responses to alcohol in pregnancy can be explained by the fact that both alcohol and acetaldehyde metabolism are partly genetically determined. Twin studies show a greater correlation in the metabolism of a 1 ml/kg oral dose of 95% ethanol between identical than between fraternal twins. But what are the implications of this for the fetus? Rapid metabolism of alcohol will benefit the fetus if alcohol is the teratogen. If, however, the main teratogen is acetaldehyde, rapid metabolism of alcohol will present the fetal tissues with a large load of acetaldehyde which could accumulate to toxic levels. Genetic differences in acetaldehyde metabolism also occur. Alcoholics have a tendency for low levels of the cytosolic component of acetaldehyde dehydrogenase (Jenkins & Peters, 1980) but no correlation has yet been shown between rates of maternal alcohol metabolism and the risk of FAS. Such a study might not be informative anyway, since the ability of the fetus, rather than that of the mother, to cope with alcohol and its metabolites may be the critical factor.

It is not necessary to explain FAS on the effects of one single teratogenic factor. The varied manifestations of FAS may result from several teratogenic mechanisms which include alcohol, its metabolites, and genetic and nutritional factors.

In postnatal life the dangers of a heavy alcohol consumption include the potentiation of other drug effects. Potentiation with alcohol is particularly likely for drugs acting on the CNS. Many alcoholic women are epileptic or depressed and are taking drugs as treatment. Others may take illicit drugs and potentiation of the metabolic or teratogenic effect of alcohol by drugs may account for some of the more bizarre manifestations of FAS (Poskitt et al, 1982). Smoking also increases the risk of spontaneous abortion or other adverse outcome to pregnancy in chronic alcoholism (Sokol et al, 1980).

PREVENTION OF FAS

Complete prevention of FAS is only possible if all women abstain from all alcohol throughout their childbearing years. This is not a particularly attractive preventive measure and is probably more extreme than necessary (Anon, 1981). How much alcohol is necessary for the fetus to be harmed? Regular or occasional ingestion of the equivalent of less than 30 ml absolute alcohol (about one and a half wine glasses, 700 ml of beer or 70 ml of spirits) per day, probably carries little risk for the fetus though proof of this remains uncertain. Levels above this seem to carry an increasing risk of abnormality, growth retardation and low IQ. Whether irregular but higher levels of alcohol consumption are equally teratogenic to steady moderate drinking is not certain, but the effect of high doses of alcohol on abortion suggests they are (Kline et al, 1980). Thus 'binge' drinking should be avoided by all women of childbearing years and women proposing to have children should avoid ingesting more than the equivalent of 30 ml absolute alcohol daily. Women who smoke or take other drugs, particularly anticonvulsants and antidepressants, should probably abjure all alcohol (and where possible abjure other drugs and cigarettes as well).

Education of the public is an essential part of reducing the prevalence of

FAS. The importance of alcohol as a teratogen and inhibitor of fetal growth throughout pregnancy needs to be stressed. Many women reduce their alcohol intake apparently spontaneously in early pregnancy, but by then fetal damage has occurred. Maternal alcohol consumption in early pregnancy may be underestimated if the intake in late pregnancy is the only intake recalled. A high alcohol consumption at any stage in pregnancy is dangerous to the fetus, but a reduction in alcohol intake at any stage can improve the outlook for the fetus (Little, 1977; Rosett et al, 1978).

We do not know how commonly fetal damage due to alcohol occurs in Britain. This author's experiences suggest that the full FAS is more frequent than one case per 2500 births in an inner city area. Studies in the US and Sweden suggest an incidence of one or two cases of FAS per thousand births with a more frequent occurrence of fetal alcohol effects (Clarren & Smith, 1978; Olegard et al, 1979). In the USA approximately 5–10% of women drink at a level that places the fetus at risk (Rosett & Weiner, 1982). Particular attention should be paid to the nutrition of these women during and prior to pregnancy and they should not only be advised to reduce their alcohol intake but to avoid cigarettes and, where medically possible, other drugs. Infants born to families where there is a risk of FAS should be monitored postnatally for behavioural and social problems that may exacerbate the handicap of a mildly brain-damaged child.

It is easy to state that education of the public and encouragement of those women with drink problems to stop drinking lead to prevention of FAS. It is more difficult to state how these things can be done successfully as we know already from the 'smoking' literature that it is very difficult to change behaviours which are often dependent on a multitude of social, economic and psychological factors. The mother with a recognised alcohol problem should be referred for psychiatric or community help. Counselling for chronic alcoholic women should be coupled with the offer of hospital admission for alcohol withdrawal. It is however relatively rare for the heavy drinker to be accurate and explicit about her alcohol consumption when questioned in an obstetric clinic (Little et al, 1976). Thus health education of school children and pre-conception counselling on the adverse effects of alcohol are important in helping prevent addiction.

It is obviously important to recognise the middle class women who 'take to the bottle' secretly whilst their husbands are out at work or who become dangerously heavy drinkers through frequent cocktail and dinner parties. Such women are likely to be reached by health education programmes although they may not be prepared to acknowledge their problems. More worrying perhaps are the heavy drinking, heavy smoking and poorly nourished women from stressful and deprived environments who have a poor record of attendance for antenatal care. Their infants are not only at risk between conception and birth but are postnatally disadvantaged by the environment as well. There may be little opportunity in postnatal life to overcome or minimise antenatal damage from alcohol. If we only knew how

to improve the environment, lifestyle and nutritional habits of this fraction
of society we might reduce the prevalence of many health problems as well
as those resulting from the effects of alcohol on the unborn child.

REFERENCES

Ammann A J, Wara D W, Cowan M J, Barrett D J, Stiehm E R 1982 The DiGeorge
syndrome and the fetal alcohol syndrome. American Journal of Diseases of Children
136: 906–908

Anon 1981 Fetal alcohol advisory debated. Science 214: 642–644

Christoffel K K, Salafsky J 1975 Fetal alcohol syndrome in dizygotic twins. Journal of
Pediatrics 87: 963–967

Clarren S K, Smith D W 1978 The fetal alcohol syndrome. New England Journal of
Medicine 298: 1063–1067

Clarren S K, Alvord E C Jr, Sumi S M, Streissguth A P, Smith D W 1978 Brain
malformations related to prenatal exposure to ethanol. Journal of Pediatrics 92: 64–67

Cremin B J, Jaffer Z 1981 Radiological aspects of the fetal alcohol syndrome. Pediatric
Radiology 11: 151–153

Fox H E, Steinbrecher M, Pessel D, Inglis J, Medvid L, Angel E 1978 Maternal ethanol
ingestion and the occurrence of human fetal breathing movements. American Journal of
Obstetrics and Gynecology 132: 354–358

Friedman J M 1982 Can maternal alcohol ingestion cause neural tube defects? Journal of
Pediatrics 101: 232–234

Goodwin D W, Schulsinger F, Hermansen L, Guze S B, Winokur G 1975 Alcoholism and
the hyperactive child syndrome. Journal of Nervous and Mental Disease 160: 349–353

Hammer R P Jr, Schiebel A B 1981 Morphologic evidence for a delay in neuronal maturation
in fetal alcohol exposure. Experimental Neurology 74: 587–596

Harlap S, Shiono P H 1980 Alcohol, smoking and incidence of spontaneous abortion in first
and second trimester. Lancet ii: 173–176

Havlicek V, Childaeva R 1976 EEG component of fetal alcohol syndrome. Lancet ii: 477

Hermann J, Pallister P D, Opitz J M 1980 Tetraectrodactyly and other skeletal
manifestations in the fetal alcohol syndrome. European Journal of Pediatrics 133: 221–226

Hill R M 1976 Fetal malformations and antiepileptic drugs. American Journal of Diseases of
Children 130: 923–925

Iosub S, Fuchs M, Bingol N, Gromisch D S 1981 Fetal alcohol syndrome revisited.
Pediatrics 68: 475–479

Jaffer Z, Nelson M, Beighton P 1981 Bone fusion in the fetal alcohol syndrome. Journal of
Bone and Joint Surgery 63B: 569–571

Jenkins W J, Peters T J 1980 Selectively reduced hepatic acetaldehyde dehydrogenase in
alcoholics. Lancet i: 628–629

Johnson S, Knight R, Marmer D J, Steele R W 1981 Immune deficiency in fetal alcohol
syndrome. Pediatric Research 15: 908–911

Jones K L, Smith D W 1975 The fetal alcohol syndrome. Teratology 12: 1–10

Jones K J, Smith D W, Ulleland C N, Streissguth A P 1973 Pattern of malformation in
offspring of chronic alcoholic mothers. Lancet i: 1267–1271

Kline J, Shrout P, Stein Z, Susser M, Warburton D 1980 Drinking during pregnancy and
spontaneous abortion. Lancet ii: 176–180

Krous H F 1981 Fetal alcohol syndrome: a dilemma of maternal alcoholism. Pathology
Annual 16 Part B: 295–311

Lewis P J, Boylan P 1979 Alcohol and fetal breathing. Lancet i: 388

Little R E 1977 Moderate alcohol use during pregnancy and decreased infant birth weight.
American Journal of Public Health 67: 1154–1156

Little R E, Schultz F A, Mandell W 1976 Drinking during pregnancy. Journal of Studies on
Alcohol 37: 375–379

Little R E, Streissguth A P, Barr H M, Herman C S 1980 Decreased birth weight in infants
of alcoholic women who abstained during pregnancy. Journal of Pediatrics 96:974–977

Nichols M M 1967 Acute alcoholic withdrawal symptoms in a newborn. American Journal of
Diseases of Children 113: 714–715

Nora A H, Nora J J, Blu 1977 Limb reduction anomalies in infants born to disulfiram treated alcoholic mothers. Lancet ii:664

Olegård et al 1979 Effects on the child of alcohol abuse during pregnancy. Acta Paediatrica Scandinavica Supplement 275: 112–121

Ouellette E M, Rosett H L, Rosman N P, Weiner L 1977 Adverse effects on offspring of maternal alcohol abuse during pregnancy. New England Journal of Medicine 297: 528–530

Palmer R H, Ouellette E M, Warner M S W, Leichtman S R 1974 Congenital malformations in offspring of a chronic alcoholic mother. Pediatrics 53: 490–494

Poskitt E M E, Hensey O J, Smith C S 1982 Alcohol, other drugs and the fetus. Developmental Medicine and Child Neurology 24: 596–602

Pratt O E 1982 Alcohol and the developing fetus. British Medical Bulletin 38: 48–52

Root A W, Reiter E O, Andriola M, Duckett G 1975 Hypothalamic pituitary function in the fetal alcohol syndrome. Journal of Pediatrics 87: 585–588

Rosett H L, Weiner L 1982 Prevention of fetal alcohol effects. Pediatrics 69: 813–816

Rosett H L, Weiner L, Edelin K C 1981 Strategies for prevention of fetal alcohol effects. Obstetrics and Gynecology 57: 1–7

Rosett H L, Ouellette E M, Weiner L, Owens E 1978 Therapy of heavy drinking in pregnancy. Obstetrics and Gynecology 51: 41–46

Rosett et al 1979 Effects of maternal drinking on neonatal state regulation. Developmental Medicine and Child Neurology 21: 464–473

Sandor G C S, Smith D F, MacLeod P M 1981 Cardiac malformation in the fetal alcohol syndrome. Journal of Pediatrics 98: 771–773

Shaywitz S E, Cohen D J, Shaywitz B A 1978 The expanded FAS (EFAS)—behavioral and learning deficits in children with normal intelligence. Pediatric Research 12: 375

Smith C A 1947 Effects of maternal undernutrition upon the newborn infant in Holland 1944–1945. Journal of Pediatrics 30: 229–243

Smithells R W, Sheppard S, Schorah C J 1976 Vitamin deficiencies and neural tube defects. Archives of Disease in Childhood 51: 944–950

Sokol R J, Miller S I, Reed G 1980 Alcohol abuse during pregnancy: an epidemiological model. Alcoholism: Clinical and Experimental Research 4: 135–145

Spiegel P G, Pekman W M, Rich B H, Versteeg C N, Nelson V, Dudniknov M 1979 The orthopedic aspects of the fetal alcohol syndrome. Clinical Orthopaedics and Related Research 139: 58–63

Stein Z, Susser M 1976 Maternal starvation and birth defects. In: Kelly S, Hook E B, Janerich D T, Porter I H (eds) Birth defects. Risks and Consequences, pp 205–220. Academic Press, New York

Streissguth A P 1976 Psychologic handicaps in children with the fetal alcohol syndrome. Annals of the New York Academy of Science 273: 140–145

Streissguth A P, Herman C S, Smith D W 1978 Intelligence, behavior and dysmorphogenesis in the fetal alcohol syndrome: a report on twenty patients. Journal of Pediatrics 92: 363–367

Tze W J, Friesen H G, MacLeod P M 1976 Growth hormone response in fetal alcohol syndrome. Archives of Disease in Childhood 51: 703–706

Warner R H, Rosett H L 1975 The effects of drinking on the offspring. An historical survey of the American and British literature. Journal of Studies on Alcohol 36: 1395–1420

Squints—a sideways look

THE DILEMMA

Jonathan was just 2 when the health visitor called to see his newborn sister. 'He has got a squint' she pronounced after a cursory inspection. 'You had better tell your doctor to send him onto the hospital. Squints can cause serious vision problems' she said conscientiously. An appointment was made for 4 months time and after many sleepless nights dreaming of unpleasant eye surgery and guide dogs, Jonathan's mother was eventually prescribed valium. At the Eye Unit it was found that the eyes were perfectly normal and that the apparent squint or 'pseudo squint' was a result of a combination of wide nasal bridge and epicanthus which partly hid one of the eyes when looking sideways.

Mary was exhausted at the end of a long drive home from holiday. It was then that her bespectacled mother thought she was squinting. As Mary approached her third birthday the squint became more frequent, particularly at the end of the day. Remembering the problems that she had had as a child, her mother was keen to seek medical attention. However, when her general practitioner shone a light into Mary's eyes they seemed perfectly straight. He told her mother not to worry, that she would probably grow out of it and that anyway she was a bit young for treatment.

Eighteen months later Mary 'passed' her preschool eye-test because she managed to 'peep' with her left eye while the right was being tested. Eventually Mary's school teacher pressurised her mother to go back and ask for a retest, as a right convergent squint was now clearly present. At the hospital the squinting eye was found to be densely amblyopic. Orthoptic exercises and surgery failed to restore binocular vision and visual acuity to a reasonable level. For the rest of her life, Mary would only have one good eye. Had orthoptic treatment been started earlier, Mary would have had a good chance of maintaining good acuity and binocular vision.

Here then are the two ends of the spectrum of childhood squint or strabismus; the tragedy of delayed diagnosis and treatment and the futility and cost of false positive pseudo squints. How in the child health service are we to strike a reasonable balance between over-zealousness on the one hand and misplaced conservatism on the other? This chapter seeks to review the scale and nature of the problem, how a reasonable squint assessment can be made at primary care level, what treatment is available and how effective it is and what we should be doing to improve the preventive services.

Supporting evidence is drawn from a study in Southampton on the epidemiology and outcome of visual disorders in children (Catford et al, 1983). A cohort of all Southampton District children born in 1970 who had attended Southampton Eye Hospital before the age of 8 years was constructed from orthoptic records. 624 case notes were abstracted for information concerning diagnoses, treatment and visual function such that the outcome for each diagnostic group at age 8 or on discharge was known. Special attempts were made to include defaulters and those who had moved away. Outcome information was available for 86% of the cohort. Since the Eye Hospital was the only referral centre in the District, the denominator used in the rates calculation was the number of live births in the District in 1970. Although migration out of the District has been small since then, the incidence of visual disorders may be slightly underestimated.

THE SCALE OF THE PROBLEM

Visual disorders are one of the commonest problems in childhood. In Southampton, by the age of 8 years, one in every ten children will have been up to the Eye Hospital and this proportion excludes those who have gone direct to opticians and have not subsequently been referred. Table 4.1 shows the referral rates for the 1970 cohort. Approximately 4% of all children will have been seen by their 8th birthday for a convergent squint and almost 1% for a divergent squint. Another 4% of children referred turned out to have 'pseudo squint' with normal vision.

Figure 4.1 shows the referral rates by age for both convergent and divergent squints and the proportion undergoing surgery. The commonest age is between 1 and 5 years. By far the majority of squints when detected receive surgery in addition to occlusion therapy. Squint surgery in fact, along with circumcision and hernioraphy, is the commonest operation now for children

Table 4.1 Referral rate of children aged up to 8 years to Southampton Eye Hospital for visual disorders

Diagnosis	cases/1000 children
Convergent squint	41.2
No abnormality found/pseudosquint	38.6
Refractive error*	14.0
Divergent Squint	7.8
Nystagmus	2.6
Other visual disorders	2.0
Total referrals	106.2

* Other cases may have been seen outside the hospital service

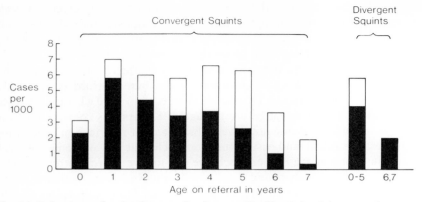

Fig. 4.1 Referral rate of squints by age to Southampton Eye Hospital and the proportion undergoing surgery (shown by solid columns)

aged 0 to 4. Cases of squint have, therefore, a considerable impact on the hospital services both as in-patients and out-patients.

NATURAL HISTORY

Squint or strabismus is a condition in which only one of the visual axes is directed towards the object of regard, the other deviating away from this point. This occurs when a tendency for the eyes to deviate is not corrected by the strong CNS fusion mechanism which seeks to obtain binocular single vision (BSV). This is the co-ordinated use of the two eyes to produce a single mental impression which helps in the judgement of distance.

Squints can be categorised according to their aetiology, onset, severity and clinical types, as summarised below.

Aetiology: *paralytic*—disturbance of eye muscles or nerves
              non-paralytic—defects in the afferent pathways or centrally. The most common form in childhood
              concomitant—angle of squint remains constant whatever the direction of gaze
              incomitant—angle of squint varies with the direction of gaze, eg in paralytic squint

Onset: *congenital*—genetic or following birth trauma
              acquired—the most common form in childhood

Severity: *manifest* (tropia)—fusion mechanism not achieving BSV
              latent (phoria)—BSV is achieved by the fusion mechanism controlling the deviation

Clinical types: *horizontal*—convergent (Eso)
                          —divergent (Exo)
                vertical (Hyper or Hypo)

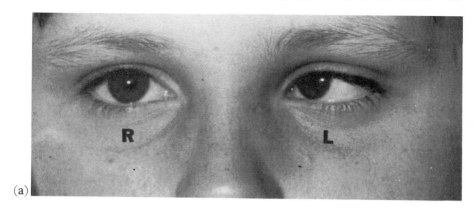

(a)

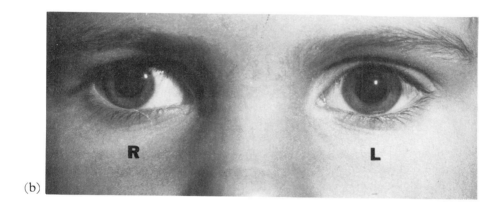

(b)

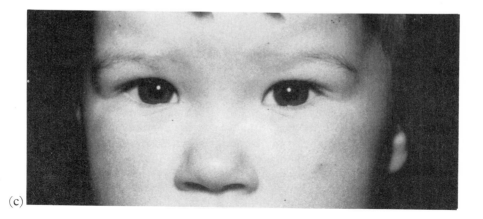

(c)

Fig. 4.2 Examples of strabismus. (a) Left concomitant convergent squint (esotropia); (b) right concomitant divergent squint (exotropia); (c) pseudosquint with epicanthus

Figure 4.2 gives examples of a convergent and divergent squint together with a pseudo squint.

Non-paralytic squints are by far the commonest in childhood and may result from a refractive error which will need treatment with spectacles. Initially squints produce diplopia—'double vision'. However, infants and children rapidly learn to suppress the central vision of the squinting eye and if this is maintained, suppression results in amblyopia (literally blunted sight). If caught at an early stage the amblyopia is reversible but the longer it is left and the earlier the onset, the more profound and irreversible it becomes.

Beyond the age of about 8 years, amblyopia which has not responded to treatment is considered to be irreversible. This is the reason why ophthalmologists have kept on emphasising the importance of early recognition allowing early correction of visual defects by spectacles, occlusion therapy and surgical straightening (Fells, 1978). On the other hand, squint arising after the age of 8 does not lead to amblyopia.

Some children attempt to overcome their squint by adopting a head posture which brings the two eyes back into parallel. This is an important telltale sign of strabismus and a case is demonstrated in Figure 4.3. Loss of binocular single vision will not only make distance judgement difficult but in later life certain occupations will be prohibited for the affected adult. These are ones that require binocular single vision such as flying, surgery using binocular microscopes, precision electronic engineering and microcircuit factory work.

HISTORY AND EXAMINATION

A careful history is a great aid in the diagnosis, treatment and prognosis of squint. Prematurity or a strong family history of refractive errors or strabismus is frequently present. Autosomal dominant inheritance is common. The age at onset is the single most important factor in prognosis. As will be shown later, the earlier the onset the worse the prognosis for fusion. The type of onset (gradual, sudden, intermittent, etc) and the conditions under which the squint appears are also important to note.

Examination of the eyes depends very much on the age, intelligence and co-operation of the child. Table 4.2 describes the procedures that health visitors, general practitioners and clinic doctors could undertake with the minimum of equipment in order to decide whether to refer a child. In the school setting the testing is made easier because the child is co-operative and more sophisticated equipment, such as the Keystone apparatus, can be used.

Whereas examination of eye movements and corneal light reflexes are comparatively easy, great difficulty is found in applying the cover tests. However the latter are really the definitive examinations for squint. If they were applied competently, the quality of referrals would be greatly

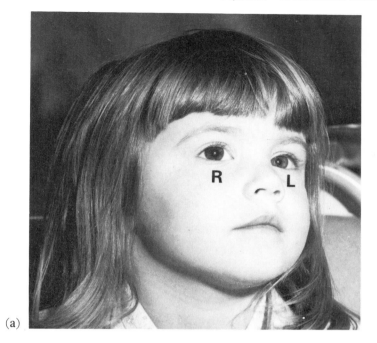

(a)

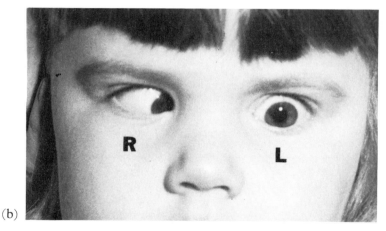

(b)

Fig. 4.3 Compensatory head posture in a case of left convergent squint (Duane's Retraction Syndrome). (a) BSV achieved with face turned to left and chin raised; (b) looking to the left: right eye normal and left eye restricted

improved—pseudo squints would be syphoned off and intermittent/latent squints would be detected.

Assessing visual acuity accurately at primary care level in pre-school children is extremely difficult unless there is severe visual loss. This is because the tests are not sensitive enough to detect milder defects of vision, which

Table 4.2 Procedure for testing children for squint and visual defect at primary care level

---

History and observation
Be very suspicious if
    (a) mother suspects a squint (parents are frequently right)
    (b) there were visual problems in the immediate family from an early age (there is often a strong family history)
    (c) the child was born prematurely or has congenital disorders such as hydrocephalus, cerebral palsy (they are a common association)
    (d) there are abnormal head positions or body postures (this is a tell-tale sign of eye movement problems)

Examination
    (a) *Perform Tests One, Two and Three* If the result is 'Yes' to all of them, carry out Test Four. If the result is 'No' to any of them REFER.

Test One:
    Check eye positions with child's head and eyes directed straight at you (primary position):
    Are the eyes straight and do they remain aligned in the other eight positions of gaze (up, down, right, left, upright, upleft, downright, downleft)?
Note: Be aware of being misled by a wide nasal bridge or epicanthic fold causing a pseudo squint which alone does not require referral.

Test Two:
    Test corneal light reflexes:
    Are they symmetrical?

Test Three:
    Perform cover/uncover and alternate cover tests (In infants the latter may only be possible):
    Do both eyes remain stationary?
    (b) *Perform Test Four if the child passed Tests One, Two and Three*
Choose the appropriate test according to age and concentration ability. If the result is 'Yes' inform parents that a squint has not been detected and advise on retesting policy. If the result is 'No' REFER.

Test Four:
    (i) Under 2 years old (and older children with poor concentration). Check for severe visual loss (one eye covered at a time): Can they fix on and preferably pick up 'hundreds and thousands' (minute sweets)?
    (ii) 2–3 years old (and older children with poor concentration). Check approximate visual acuity (one eye covered at a time): Using the Sheridan-Gardiner matching letter test at 6 metres, is the vision 6/9 or better in each eye and are they the same?
    (iii) 4 years and over. Check visual acuity (one eye covered at a time): Using the Snellen 6 m chart with key cards, is the vision 6/9 or better in each eye and are they the same?

---

require refraction for diagnosis. However, refraction of all children is not yet a practical possibility at primary care level. Everyone involved in the work should be aware of the danger of overlooking milder vision defects, and should report *all* doubtful results, however slight or borderline.

When a squint is found, it is important to exclude secondary causes. These were found in five children in the present study (2% of all squint cases): two had congenital cataracts, two optic atrophy and there was one albino. The most important cause of secondary squint to exclude is the very rare malignant and sometimes hereditary neoplasm, retinoblastoma. Emergency enucleation of the eye for this can be lifesaving. Inspection of the retina is therefore desirable in squint cases. In the early stages, small, yellowish white nodular masses may be seen protruding into the vitreous from the retina.

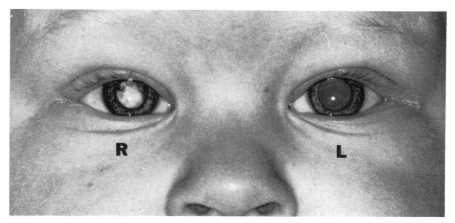

Fig. 4.4 Retinoblastoma in right eye showing white pupil

Later on the mass grows to produce a white pupil and proptosis as shown in Figure 4.4.

The cover tests

To perform the cover tests, the child is asked to look at a near fixation object. An interesting face stuck onto the end of a lollypop stick is very suitable. If binocular single vision is being maintained, both foveae will be directed towards this. To check this the examiner covers one eye while closely watching the other to see if it moves. If it does then a manifest squint is present. This 'cover/uncover' test is then repeated on the other eye.

   The presence of a latent squint is now assessed. In this condition the visual axes are held in parallel by the power of fusion. On dissociation the stimulus to maintain BSV is removed, and the non-fixing eye deviates away from the straight position. When dissociation ceases the deviating eye will move to restore bi-foveal fixation, and BSV is re-established. To demonstrate this the child remains fixing on the near object while the right eye is occluded for a few seconds. On removing the cover the right eye will be seen to move:
(a) outwards, indicating a latent convergent deviation under the cover
or
(b) inwards, indicating a latent divergent deviation under the cover
or
(c) upwards or downwards, indicating a latent vertical deviation under the cover.
This 'cover/uncover' test is then repeated on the left eye. If neither the manifest nor latent cover tests are conclusive then the alternate cover test may be performed. In this the child remains fixing on the near object while one eye and then the other is occluded alternately in quick succession while watching to see if the eye being uncovered moves to take up fixation. If so a squint is present, latent or manifest. (For further details see Cashell & Durran, 1980).

FORMS OF MANAGEMENT

The treatment of a squint aims to overcome amblyopia and restore binocular vision, and should always be carried out in the local Ophthalmic Unit. Refraction is performed under cyclopegia to detect any error (chiefly hypermetropia) which may be contributing to or causing the squint. Appropriate spectacles are prescribed and occlusion of the non-squinting eye by a patch is performed by the orthoptist in order to improve the vision of the squinting eye. The shorter the interval between onset and treatment and the older the child at onset, the better the result. Children with early onset squint, in whom treatment is delayed until after the age of 8, do not obtain improvement in their vision. Regular supervision is necessary to ensure compliance and to check the visual acuity in both eyes. Even if the vision is restored, occlusion may still have to be continued intermittently to keep it so. Other treatments for amblyopia may be used but appear to have few additional benefits over occlusion therapy. Once the best vision is obtained then surgical straightening of the squint can be considered; surgery alone will not restore binocular vision or overcome amblyopia, even though a cosmetic result is achieved. Operations consist of lengthening, shortening or moving the insertions of relevant muscles, e.g. the medial and lateral recti in convergent and divergent squints. Once the eyes are straight binocular vision may be strengthened by orthoptic treatment.

Follow-up should continue until the visual development is complete. Normally this is reached by the age of 7 or 8 but sometimes sooner. After 8 years it is believed that the ability to influence binocular vision and untreated amblyopia is lost. However, cosmetic surgery may be undertaken at any age.

OUTCOME STUDIES

There are relatively few outcome studies of the results of intervention in squint. In Southampton we followed the cohort of children born in 1970 with squint until they were 8 years of age or were discharged. Comparisons were made of the state of amblyopia on referral and after treatment (the best result).

The findings are presented in Table 4.3 by age on referral. It is apparent that treatment is effective for some cases of convergent squint whatever the age on referral. However the results improve dramatically as the age of referral increases. After the age of 2, it is most unlikely for convergent squints to remain densely amblyopic. Over 50% will achieve satisfactory visual acuity in both eyes by the age of 8 and the remainder, although mildly amblyopic, will have some useful vision in the squinting eye.

The prognosis for divergent squint is very different. No overall improvements were found in the mildly amblyopic group but on the whole divergent squints are less handicapped visually. There were no densely amblyopic children before or after treatment.

Table 4.3 Amblyopia before and after treatment

	Age on referral in years									
	Convergent squints								Divergent squints	
Visual Status	0	1	2	3	4	5	6	7	0–5	6,7
No amblyopia										
% on referral	27	42	26	17	25	29	29	36	73	92
%after treatment	40	47	59	66	53	58	53	55	73	83
Mild amblyopia*										
% on referral	40	33	53	59	44	45	53	55	27	8
% after treatment	40	39	41	34	36	42	47	45	27	17
Dense amblyopia**										
% on referral	33	25	21	24	31	26	18	9	0	0
% after treatment	20	14	0	0	11	0	0	0	0	0
Number of cases	15	36	34	29	36	31	17	11	26	12

* defined as amblyopic eye better than 6/36, less than 5 lines difference
** defined as amblyopic eye 6/36 or worse, 5 lines or more difference

Table 4.4 Binocular single vision after treatment. Percentage with constant or intermittent BSV in at least the primary position

	Age on referral in years									
	Convergent squints								Divergent squints	
Position of objects	0	1	2	3	4	5	6	7	0–5	6, 7
Near	27	22	35	52	56	65	59	82	92	100
Distant	27	28	35	48	56	65	59	82	77	87

Table 4.4 presents the state of binocular single vision (BSV) after treatment at age 8 years or on discharge. It was not always possible to assess the state of BSV at referral as the children were either too young or unco-operative. As with amblyopia the prognosis for convergent squints improves with the age of onset (indicated by age at referral). Over 50% of children had useful BSV over the age of 3 years and 80% at age 7. It is disappointing that of those seen in the first year of life, only a quarter had a good result. The prognosis in divergent squints is excellent, over 90% had some useful binocular vision.

It would be quite wrong to conclude from our study that it is better to refer children at a later age. The improved outcome observed with increasing age on referral is accounted for by the later age of onset. This was demonstrated by a sub-study which showed that there was a relatively short period between onset and referral. A sample of 103 recent admissions for surgery were sent a questionnaire enquiring about the history and origin of referral, to comp-lement information in the case notes. Sixty-nine per cent reported receiving ophthalmic attention within 3 months of onset of the squint; 8% of mothers admitted to not seeking medical advice for more than 3 months after onset; 23% of cases were delayed for more than 3 months by the general practitioner or health visitor and these were often the ones with the worst outcome.

We have concluded, therefore, that:

1. The prognosis for amblyopia and BSV in convergent squints is good in many cases where treatment commences soon after onset.

2. The prognosis for BSV in divergent squints is excellent but treatment does not appear to make an impact on amblyopia.

3. The prognosis for amblyopia and BSV in convergent and divergent squints improves with the age of onset.

We would emphasise therefore that *early referral* of any child with squint or visual defect *is mandatory*.

CONCLUSION

The earlier treatment is commenced for squint, the greater is the chance of achieving useful binocular vision and preventing long-term amblyopia. This principle has been so much publicised in recent years in the Southampton area such that referrals to ophthalmologists have increased dramatically. However in 1978/79, 51% of suspected squints were found to be normal. Although true cases were referred earlier, much of the advantage was lost as a result of increased waiting times for appointments due to increased workload.

We see improvements in the early detection and treatment of squint following a logical pattern which depends very much on the commitment of those involved and the resources available. The premise we have followed, perhaps somewhat conservatively, is that certainly as many as 50% of squints can be detected early enough by informed parents. In fact only 6% of squints in our questionnaire study were spotted by health professionals before the family. The emphasis, therefore, should initially be on improving clinical skills at primary level (that is amongst clinical medical officers, GPs, health visitors and school nurses). In health educating it should be stressed that a child suspected of squint should receive immediate medical advice. The process of referral should be speeded up before costly screening programmes are undertaken. The importance of history taking and recognition of the fact that parents are often right needs to be emphasised. Above all, the method of cover testing must be learnt and practised, possibly with the help of the local orthoptic department.

We are now convinced that an intermediate diagnostic clinic run by orthoptists and a medical refractionist is the best way to avoid unnecessary referrals to hard pressed consultant opthalmologists. A number of schemes have been described in the literature (Gardiner, 1974; MacLellan & Harker, 1979). The preliminary results of such a clinic set up recently in Southampton are promising.

By the age of 5 there is less likelihood that long standing squints will respond to treatment. However, examination at school entry affords the ideal opportunity to examine less privileged groups who may not have fully used the primary care services. Ingram (1973) reported in a study of Northamptonshire schools that there was an appreciable number of undiagnosed squints detected at the primary school stage, many of whom were aged under 8, when treatment might be effective. This was because some squints did not produce a dramatic enough cosmetic deformity to be noticed. He found that 43% of children with squints referred to the school eye clinics were over 7 years when first detected.

We would wish to see pre-school vision screening improved to achieve 100% coverage in both the state and private systems, using the procedures outlined in Table 4.2. In subsequent school vision tests the Keystone Apparatus may also be useful.

Should resources permit an extension of this programme, then we would favour starting with the population most at risk, namely, those who were premature or have a positive family history. Registers of 'visually at risk' children could be set up by general practices. Refractionists and orthoptists could attend the surgery or health clinic to see groups of children by prior arrangement. Probably 3 to $3\frac{1}{2}$ is the best age, as the children will be young enough to have a reasonable chance of benefiting from treatment and yet old enough for the examination to give accurate results. If this method proves successful (we are unaware of any published studies), the scheme could be extended to all children. In Ayrshire (Cameron & Cameron, 1978) a comprehensive programme has been reported as being feasible and of value. However, there are considerable resource implications not the least concerning the availability of sufficient refractionist and orthoptist manpower.

Alternative methods of screening are also being considered. One concerns the analysis of stereoscopic photographs of the eyes and is being investigated in Cambridge. In Nottingham, Ingram (1977) has found that refractive errors in the under two's are a good predictor of squint and amblyopia. Refraction also has the advantage of picking up the much rarer condition of straight-eyed amblyopia which the cover tests cannot reveal. Nevertheless there are considerable practical difficulties in refracting large numbers of children. We await with interest the results of Ingram's treatment of his series of cases. Outcome expressed in terms of visual acuity and binocular function will indicate whether there is any advantage over the more traditional methods.

REFERENCES

Cashell G T W, Durran I M 1980. The Cover Test. In: Handbook of Orthoptic Principles, 4th edn, Ch. 2 pp 14–22. Churchill Livingstone, Edinburgh

Catford J C, Absolon M J, Millo A 1983 The epidemiology and outcome of visual disorders in Childhood. (in preparation)

Cameron J H, Cameron M 1978 Visual screening of pre-school children. British Medical Journal ii: 1693–1694

Fells P 1978 Recognition and management of squints. Journal of Maternal and Child Health
    3: 8–14
Gardiner P A 1974 Squint Diagnostic Clinics. Transactions of Ophthalmological Society UK
    94: 280–282
Ingram R M 1973 Role of the School Eye Clinic in Modern Ophthalmology. British Medical
    Journal i: 278–280
Ingram R M 1977 Refraction as a basis for screening children for Squint and Amblyopia.
    British Journal of Ophthalmology 61: 8–15
MacLellan A V, Harker P 1979 Mobile Orthoptic service for primary screening of visual
    disorder in young children. British Medical Journal i: 994–995

Defective colour vision in children

Effects on education

Defective colour vision is a disability of the colour sense in which certain colours are perceived abnormally and confusions between colours can arise due to a reduced colour discrimination ability. The severity of this disability depends upon the nature of the defective colour vision and there is growing concern amongst educationalists that it could give rise to specific learning difficulties. In primary schools, for example, there is an increasing use of colour coded material to aid teaching in the basic concepts of numeracy and literacy. Confusions between the colour codes used in these teaching aids could impair learning progress at an important age in educational development.

As with any other childhood disability, there is now a legal requirement in Britain (Education Act, 1981) for special provision to be made for the educational needs of disabled children. Although the social principles behind this improved Education Act are commendable, the Warnock Report recommendations which preceded its drafting makes the implicit assumption that there is a known and established relationship between all clinically definable disabilities and learning progress. Clinical and educational sciences are far from such a state of certainty. This is principally because there are considerable difficulties associated with the reliable measurement of motor and sensory function in the young child and also of learning progress. Consequently, where there is uncertainty concerning the effect of a disability on learning progress, it is important to be vigilant to such possibilities and make allowance in the educational methods to be adopted for that child.

Defective colour vision is one of the minor sensory disabilities for which there is no clear evidence that sufferers are poorer educational achievers than their colleagues who have normal colour vision. While it is not unreasonable to postulate a possible relationship between learning disabilities and defective colour vision, the published literature on this topic is sparse and somewhat conflicting. Almost as many authors claim that colour vision deficiencies have no effect on academic achievement (e.g. Waddington, 1965; Mandola, 1969;

Lampe et al, 1973) as those who report a measureable relationship. Amongst this latter group of investigators Espinda (1971), for example, reported the results of a study which indicated that colour defective children have a lower school grade point average than children with normal colour vision. In a subsequent study, also on an American child population, Espinda (1973) reported that there were more than the expected number of colour vision defectives amongst referrals to special programmes for the learning disabled. Furthermore, a poorer primary school reading performance amongst colour defective children has been reported by Grosvenor (1977). More specifically, in a study involving secondary school children, Dannemaier (1972) found that pupils with defective colour vision had greater difficulty with the school biology course and were generally poorer achievers in this subject.

The confusion produced by these conflicting reports is almost certainly due to problems of methodology concerning use of the tests employed to define and measure defective colour vision. For example, Cox (1971) has shown that there is a low test—retest reliability for performance on the wavy line plates of the Ishihara test (see Appendix) when assessed at pre-school age and again on the same children when in the third primary school grade (8 years). Further evidence which highlights such measurement problems has been provided by Cohen (1976). In an attempt to test the hypothesis that there was a higher incidence of colour vision deficiencies amongst children with known learning disabilities, he found that over 80% of the children classified as 'deficient' on one test (ie the Farnsworth Panel D–15) were classified as 'normal' by a second test (ie the HRR pseudo-isochromatic plates) (see Appendix for a description of these tests). Such findings were clearly a consequence of the different conceptual and perceptual-motor skills required in performing different tests for defective colour vision. The recognition of this problem is important if decisions have to be made about colour vision which are independent of and therefore uninfluenced by learning development. It should be realised that children with learning difficulties are generally of average intelligence but their learning is impaired usually because their methods of learning are different from those of the majority of children. Nevertheless, learning difficulties could be associated with low intelligence.

In addition to the educational problems associated with defective colour vision, there are factors which could influence the psychological development of a child. The child whose colour vision defect is unknown is often accused of carelessness by his teacher which could lead to some feelings of inferiority. Indeed, the colour defective child has an unstable reference in the development of his language and visual associations as a consequence of persistent and apparently contradictory correction by adults in the use of colour names. Such frequent confusions can not only affect learning progress but also personality development, such as has been demonstrated for example by Bacon (1971) and Snyder (1973).

Effects on employment

Whereas learning disability is frequently difficult to demonstrate as a consequence of defective colour vision, it is indisputable that colour vision defectives are excluded by selection from several vocational occupations (Taylor, 1971). The reason for such discrimination is usually that of safety to avoid injury to the affected individual or to others, which could occur from a failure to recognise or confuse potentially hazardous colour coded systems or warning devices (e.g. electrical or electronics industry, or air crew in aviation industry). There are also occupations from which colour defectives are barred entry where errors of colour perception would result in considerable expense to the employer through damaged materials and subsequent loss of productivity (e.g. chemical and textile industries using colour dying procedures). Although instrumentation is gaining more widespread acceptance in some industries for monitoring and control of a product colour, few have yet equalled the sensitivity of the human eye with normal colour vision for discriminating small colour differences or making judgements of perceived colour equality. It is evident, therefore, that since there are somewhat restricted career opportunities for colour defectives, clear and appropriate guidance must be given on career choice as well as on subject selection at secondary school level. Although many jobs are open to colour defectives they would be well advised to avoid those occupations which involve accurate colour judgement or colour matching.

It is usually the more marked colour vision defects where employment difficulties arise, as is also undoubtedly the case with learning disabilities. Therefore, before specific advice can be given concerning the capabilities of a colour defective child, it is essential that a detailed examination is undertaken to determine the type and severity of the defect (Taylor, 1966). Where an obvious problem exists requiring guidance it is wise not only to inform the parents and classroom teacher but also to advise the child. When a child knows of their colour defect, they can more easily learn to compensate for it by maximising on other perceptual cues, and can therefore plan more wisely for a future career.

When to test

Clinically it is only of value to screen for a deficiency where some action can be taken which is beneficial to the individual. While it is not possible to correct defective colour vision, advice can be given at the appropriate age to help the child cope more effectively with the disability. In view of the reasonable possibility that defective colour vision affects learning development, it would seem desirable to provide for the detection of colour vision abnormalities at the start of formal primary school education (4–5 years). While many investigators cautiously advise that this age is too young to obtain satisfactory and meaningful performance due to the child's inability to understand the test instructions (e.g. Verriest, 1981), a proposal is outlined here which provides a solution, at least in part, to this problem. However, if this part solution for screening the colour vision of children at the start of primary school is considered unacceptable, then it should be realised that there would be little benefit from a mass colour vision screening programme of children until the next critical age at which appropriate action could be taken in the educational guidance of an affected child. This would occur at the start of secondary school education (10–11 years). But if general colour vision screening is left until this age, it is important not to overlook the problems which can accrue from an undetected colour vision deficiency. If, for example, a child is found to be having learning difficulties in primary school, then one of the tests which should be considered while investigating the causes for that problem should be an assessment of colour vision. If this is not possible, then an enquiry into family history may be revealing.

The age at which it is most effective to screen for defective colour vision depends not only on the cognitive skills demanded of the testee but also the attributes of test sensitivity and specificity when considered in conjunction with the rationale of the screening programme. For example, because of the marked trade-off between false-positive and false-negative error rates on most tests, it is important to decide at the onset of a screening programme whether the test is designed to detect colour defectives or to identify colour normals. It should be realised that the function of most medical screening programmes is to identify the normal with respect to a disease or defect and consequently the rationale is to distinguish between those individuals who would benefit from further examination and those who need no further examination (Aspinall & Hill, 1983). This principle is particularly applicable to screening for defective colour vision in children. But before discussing the factors which it is necessary to consider in setting up a colour vision screening programme, it will be helpful to describe the characteristics and population distribution of normal and defective colour vision.

Characteristics of normal colour vision

The first stage of colour differentiation in the visual system occurs within the retina, particularly the receptors known as the cones. Although there is evidence of some minor modifications to the colour component of the signal both within the neural layers of the retina and at other stages in the visual pathways (i.e. the lateral geniculate nucleus and visual cortex), the photo-pigments in the retinal cones appear to play the major role. There is now ample evidence to indicate that three different photopigments are involved and that these are contained in separate cones distributed throughout the retina. Because it is possible to match any perceived colour by a mixture of three defined colour primaries, normal colour vision is known as trichromatic.

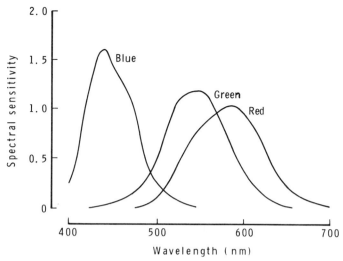

Fig. 5.1 A possible set of spectral sensitivity curves for the three receptor processes believed to be responsible for colour vision. In the trichromatic theory of colour vision they are referred to as the red (R), green (G) and blue (B) systems and they behave in an additive principle to produce the wide range of differentiated colours perceived in the visible spectrum

The three cone pigments each have different spectral absorption characteristics the specific details of which are still somewhat speculative (Fig. 5.1). They provide for colour differentiation of incident white light in much the same way as the spectral emission curves of the 'red', 'green' and 'blue' phosphors used in colour television. Each wavelength of light absorbed by the cone pigments provides for a unique response triplet giving a differential signal along the nerve pathways to the visual cortex where this is then converted into the sensation of colour. (In practice the threshold for wavelength discrimination in the normal eye varies between 1 nm and 2 nm over most of the spectral range and gets progressively poorer at the limits of the visible spectrum.) The colours associated with each wavelength are therefore the result of different proportional response outputs from the three types of retinal cone. The more incident light that is absorbed by each photopigment, the greater is the resultant signal strength. The total combined signal output from the three cone types provides information about the intensity of the stimulus. Since this is a combined or summed response from the three cone types, the average spectral sensitivity of the eye will be represented by a single response curve the characteristics of which will differ depending on whether the eye has normal or defective colour vision (Fig. 5.2).

The maximum concentration of cones occurs in the central region of the retina around the fovea centralis, whereas towards the periphery there is a predominance of a different type of receptor known as a rod. Rods contain a different photopigment and since they are more sensitive than cones they

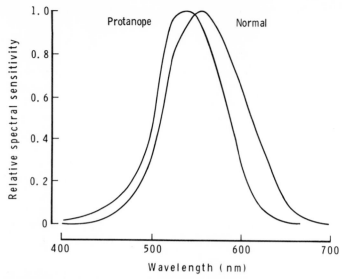

Fig. 5.2 The averaged total spectral sensitivity curve for a subject with normal colour vision and a red blind colour defective (Protanope). The normal curve is based upon the sum of the three cone spectral sensitivity curves represented in Fig. 5.1, somewhat modified by neural processing within the retina. For the protanope, the R receptor process is missing which is why their overall sensitivity curve is lower at the red end of the spectrum by comparision with the normal

are responsible for vision in low illuminances. At very low illuminance, such as moonlight, vision is without colour differentiation since only one pigment is being used. Normal rod vision is therefore said to be achromatic and since there are no rods at the fovea our central vision is very poor in moonlight. As the light levels increase so the cones begin to come into play and the visual scene gradually acquires colour until at high illuminances, such as in day-light, we achieve maximum colour discrimination.

Characteristics of defective colour vision

Normal colour vision involves three cone types and permits the matching of any perceived colour by a mixture of three defined primaries. It is therefore termed trichromatic. If there is a disturbance to the spectral response curves of any of the three cone types, then clearly the differential output signal arising from a stimulus of any given wavelength will not be the same as in the normal eye. The resultant colour percept will therefore be anomalous. Such disturbances, if they exceed normal biological variation, result in defective colour vision. In the extreme form of the deficiency all the cones are either absent or they provide no differential signal. This is the only form of total colour blindness and is known as monochromatic vision or achromatopsia. To the affected person the world appears in terms of light and shade only, much as on a black and white television picture. Fortunately, this is an extremely rare condition with an estimated incidence of only three in 100 000.

More commonly occuring colour vision deficiencies are due to anomalies of one of the cone photopigments. This may take the form either of a reduced sensitivity from one of the cone types, an alteration of the spectral absorption properties of one of the pigments, or an absence of one of the pigments. The first two possibilities produce varying states of anomalous trichromacy. Where there are only two cone pigments present, vision is said to be dichromatic because any colour percept may be matched by a mixture of only two rather than three defined colour primaries. It will be evident from Fig. 5.1 that if one of the three responses curves is absent there will be a range of several wavelengths which will provide the same proportional output signal from the two remaining cone types. Such wavelengths will be indistinguishable from each other in terms of the colour they evoke. Consequently, in dichromatic vision, colour discrimination is very poor in selected regions of the visible spectrum as well as there being a distortion of colour perception. The parts of the spectrum which will be affected depends upon which cone type is missing. There are, therefore, three major types of defective colour vision.

Depending on whether the 'red', 'green' or 'blue' cone system is missing, the resultant dichromatic vision has been given the names protanopia, deuteranopia and tritanopia respectively. The nomenclature, which is based upon Greek words, simply reflects the order in which the different defects were described historically. The approximate effects of these characteristi- cally different forms of dichromatic vision can perhaps best be simulated on a colour television. Switching off the 'red' electron gun will simulate the visual scene perceived by a protanope, elimination of the 'green' gun for a deuteranope and elimination of the 'blue' gun for a tritanope. This is fairly realistic because the spectral emission characteristics of the 'red', 'green' and 'blue' phosphors on a colour television screen match reasonably closely the spectral characteristics of the three postulated cone sensitivity curves of the eye (Fig. 5.1).

Whereas protanopia, deuteranopia and tritanopia are sometimes mislead- ingly refered to as 'red-blind', 'green-blind' and 'blue-blind' (terms which are strongly depricated), there is a further group of colour vision deficiencies in which all three pigments are present but of which one gives an altered response sensitivity curve. This group of deficiencies is refered to as anom- alous trichromatic vision. Depending upon which cone pigment is affected there are three forms of anomalous trichromacy. These are protanomaly, deuteranomaly and tritanomaly, refering respectively to an anomalous 'red', 'green' or 'blue' system. Again, the colour television can be used to give an approximate simulation of varying degrees of anomalous trichromacy (from mild to extreme) simply by altering the amount of 'red', 'green' or 'blue' signal present in the picture.

An indication of the colour names given to different parts of the visible spectrum by each type of colour defective person is given in Table 5.1.

Table 5.1 Typical colour names associated with different isolated parts of the visible spectrum given by the various types of colour vision defectives. (When the spectrum is seen in full, the colour defective may make minimal or no naming errors due to contextual association cues being present.)

Normal description	Dark red	Red	Orange	Yellow	Green	Blue/ green	Blue	Violet
Red deficiencies Protanopia	dark grey	brown	brownish/ yellow	yellow	grey	grey	blue	dark blue
Protanomalous	dark brown	dark red	orange	yellow	grey/ green	bluish	blue	violet
Green deficiencies Deuteranopia	brown	red	green	yellow	brown/ green	bluish	blue	dark red
Deuteranomalous	dark red	red	orange	yellow	greenish	blue	blue	dark violet
Blue deficiencies Tritanopia	dark red	red	pinkish	grey	green	green	blue/ green	violet
Tritanomalous	dark red	red	mauve	palish/ yellow	green	greenish/ blue	blue	bluish purple
Total colour blindness (Achromatopsia)	very dark	dark grey	grey	light/ yellow	light/ grey	grey	dark grey	very dark

Infant and childhood colour vision

The above classification is based upon the characteristics of congenitally defective colour vision which remain unaltered throughout life. However, there is recent evidence suggestive of developmental changes in colour vision which appear to occur during the first few months of life and possibly extending into the early years of infancy.

The question is often raised, 'Does the newly born baby perceive colour?'. This question is difficult to answer in detail but there is evidence to indicate that some colour processing is taking place within the first 4 weeks. Using operant conditioning procedures, Peebles & Teller (1975) and Bornstein (1976) were able to show that by 2 and 3 months post-natal, most infants can make some discriminations solely on the basis of wavelength differences. Thus 2–3-month-old infants must at least be dichromats. But their status as normal trichromats is far from established because of an inability to make certain discriminations which are easy for colour normal adults (Teller et al, 1978). Using a forced choice preferential looking technique (which involves presenting the infant with a coloured visual stimulus that appears randomly on either the right or left side in an otherwise homogenous field), Hamer et al (1982) have extended this work to show that wavelength discrimination is possible even at 4 weeks. They further demonstrated that there is a significant improvement and systematic change in the nature of the colour vision up to 3 months of age. It has been suggested that infants are essentially without a functional fovea before 3 months of age (Bronson, 1974), hence this developmental change in colour vision when combined with other known functional changes in infant foveal vision, points to an immaturity of neural processing. More specifically, Hamer et al (1982) suggest that the immature infant retina shares many of the functional properties of adult peripheral vision.

The nature of this immaturity of an infant's colour vision is in the form of a slight protanomaly or weakened red sensitivity. A similar small weakened red response has also been observed in children between the ages of 4 and 11 years compared with the performance of an adult population on a colour matching test using an anomaloscope (data of Hill et al, 1982). Furthermore, in a study of incremental colour thresholds Verriest & Uvijls (1977) have shown that the fovea (i.e. central vision) in young adolescents from the age of 10 years is less sensitive both for the shorter (i.e. blue) and longer (i.e. red) wavelengths than in adults. These differences in colour vision between childhood and young adults cannot be explained in terms of the known changes in absorbance of the crystalline lens of the eye which generally occurs after the fourth decade. Whether they are due to a developmental change in one or more of the receptor types or to a developmental change of neural processing remains to be established. The measured deviations from the adult norm, although stastically significant are nevertheless small and unlikely to affect performance on any of the standard colour vision screening tests.

Modes of inheritance

The red (protan) and green (deutan) type of congenital colour vision deficiencies are transmitted by a recessive X-linked mode of inheritance. The blue (tritan) deficiencies, on the other hand, are thought to be incompletely autosomal-dominant although their hereditary transmission is not yet fully explored. This is largely because tritan defects have a particularly low incidence of between 0.002% and 0.007%. The incidence of the different defective colour vision genotypes is summarised in Table 5.2.

Red-green colour deficiencies, like haemophilia, are a classical example of X-linked inheritance since there are very few deviations from the rules for its mode of transmission. The defective gene is located on the X-chromosome and since it has a recessive trait the normal allele is always dominant. Males, therefore, who have only one X-chromosome are colour defective if that chromosome contains the defective gene. They are said to be hemizygous for that gene. Females, however, who have two X-chromosomes are only colour blind if both X-chromosomes contain the defective gene (i.e. homozygous for that gene) but are phenotypically normal and a carrier for colour deficiency if only one X-chromosome is affected (i.e. heterozygous for that gene). The various gametic combinations for this mode of inheritance are illustrated in the theoretical pedigrees in Fig. 5.3.

Since the defective genes for protan and deutan deficiencies occur at different loci on the X-chromosome, they are non-allelic. The rules of trans-

Table 5.2 Incidence and mode of inheritance of the major types of congenital colour vision defects amongst Caucasian Europeans

Type	Incidence (%)		Mode of inheritance
	Males	Females*	
Red deficiencies			
Protanopia	1.0	0.01	X-linked recessive
Protanomaly	1.0	0.03	
Green deficiencies			
Deuteranopia	1.0	0.01	X-linked recessive
Deuteranomaly	5.0	0.35	
Blue deficiencies			
Tritanopoa	0.005	0.005	Autosomal dominant
Tritanomaly	?	?	
Total colour blindness (Achromatopsia)			
With reduced visual acuity	0.003	0.003	Autosomal recessive
With normal visual acuity	0.000001	0.000001	

* The figures for red and green deficiencies amongst females are for allelic compounds. The non-allelic compounds in females, having a protan defective gene on one X chromosome and a deutan defective gene on the other, manifest as varying atypical forms of defective colour vision with a total incidence of 0.24%.

mission in Fig. 5.3 are therefore only applicable if the same class of deficiency is involved. In this instance there will be intrafamilial stability, although there is likely to be some irregular alternation between generations for the different alleles (i.e. for dichromacy or anomalous trichromacy) of the same series. Typically the minor disturbances are more prevalent than the more serious defects, hence anomalous trichromacy is likely to occur with greater frequency. The incidence of the different biotypes of defective colour vision are given in Table 5.2. These figures are for European races. There are however, known small variations demographically within Britain (with the lowest incidence amongst males in Scotland at about 5.0%) as well as large variations occuring in different populations throughout the world, the lowest being approximately 2.5% in the American Indians (Cruz-Coke, 1970).

It will be noticed from Table 5.2 that there is a discrepancy between the observed incidence of colour deficiency amongst females compared with the theoretically expected value which should be 0.08 squared (i.e. 0.0064 or 0.64%). This is because where crossing-over occurs with the exchange by recombination of genetic material between the defective genes for protan and deutan deficiencies, the resultant colour vision of such non-allelic compounds is phenotypically normal. Occasionally, however, an atypically deviant phenotype may occur (Hill & Aspinall, 1982b). The 'missing' 0.24% in the female totals of Table 5.2 are the non-allelic compounds.

Acquired colour deficiencies and pathology

It is important to realise that defective colour vision can occur as a conse-

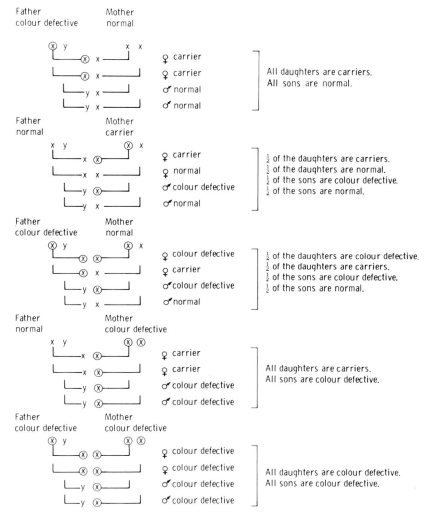

Fig. 5.3 The main hereditary patterns of X-linked recessive transmission of red and green defective colour vision. The symbol for the affected chromosome has been encircled to show whether its presence in an offspring has originated from the father or mother

quence of pathology. While this is mostly a problem associated with certain ocular pathology in adults, it can also occur in childhood. For example, it can appear as a characteristic in infantile optic atrophy or as a result of damage to the retina from neuro-toxic agents. In the early stages of a degenerative condition, the acquired colour vision deficiency may resemble a congenital deficiency. But whereas congenital colour vision defects are stable, the acquired deficiency will vary with the progression of the disease. If, therefore, pathology is suspected as the cause of the colour vision deficiency, then the child should be given a full ophthalmological examination.

Diabetes in childhood presents special problems with respect to defective colour vision. While the acquired colour vision losses associated with the condition do not usually manifest until several years duration of the disease, affected children or their parents are frequently required to monitor the urine glucose level until a stable treatment regime is obtained. The test most typically used for this home monitoring involves visual colour matching (e.g. Clinitest). If the person who uses the test is colour defective then problems will certainly arise in the correct interpretation of the results (Aspinall et al, 1980). Before issuing a child with such a test it is essential, therefore, to ensure that the user can perform the test adequately and correctly. For this it is not necessary to assess the colour vision of the user but rather to arrange a practical means of evaluating their ability to perform the urine colour matching test itself. This can be achieved with standard preparations of urine having known glucose concentrations which are matched in turn against the reference colour by the user.

Most colour vision tests are designed on the basis of classically established colour confusions found in congenital colour vision deficiencies, although many are also used with varying degrees of efficiency for the detection and investigation of acquired colour losses. It should be appreciated that acquired colour vision deficiencies are somewhat more variable in expression than congenital deficiencies and therefore, when of only mild severity, they could go undetected by some of the simple screening tests. However, since most childhood ocular pathologies are accompanied by other functional deficits of vision (e.g. reduced visual acuity or nystagmus etc), an acquired colour vision deficiency is unlikely to be of primary clinical significance. Furthermore, without special testing facilities it is frequently difficult to provide a differential diagnosis between an acquired and congenital colour defect (Pokorny et al, 1979), although if the deficiency is confined to one eye (i.e. monocular) then it is almost certainly of an acquired nature. With only extremely rare exceptions, congenital colour deficiencies are binocular.

Colour vision tests for children

Of the large number of commercially available colour vision tests, few have been designed specifically for use by young children. Recently, some novel proposals have been made by Verriest (1981) for tests based upon the principle of colour matching domino and lotto games. These tests were intended for use by 3–6-year-old children but were found unsuccessful in evaluation due to a child's difficulty in understanding the instructions. Clearly, in designing or selecting a colour vision test for use on young children, careful consideration has to be given both to the cognitive demand of the test in addition to the perceptual and motor skills required of the child to perform that task.

Since children encode reality in different ways at different stages of development (Bruner, 1966) it is helpful to attempt a classification of colour vision tests according to the complexity of the perceptual task involved. A simple hierarchical order of perceptual segregation is through the following five identifiable stages:

detection of the presence of a stimulus

discrimination of a figural unity as separate from the background

resolution of finer details providing a differentiated figure

identification or recognition of a form or pattern

interpretation of this identified form

Each successive stage in this hierarchy involves the extraction of progressively more information from the stimulus in the perceptual task. It will be clear that this order reflects the increasing role of experiential and psychological factors in perception. The higher-order tasks of identification and interpretation demand not only greater intelligence for their understanding but also a greater familiarity of the particular type of material and situation for their performance.

It is possible, therefore, to classify groups of different colour vison tests, from the simplest to the most complex, according to such a hierarchy of perceptual complexity (Table 5.3). While it is appreciated that the perceptual subtasks implied by each group of colour vision test examples given here are not 'pure', they provide a useful framework for the classification of tests. The HRR and F2 pseudo-isochromatic tests (see Appendix), for example, could also be classed as more of a 'resolution task' if their mode of use involved the tracing of geometric shapes rather than matching with cut-out templates

Table 5.3 Classification of colour vision tests for children using a hierarchy of perceptual complexity

Perceptual level	Colour vision related task	Colour vision test (selected samples)	Suggested minimum age for test group
Detection	Gaze preference Induced OKN[1] Pattern VEP[2]	Special laboratory based tests	3 months
Discrimination	Colour differentiation	Anomaloscope ('same' versus 'different')	4 years
Resolution	Tracing	*Ishihara (wavy line)	8 years
Identification	Object matching	*Velhagen (illiterate E matching) *Guys (letter matching) *HRR (shape matching) *F2 (shape matching)	10 years
Interpretation	Manipulating stimulus properties including colour naming and problem solving	*Matsubara (object patterns) *Ishihara (letters) *City (estimate of colour difference) Panel D-15 (colour order) FM 100 hue (colour order)	12 years

* These are all different pseudo-isochromatic plates. See Appendix for test descriptions [1] Induced opto-kinetic nystagmus; [2] Pattern visual evoked potential.

requiring prior identification. On the other hand, the numeral plates of the Ishihara test are a particularly complex task requiring the interpretation of an embedded figure against a patterned background. Although the minimum ages recommended in the last column of Table 5.3 may surprise some colour vision test users, they are based upon experimental evidence. They are the ages at which children with normal colour vision can pass the tests within an acceptable false-positive error rate (Hill et al, 1982). As such, they are operationally minimum ages for the set of colour vision tests indicated. The classification of colour vision tests in this way is based upon their content validity and therefore, the correlation between perceptual complexity and test performance is accidental rather than real. It is more a consequence of the design limitations of the test used than of a limited understanding of perceptual development in children. In this respect it should be realised that with appropriately presented test material and instructions, young children of 4 years can satisfactorily carry out tests of identification or interpretation (Donaldson, 1978). So far, however, no acceptable colour vision test satisfying such design criteria for children of this age has been made commercially available. Until then, guidance should be based upon the recommendations of Table 5.3.

In summary, the lower down the heirarchy of tasks, the less influenced will be the test result by factors other than of colour perception. Recent findings by Hill et al (1982) from a comparative evaluation of different colour vision tests for children tends to support the rationale of such a classification. The only colour vision tests relatively uninfluenced by psychological and behavioural factors are the laboratory based tests of opto-kinetic nystagmus (Moreland et al, 1976) and pattern visual evoked potential (Kinney & Mckay, 1974) but unfortunately these are quite impractical as clinical tests and present problems of instrumental resolution.

Which test to choose

A review of the literature by Alexander (1975) on colour vision testing in children revealed extremely varied results, making recommendations on test selection particularly difficult. Verriest (1981) has extended this literature review with an evaluation of the reliability of several colour vision tests used by children, concluding that few tests provide for a satisfactory performance below the age of 10 years (i.e. Ishihara and HRR tests). Since then, Hill et al (1982) have validated four colour vision tests, including the two recommended by Verriest (1981), on a population of children between the ages 4 and 11 years.

The validation of any test or test procedure implies that there exists an agreed validating criterion against which to evaluate the predictor test performance. In clinical colour vision testing that validating criterion is an anomaloscope. This instrument requires the testee (or patient) to make a judgement of 'same' or 'different' for a pair of coloured lights presented in a split field, one half of which is a standard reference colour. Such instruments require skilled operation by the examiner and are therefore best reserved for use in the clinic. Essentially, there are two types of anomaloscope instrument; those requiring the colours to be viewed through a telescope and those providing for a direct view of the colour field. Although the colours in each type of instrument are produced in different ways (the former with narrow band and the latter with broad band range of wavelengths), Verriest (1981) has shown that a telescopic viewing system as in the Nagel anomaloscope is too difficult to use satisfactorily by children any younger than 12 years of age. The direct viewing principle of the Pickford-Nicolson anomaloscope, however, has considerable advantages in simplicity of use and has been successfully used for the examination of children as young as 4 years (Hill et al, 1982). It has also proved satisfactory for the assessment of defective colour vision amongst mentally retarded children where the incidence of red and green colour deficiencies was found by Salvia & Ysseldyke (1971) to be 8.7% amongst boys. This is very similar to the incidence to be found in an unselected European male population. Not surprisingly, pseudo-isochromatic plates such as the Ishihara test give a very high false-positive error rate among mentally retarded (suggesting an apparent incidence of up to 30% colour defective males), with extremely poor inter-test correlations. For practical reasons, therefore, it would seem sensible to designate a direct view anomaloscope (e.g. Pickford-Nicolson anomaloscope) as the clinical validating criterion for defining the presence or absence of defective colour vision in children and against which to assess the performance of rapid screening tests. It has already gained wide acceptance as a validating instrument for adult populations (e.g. see Pokorny et al, 1979), and norms have been published by Lakowski (1971).

Hill et al (1982) used the Pickford-Nicolson anomaloscope to validate four pseudo-isochromatic colour vision screening tests on 440 boys between the ages of 4 and 11 years. The screening tests were: the Ishihara (tracing wavy lines), the HRR (matching geometric shapes with a template), Guys (matching letter with template) and Matsubara (simple object naming of animals, insects etc). A description of these tests is given in the Appendix. The latter two tests had been specifically designed for use by children. Fig. 5.4 shows the extremely high false-positive error rates with the younger age groups by comparison with adults. The rank order of increasing false-positive error rate on these four tests at any age, is in close agreement with what would be expected from their relative task complexities indicated in Table 5.3. At all age levels, the classical Ishihara test provides both for the lowest false-positives and also the smallest false-negative misclassifications at any school age, consequently this is the screening test of choice for children.

Setting pass/fail criteria

For reasons discussed earlier concerning the problems of perceptual task

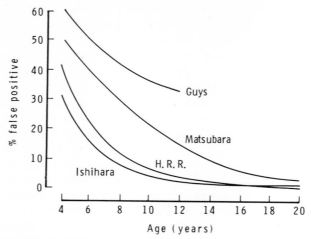

Fig. 5.4 Variation in the false-positive error rate expressed as a function of age for four pseudoisochromatic colour vision screening tests. The curves are based on data from 1361 colour normal subjects including, 411 children aged 4–11 years validated by the Pickford-Nicolson anomaloscope (Adapted from Hill et al, 1982)

complexity facing the person performing a colour vision test, there is a high false-positive error rate associated with most screening tests (i.e. several individuals with normal colour vision will fail the test and will be inappropriately classified as colour defective). This is particularly so with young children but is also found amongst the test performance of adults. These error rates, when combined with the low incidence of defective colour vision in an unselected population, will affect the confidence with which a user can make decisions of colour normal or defective from a test result. For example, it has been shown (Hill & Aspinall, 1980) from an evaluation of seven colour vision tests on an adult population and using single pass/fail cut-off criteria the confidence with which decisions of colour normal can be made is always greater than that for decisions of colour defective. Low error rates combined with low prevalence of the deficiency found in female adults, has a similar consequence on decisions for colour defective as does the combined effect of high error rates and greater prevalence found amongst young boys aged 4–11 years. Both these factors of variable error rate as a function of age and differing incidence values for males and females should therefore be taken into account when establishing satisfactory cut-off criteria for pass/fail decisions on any test. What is important is that the minimum confidence levels required for decisions of colour normal and colour defective are defined by the test user. These may be generated by the same methods as for any subjective probabilities (see Aspinall & Hill, 1983). In the absence of specific data on such estimates for colour vision testing, it is assumed that confidence levels typically found in scientific enquiry of $P = 0.95$ or $P = 0.99$ are likely to be required.

Using Bayesian inferential statistics it is possible to calculate the pass and fail criteria associated with these two levels of confidence both for males and females at two age groups using the data obtained from sample populations of children and young adults. Tables 5.4 and 5.5 provide a summary of the pass/fail criteria on the Ishihara test for each of these identified groups. These tables show that different cut-off values (expressed in terms of the number of plate errors on the test) are required for comparable confidence levels in decisions of colour normal or colour defective for the different population groups. It is clearly not possible to recommend a single criterion to be used on the test for all eventualities. Whereas many view clinical tests as being based upon an all or none classification procedure, with the Bayesian approach to analysis there are many surprises which become apparent to the user. One of these is the need for a sliding criterion. This is a logical consequence of the Bayesian approach to decision analysis and as such the principles are not in question, (Aspinall & Hill, 1983). Nevertheless, the consequences in terms of specific test recommendations may surprise those who seek a simple practical solution for a single pass/fail criterion.

As with other applications of mass screening, the objective in a mass colour vision screening programme should be to identify the normal and detect those who would benefit from further examination. Screening, therefore, should not be aimed at detecting the defective. In colour vision assessment, decisions for defective should always be based upon subsequent testing either with the same test or preferably with an anomaloscope. The maximum number of plate errors to be used as a pass criterion on the Ishihara test which provide for decisions of colour normal are given in Tables 5.4a and 5.5a. For males and females of both age groups it will be seen that these criteria all give a high specificity (i.e. proportion of colour normals who are correctly identified). For young children, however, it is possible for girls to make errors on all 12 of the wavy line plates and a decision for colour normal is still more probable than that for colour defective. This is because of the low incidence of defective colour vision in females and means that there is little value in using a single Ishihara test to screen for the condition amongst young girls. Where there is doubt about the colour vision of a young girl, one of two approaches should be taken. The colour vision should either be assessed on an anomaloscope, or additional familial evidence should be sought prior to re-testing with the Ishihara. If the latter approach is taken, then it is necessary to assess the colour vision of the parents (or other family members) of propositus. Since the deficiency is sex linked, it will be seen from Fig. 5.3 that there are only two parental combinations of relevance and in both instances the father will be colour defective. If the mother is also colour defective then it is almost certain that any daughters will be defective. However, if the mother is a carrier of the defective gene (as demonstrated by examining other appropriate family members), then there is a 50% chance that any daughters are also affected. The recommended pass/fail criteria given in Tables 5.4 and 5.5 where familial evidence is present are based upon

68 PROGRESS IN CHILD HEALTH

Table 5.4 Pass/fail criteria for decisions of colour normal and colour defective with corresponding levels of test specificity and sensitivity when using the Ishihara Test (wavy line trials) on children aged from 4–11 years at two decision confidence levels (based on a sample size n = 440). Values are for the 38 plate edition of the test
(a) *Maximum* permissible number of plate errors for a pass criterion giving decisions of colour normal

		Males (P = 0.08)		Females (P = 0.0044)		Familial evidence	
		Max plate errors	Spec %	Max plate errors	Spec %	Max plate errors	Spec %
P(Normal/Pass) Decision confidence level	0.95	8	98.8	12	99.9	3 (×2)	96.6
	0.99	1	92.9	12	99.9	3 (×2)	96.6

(b) *Minimum* permissible number of plate errors for a fail criterion giving decisions of colour defective

		Males (P = 0.08)		Females (P = 0.0044)		Familial evidence	
		Min plate errors	Sens %	Min plate errors	Sens %	Min plate errors	Sens %
P(Defective/Fail) Decision confidence level	0.95	4 (×2)	71.4	9 (×2)	50.0	3	71.4
	0.99	6 (×2)	71.4			9	50.0

Notes. (a) The prior probabilities used for calculating pass/fail criteria in instances where there is positive familial evidence for defective colour vision were P(D) = P(N) = 0.5. (b) A blank in the table means that the criterion is not attainable. (c) (×2) means that the test should be presented twice with the specified number of errors on each presentation (see page 69 for discussions).

Table 5.5 Pass/fail criteria for decision of colour normal and colour defective with corresponding levels of test specificity and sensitivity when using the Ishihara Test (numerals) on children and adults aged over 12 years at two decision confidence levels (based on a sample size n = 1000). Values are for the 38 plate edition of the test
(a) *Maximum* permissible number of plate errors for a pass criterion giving decisions of colour normal

		Males (P = 0.08)		Females (P = 0.0044)		Familial evidence	
		Max plate errors	Spec %	Max plate errors	Spec %	Max plate errors	Spec %
P (Normal/Pass) Decision confidence level	0.95	4	99.9	6	99.9	1	85.2
	0.99	2	94.6	6	99.9		

(b) *Minimum* permissible number of plate errors for a fail criterion giving decisions of colour defective

		Males (P = 0.08)		Females (P = 0.0044)		Familial evidence	
		Min plate errors	Sens %	Min plate errors	Sens %	Min plate errors	Sens %
P(Defective/Fail) Decision confidence level	0.95	5	70.0	7	66.0	4	84.0
	0.99	7	66.0	7	66.0	5	70.0

See Table 5.4 for notes

this revised prior probability of $P = 0.5$. In such instances a decision of colour normal for a young girl can be made if the child makes no more than three plate errors on each of two successive presentations of the Ishihara test.

Whereas the question of achieving a given level of confidence for a single test performance is not so important as the decision to use multiple tests, there are precautions to be taken in making inferences from multiple test data. When combined tests are used, they should not be highly correlated. Using the same test twice, therefore, can present difficulties. Unfortunately, of the four tests evaluated by Hill et al (1982) for use on children the second best (i.e. HRR) is now out of print. Those who possess a copy of this test should therefore use it with the Ishihara in preference to a double presentation of the Ishihara itself where evidence from more than one test is required. If, however, it is required to present the Ishihara twice to the same child, then it is necessary to allow both a short time delay of a few minutes between presentations and to ensure that the plates are shown in a different random order on each occasion. Obvious correlations will therefore be minimised.

There is one further feature evident from the recommendations given in Tables 5.4 and 5.5. There is rarely continuity between the criteria for pass and those for fail within a population group. Hence, where test performance falls between two criteria there is genuine decision uncertainty and further testing is required. For example, if any male over the age of 12 years makes between three and six errors on the Ishihara, then neither the pass nor fail decisions are reached at the $P = 0.99$ level. A zone of indecision is common to most clinical tests and accords with the recommendations in the latest editions of the Ishihara test user's manual (Hill & Aspinall, 1982a).

Practical guidance on screening and testing

There are essentially three instances in which it may be necessary to use colour vision testing in children. These may be identified as:
1. screening
2. detailed clinical investigation
3. vocational selection

Some tests recommended for use according to each of these functions are summarised in Table 5.6.

In all instances it is essential that the room illumination is controlled since this could affect performance on the tests. For tests based upon printed colour materials it is preferable to use artificial daylight fluorescent lamps producing a minimum illuminance of 300 lux (Hill et al, 1978). In most schools or consulting rooms, however, such lamps are rarely in use so emphasis should be placed on natural daylight avoiding direct sunlight. Viewing of the tests under tungsten lamps should be avoided since this will alter the false-positive and false-negative misclassifications due to changes in colour appearance of the plates. It is also important to avoid undue exposure

Table 5.6 Suggested tests for different applications of colour vision assessment in children

Test application	Age in years	
	4–11	12 +
Screening	Ishihara (wavy lines)	Ishihara (numerals)
Clinical investigation and diagnosis	P–N anomaloscope	P–N or Nagel anomaloscope FM 100 hue Panel D-15
Vocational selection	—	As above, plus special colour naming or colour discrimination tasks

of the test plates to sunlight since this will cause fading of the colours and consequently affect the test efficiency.

In detailed clinical investigation, colour discrimination tests are sometimes used as an alternative or in addition to the anomaloscope. The most popular of such tests for adults is the FM-100 hue (see Appendix). Verriest et al (1982) has established age norms for this discrimination test down to the age of 6 years but concluded that the extremely wide normal range of numerical error scores meant that the test had little clinical value below the age of 10 years. This was due primarily to an inability of children to understand the task, a problem which has also been found in children using the FM D-15 test (see Appendix). Both tests involve an understanding and manipulation of the difficult concept of colour order.

Where conventional clinical tests prove inadequate for vocational selection some guidance may be obtained for specified occupations in a discussion of the subject by Voke (1980). Frequently, a satisfactory indication of the adequacy of a person's colour vision can be obtained by using colour sorting or colour naming tasks based upon material specific to the occupation.

REFERENCES

Alexander K R 1975 Colour vision testing in young children: a review. American Journal of Optometry and Physiological Optics, 52: 332–377

Aspinall P, Hill A R, Cameron D 1980 An evaluation of the Ames' Clinitest. In: G Verriest, (ed) Colour Vision Deficiencies V. Adam Hilger, Bristol

Aspinall P A, Hill A R 1983 Is screening worthwhile? In: A MacFarlane, (ed) Progress in Child Health. Churchill Livingstone, Edinburgh

Bacon L 1971 Colour vision defect—an educational handicap. Medical Officer, 125: 199–209

Bornstein M 1976 Infants are trichromats. Journal of Experimental Child Psychology 21: 425–445

Bronson G W 1974 The post natal growth of visual capacity. Child Development 45: 873–890

Bruner J S 1966 Studies in Cognitive Growth. John Wiley and Sons, New York

Cohen J D 1976 Diagnosis of color vision deficiencies in learning-disabled children. Modern Problems of Ophthalmology 17: 364–367

Cox B J 1971 Validity of a preschool colour vision test. Journal of School Health 41: 163–165

Cruz-Coke R 1970 Color Blindness. An Evolutionary Approach. Charles C Thomas, Springfield

Dannemaier W 1972 The effects of color perception on success in high school biology. Journal of Experimental Education 41: 15–17

Donaldson M 1978 Children's Minds. Fontana, London

Espinda S D 1971 Color vision deficiency in third and sixth grade boys in association to academic achievement and descriptive behavioral patterns. Dissertation Abstracts International, 32: 786

Espinda S D 1973 Color vision deficiency: a learning disability? Journal of Learning Disabilities 6: 163–166

Grosvenor T 1977 Are visual anomalies related to reading ability? Journal of the American Optomeric Association 48: 510–517

Hamer R D, Alexander K R, Teller D Y 1982 Rayleigh discriminations in young human infants. Vision Research 22: 575–587

Hill A R, Aspinall P A 1980 An application of decision analysis to colour vision testing. In: G Verriest (ed), Colour Vision Deficiencies V., pp 164–171. Adam Hilger, Bristol

Hill A R, Aspinall P A 1982a Pass/fail criteria in colour vision tests and their effect on decision confidence. Documenta Ophthalmologica, 33: 157–162

Hill A R, Aspinall P A 1982b Tetartanomoly in a mixed heterozygote. Documenta Ophthalmologica 33: 333–336

Hill A R, Connolly J E, Dundas D 1978 The performance of ten colour vision tests at three levels of illumination. Modern Problems of Ophthalmology 19: 64–66

Hill A R, Heron G, Lloyd M, Lowther P 1982 An evaluation of some colour vision tests for children. Documenta Ophthalmologica 33: 183–187

Kinney J A S, Mckay C L 1974 Test of color-defective vision using the visual evoked response. Journal of the optical society of America 64: 1244–1250

Lakowski R 1971 Calibration, validation and population norms for the Pickford-Nicolson anomaloscope. British Journal of Physiological Optics 26: 166–182

Lampe J M, Doster M E, Beal B B 1973 Summary of a 3-year study of academic and school achievement between color-deficient and normal primary age pupils. (Phase 2). Journal of School Health 43: 309–411

Mandola J 1969 The role of color vision anomalies in elementary school achievement. Journal of School Health 39: 633–636

Moreland J D, Kogan D, Smith S S 1976 Optokinetic nystagmus. An objective indicator of defective colour vision. Modern Problems of Ophthalmology 17: 220–230

Peebles D, Teller D Y 1975 Color vision and brightness discrimination in two-month old human infants. Science 189: 1102–1103

Pokorny J, Smith V C, Verriest G, Pinckers A J L G 1979 Congenital and Acquired Color Vision Defects. Grune and Stratton, New York

Salvia J A, Ysseldyke J E 1971 Validity and reliability of the red-green AO HRR pseudo-isochromatic plates with mentally retarded children. Perceptual and Motor Skills 33: 1071–1074

Snyder C 1973 The psychological implications of being colour blind. Journal of Special Education 7: 51–54

Taylor W O G 1966 An advisory clinic for colour defective children. Transactions of the Ophthalmological Society 86: 591–607

Taylor W O G 1971 Effects on employment of defects in colour vision. Brit. J. Ophthal., 55: 753–760

Teller D Y, Peeples D, Sekel M 1978 Discrimination of chromatic from white light by two-month old human infants. Vision Research 18: 41–48

Verriest G 1981 Color vision tests in children. Atti della Fondasione Giorgio Ronchi, 36: 83–119

Verriest G, van Laethem J, Uvijls A 1982 A new assessment of the normal ranges of the Farnsworth 100-hue test scores. American Journal of Ophthalmology 93: 635–642

Verriest G, Uvijls A 1977 Spectral increment thresholds on a white background in different age groups of normal subjects and in acquired ocular diseases. Documenta Ophthalmologica 43: 217–248

Voke J 1980 Colour Vision Requirements in Specific Industries and Professions. Keeler Ltd, London

Waddington M 1965 Color blindness in young children. Educational Research 7: 234–236

APPENDIX

Description of the colour vision tests refered to in this chapter.

A large variety of colour vision tests is commercially available to the user. A few examples from three types of clinical tests have been refered to in this chapter. These include anomaloscopes, pseudo-isochromatic plates and colour order tests.

Anomaloscopes

These are internally illuminated optical instruments in which the observer is required to report on the colour and brightness of one half of a coloured field as it is adjusted by an examiner to match a reference colour in the other half of the coloured field. Typically, a reference yellow is matched by a mixture of red and green light. Such tests require to be operated by a skilled examiner and are therefore reserved for use in a specialist colour vision clinic.

> *Nagel anomaloscope* is a constant deviation spectroscope in which the reference and test colours are comprised of narrow-band wavelengths of high spectral purity. The colours are viewed through a telescopic eyepiece.
> *Pickford-Nicolson anomaloscope* uses broad-band glass filters to produce the reference and test colours which are viewed directly on a diffusing opal screen.

Pseudo-isochromatic plates

The term pseudo-isochromatic means falsely appearing of the same colour. Tests designed on this principle require the detection of a coloured embedded symbol against a carefully selected coloured patterned background. The colours of the symbol and background may be selected using various criteria. The symbol may be visible to the colour normal and not to the colour defective person (vanishing type), or vice versa (hidden symbol). The symbol may appear in one form to the colour normal and in a different form to the colour defective (transformation type). Some symbols may not be visible to specific types of colour vision deficiency only; these are diagnostic plates of the vanishing type.

There are many variants of pseudo-isochromatic tests and most are presented in the form of printed books comprising several plates (i.e. pages) containing different symbols of varying colour combinations. Since each plate may sample a slightly different aspect of colour vision, it is possible to consider some multiple plate tests as simplified test batteries. Where a demonstration plate is included as part of the test, this will have been designed to be visible both to colour normals and all colour defectives, including the totally colour blind. Its utility is self-evident for detecting malingerers and those who do not comprehend the test. Failure to recognise the symbol on the demonstration plate negates the value of responses to the remaining plates of the test. In such instances, other test procedures should be adopted, preferably on a different occasion.

*AO–HRR** is a multiple plate test in which the embedded symbols are geometric shapes (e.g. circle, triangle, cross, etc) viewed against a patterned grey background. It contains screening and diagnostic plates for red, green and blue colour vision deficiencies.

*Farnsworth F2** is a single pseudo-isochromatic plate containing two overlapping coloured squares (blue and green) embedded in a purple background designed for the screening detection of red-green and blue deficiencies respectively.

Guys Hospital colour vision test is a multiple plate test in which letters of the vanishing and transformation type are embedded in a multicoloured background. It is designed for the detection of red-green deficiencies only. Cut-out templates are available for matching by the child against the recognised letter.

Ishihara test is the most widely used screening test for the detection of red and green defects. It is a multiple plate test using the three main principles of pseudo-isochromatic test design. Two-thirds of the plates contain numerals for the testing of adults and the remainder contain wavy lines which may be traced by the young child or illiterate. There are 24 and 38 plate editions of this test.

*Matsubara** colour vision test for infants is a multiple plate test for red and green defects. The embedded symbols are pictographs of objects familiar in Japanese culture (e.g. cherry blossom, flowers etc).

Velhagen colour vision test for children is a multiple plate test in which the embedded symbol is a letter E in varying orientations. A cut-out template is provided for matching against the recognised letter orientation.

Colour order tests

A number of colour vision tests employ the concept of arranging a series of colours in a specified order or estimating the relative magnitude of the colour difference between pairs of colours. Such tasks involve relatively complex perceptual judgements.

City colour vision test is a multiple item test presented in book form. Each page contains four colour samples arranged around a central colour. The task involves the judgement of relative colour differences by stating which of the four samples is closest in appearance to the central colour.

Farnsworth-Munsell (FM) 100 hue test is a colour (i.e. hue) discrimination test comprising 85 colour sample discs which have to be arranged in order such that each adjacent disc is closest in colour appearance to its neighbour.

Panel D-15 test uses 15 selected coloured discs from the FM 100-hue test. The coloured samples have to be arranged in order of closeness in colour appearance progressing through the spectrum. Only those people with marked colour vision deficiencies will make confusions of colour order on this test.

---

* This test is no longer commercially available

Contemporary issues in child abuse and neglect

INTRODUCTION

Child abuse has progressed rapidly from the early descriptions of the 'Battered Child Syndrome' of Kempe et al (1962) to a present day concern with prevention. The field of study and the spectrum of clinical concern in practice is far wider than the words 'child abuse' suggest on cursory examination, and involve the very substance and essential elements of how children are brought up by the adult caregivers in our society.

The field includes the physical and emotional neglect of children, one aspect of which is non-organic failure to thrive. It also involves the misuse of children perhaps to do adult work before their time, or to satisfy adult sexual requirements before being mature enough to refuse. These abuses of children, along with physical abuse and neglect may be seen as examples of caretaking gone astray, or having deviated from an acceptable path of development for the society concerned. Not surprisingly attempts have been made to prevent such dire consequences, hoping to ameliorate the distress caused.

PREVENTION

The consequences of child abuse are serious even where intervention and treatment has been employed (Lynch & Roberts, 1982). The death rate from child abuse is estimated to be 1% in areas having intervention and early treatment services and up to 10% in those areas without such services (Schmitt, 1978). Death is the extreme consequence but there are lesser ones. Lynch & Roberts (1982) found that almost half a group of abused children were having problems when followed up; including behaviour disturbance, problems getting on with parents and peers, poor educational performance with a minority proving too much for foster home after foster home, having no friends or attachments and trusting no-one.

Thus rehabilitation, although possible in four out of five abusing families and relatively safe from the point of view of re-abuse, is not without other consequences. We are therefore compelled to try and prevent abuse if at all possible.

What kinds of prevention are feasible? To prevent one must first predict who may be at risk. There have been several attempts to predict which newborn babies would suffer abuse. Retrospective data has suggested that the maternity hospital staff often record their concern about families who eventually did abuse their children (Lynch & Roberts, 1977). Antenatal interviews (Murphy et al, 1981; Altemeier et al, 1982), perinatal observations of how warmly or appropriately parents and child are relating (Gray et al, 1977; Ounsted et al, 1982), sometimes combined with alerting aspects of the families' histories (Lynch & Roberts, 1977) have been used to identify an 'at risk' group. In these ways half or more babies who become abused in the early years may be identified. However some babies who will be abused are not identified as newborns (false negative screening) and many families included within the 'at risk' group do well without intervention (false positive screening). So studies are needed to reduce both the false negative and false positive screening, in order to clarify who needs extra help and in what form it should be provided.

Half the children eventually to be abused cannot be identified at birth and so we must continue to search for other factors and times in a child's life which may enable abuse to be predicted. Possibilities here include the concerns of health visitors, general practitioners, and well baby clinic staff during toddler and preschool assessments; and in the field of sexual abuse, within schools (Finkelhor, 1980). Perhaps we will eventually be able to move to a more fundamental level of prevention through education of school children and parents to be.

To return to prediction of 'at risk' groups at birth, if one can predict should one intervene? Intervention is only justified (a) if no harm will follow its attempt; (b) if it will achieve anything useful; and (c) if the resources are available.

The prediction and prevention service in which the author is involved can be considered in the light of these considerations. The service was begun in 1978 and the results of the first and second years have been reported (Ounsted et al, 1982; Roberts & Ounsted, 1984).

The service consists of a regular twice weekly screening ward round of the maternity hospital. The round is conducted in a low key fashion by the head maternity social worker, accompanied by a child psychiatrist. The midwives, or occasionally medical staff refer mothers antenatally or perinatally whom they are concerned about. Their concerns, often non-specific, were fully discussed on the round and if necessary a referral made. The referral rate has remained steady at 21 per 1000 liveborn. Those referred differ from the remaining population delivered in the hospital, having babies more likely to be admitted to SCBU, higher rates of maternal psychiatric history and being more likely to be divorced, single or separated. They did not differ significantly with respect to socio-economic status.

The main reason for the midwives' concern included;

1. Doubt about the parents' ability or willingness to care for their baby (32%).

2. A psychiatric history in the mother (18%).

3. Disturbed behaviour in hospital, excluding fourth day blues (18%).

4. Families with diffuse social and medical problems, usually well known to many agencies as 'problem' families (19%) ('Diffuseness' referring to multiplicity rather than severity).

5. Previous abuse of other children (5%).

6. Marital problems, often with violence (2%).

7. Maternal physical illness of mental handicap which may interfere with parenting (2%).

8. Miscellanous, including vascillation over adoption (4%).

Intervention followed prediction and the most common action (60%) was to communicate such midwife concern to the primary health care team. The letter or telephone call to the general practitioner, or health visitor is backed up with the message that we will see the family for assessment at short notice should they be concerned about parent–child relationships. The social worker may well see a proportion of these mothers and makes a parallel contact with health visitor or community social worker. A further 26% are seen by the child psychiatrist for a single session, which is both evaluative and may introduce the parent(s) to our back-up service. Further individual or family therapy is organised as an out-patient for 9%. In 5% use is made of our in-patient Family Unit.

As far as can be judged the service does not cause harm and no short-term ill effect has resulted. The subtle effect of labelling or stigmatising a family as 'at risk', is more difficult to evaluate. The effect of 'not noticing' or averting our gaze from these families may be even more harmful. Before the preventive service began Lynch & Roberts (1977) noted in their study of abused children that in 44% concern about parenting ability had been recorded perinatally but rarely acted upon. Our emphasis is upon evaluating and responding to families' needs as opposed to alerting others to a possible gloomy outcome. We have now completed an evaluation of families identified in this way and found no evidence of harm 18 months after their referral (Roberts et al, 1984).

The question of resources is a vexed one and requires a creative use of what is available in an area rather than a blanket prescription for the optimum service. This is especially relevant at the time of writing with daily news of 'cut-backs'. Certainly co-ordination between community and hospital based services is important, yet difficult to achieve in practice. From the hospital or specialist service perspective there is a need to develop more day facilities and community orientated services in health clinics and social services settings. The practice of 'helping the helper' is a well established aspect of community mental health efforts and a psychiatric liason scheme with health visitors in Leicester was described by Clarke (1980). A specialist assessment service may prove a useful adjunct to community based help and is one feature of our service from the Park Hospital for Children. The range of resources from health, social service and voluntary sources has been reviewed by Roberts (1978).

Thus prediction is possible for a certain proportion, no harm seems to result and resources for intervention are available; but can they be effective?

The results of this preventive service, as assessed by postal questionnaire and a full search of local hospital and social service records, have shown no physical abuse in 1978 and one case from those screened in the maternity hospital in 1979. A further two children had non-organic failure to thrive in 1979. The striking finding was that roughly a quarter of the families were still causing concern to the primary health team and in one-third of these, serious concern was expressed. There were seven cases of abuse discovered in the 5246 liveborn infants not referred in 1978 and three amongst 5506 liveborns in 1979.

These findings prompted us (Roberts et al, 1983) to look in detail at a random group of referred children and their families 18 months later, comparing them with a random population sample delivered in the same hospital. The study is completed and results in preparation, but they indicate that there are still serious problems for over a third of the referred families. In the index group the children are delayed in language and social behaviour, frequently having behaviour problems, and their mothers have a high rate of psychiatric disorder, notably depressive neurosis. We have observed marked variations in mother-child attachment and interactions accompanying these problems. Frank abuse or neglect was unusual and detected in only one or two children. These problems in the families originally referred to us at birth contasted sharply with the population group, where severe problems were unusual. The research visit was often therapeutic in itself or proved to be an assessment which initiated further intervention.

In Denver, USA, similar conclusions have been reached. Those workers showed a reduced rate of child abuse and severe neglect amongst families given help, in a controlled study where half an 'at risk' group received extra help over a 2-year period and the other half did not (Gray et al, 1977). At follow-up, however, severe problems remained, as in our study.

At this toddler stage, is further screening, assessment and possibly intervention possible? Is a second tier of prediction and prevention feasible? Health visitors in particular seem to be aware of these families' problems and thus a possibility for prevention is suggested. Further studies are needed to understand what factors combine to result in a third of the families in our service having a poor outcome (even though the majority did not abuse their children). Conversely what factors protect children from such a predicament? Can certain factors whether acting for improvement or negatively, be determined at an early stage and enable us to tell which children do well and which children do not fare so happily? When these questions begin to be answered, then we can provide help to these vulnerable children.

NON-ORGANIC FAILURE TO THRIVE

Failure to thrive is not a diagnosis but a description applying to children who show a marked reduction or cessation of growth in the first 3 years of their life. Only a proportion of these children have a physical abnormality, causing them to fail to grow as normal (42%). The remainder do not grow properly because they are not adequately nurtured by their parents (30%), or because of a combination of organic and non-organic reasons (28%) (Kempe et al, 1980). 'Nurturing' includes both food itself and the emotional climate within which the food is offered. These children are also described as suffering from nutritional deprivation, emotional deprivation or maternal deprivation syndrome. Psychosocial dwarfism (Money & Wolff, 1980) or deprivation dwarfism refers to a similar condition, but is usually used to describe the older inadequately nurtured children whose short stature marks them out; many of whom were once nutritionally deprived during infancy (Elmer et al, 1969; Chase & Martin, 1970).

Unless the growth failure is sudden and severe, when the child's state is obvious to any person who cares to look, the diagnosis of growth failure requires two simple steps. First is the measurement of weight, height and head circumference, but the second is the appreciation of the significance of these figures. This can only be done by comparing the measurements with norms for the society, by plotting them on an appropriate chart, for example the Tanner chart (Tanner & Whitehouse, 1973). It is surprising how often children have their weights carefully measured, and tape measures passed around their heads, without this next obvious step being taken. Birth weight, gestation, race and parental measurements will all need to be taken into account using appropriate charts or corrections (Tanner, 1978). If there is any doubt about the explanation for the measurements obtained, referral to a paediatrician is necessary. More important, for the purpose of recognising failure to thrive is to spot an abnormally low growth velocity. Thus a fall through two percentile lines on the Tanner charts or a weight on or below the 3rd centile demands explanation. Once it is established that there is a failure of growth, and appropriate feeding advice has not resolved the problem, then hospital admission for a few days can be very revealing.

In hospital most children grow quickly, often putting on 75 g/day (Kempe, 1978). The non-organic group change from miserable, unresponsive, relatively immobile infants to normal active babies within days, but sometimes the weight gain and behavioural improvement is delayed for up to 3 weeks. Some eat ravenously, but not all—others are more delicate.

A careful medical history and a few simple routine screening tests will help to identify the organically caused group. The screening tests frequently performed are; chest X-ray, full blood count, sedimentation rate, urinalysis and microscopy and stool examination for fats and microbes. At this stage, if the history and screening tests do not point to organic illness, a full psychological and social history and evaluation should be made. It is not sensible at this stage to embark upon searches for rare metabolic disorders or malabsorption syndromes. More reasonable is to see if the baby grows when adequately fed (Kempe, 1978). In the presence of adequate growth and an unremarkable medical history with negative screening tests then non-organic failure to thrive can be diagnosed, and the psychosocial explanation sought. There will be an important group with interdependent organic and non-organic features (Kempe et al, 1980) and in these situations dualistic thinking can be harmful, with some staff seeing these families in psychiatric terms only, whilst others restrict their vision solely to physical ill-health.

The children with non-organic failure to grow now need to be understood. How has this come about? What factors have culminated in inadequate nurturing for this child? Unless one looks carefully, simple and inadequate 'causes' are blamed; for example, small teat size, 'under-educated mother', giving too little food (why?), 'feeding problem', 'doesn't agree with the milk', 'allergy' etc. etc. Repeated hospital admissions or clinic visits may then follow. The avoidance of the main issue is very understandable. The parents may seem to have over-whelming problems and they rarely seem to want help, at least in a direct way. Although they are often weary people and wearisome to be with, if their children are to grow and thrive they do need help.

The situation is all the more serious because non-organic failure to thrive is associated with both physical abuse and child neglect. So, in effect, the presentation of non-organic failure to thrive is an 'open warning' (Ounsted & Lynch, 1976) to professionals. Retrospective analysis of physical abuse cases frequently shows a premonitory failure to thrive phase occurring in the few weeks before the overt assualt.

The group is a mixed one and no one typology covers all the situations seen. Some mothers are depressed and need help, some have been deprived and were abused themselves as children. Others are unable to appreciate their 6-month-old baby's clear signals that he wants to suck more, instead the bottle is uncaringly removed and baby inappropriately 'winded'. Usually several factors combine in an individual predicament.

Assessment must be of the child within the family. A careful family history is required, with an idea of the parents' own childhood, their present relationship with each other, their other children and wider family, friends and neighbours. Housing and finances may well be relevant. The general practitioner and health visitor will often have first hand knowledge of these facts. Personal medical history should be sought with details of past illnesses and psychological problems. Information about alchohol intake, drugs (prescribed and not prescribed) and brushes with the police, help build a picture of the family. Attitudes to child rearing, immunisations, and diet can be revealing as to how closed off and inaccesible the family may be. A feeding history should be obtained in detail with a 'typical day' being carefully documented. Breaking the day up into conveniently remembered sections may aid the mother to recall the exact frequency of breast or bottle feeding.

The mother–child relationship can be observed and recorded. Sometimes the mothers seem strangely unconcerned about their infants' scrawny appearance, being more concerned to discuss themselves in avid detail with the interviewer. The babies' obvious cries for more food or to suck for longer may be quietly ignored with a subliminal battle of wits being apparent. Eventually the infant gives up asking for more and may present with a miserable and depressed face, and downturned mouth. They take a week or two to cheer up and regain their responsiveness in hospital or other safe setting. Part of the overall evaluation should be a formal developmental assessment because their language, social responsiveness and gross motor skills may all be significantly delayed.

Finally much can be learned from monitoring progress as the assessment described should progress to a management plan. Engaging the parents in treatment is often not easy; the mother may prove as resistant to the advice and helping gestures of the professionals, as she is to feeding and adequately nurturing her own baby. Therefore direct counselling alone may fail to change the situation. The development of 'foster granny' schemes to provide a mixture of counselling and a trusting supportive relationship is a most helpful approach (Kempe & Kempe, 1978). Community-based groups for parents with these and other problems with their young children, have proved effective (Roberts et al, 1977). Sometimes appropriate concern for the child may necessitate removal to a place of safety whilst matters are forced into the open and longer term plans made. However many such children can be rehabilitated within their natural families. The group in Denver, U.S.A. find a video analysis of mother and child feeding a useful adjunct in considering their management (Kempe et al, 1980).

The outcome from failure to thrive is depressing. Approximately half the children remain small and become small adults (Kempe et al, 1980). Developmental delay and school difficulties are experienced by many with lower intellectual levels than expected. A prospective 20-year follow-up of initially marasmic infants underlines how undernutrition in the first year of life severely affects later height, weight, head circumference, IQ and visuo-motor perception (Stoch et al, 1982). It is not known if careful intervention based on the assessment suggested in this chapter can alter this poor prognosis and such studies are badly needed. One problem is collecting sufficient subjects as non-organic failure to thrive forms only approximately 5% of an area's child abuse cases. The non-organic failure to thrive babies appear to contribute to the psychosocial dwarfs of later childhood. If one adds to this observation that many mothers of poorly nurtured infants had similarly depriving backgrounds themselves, the need for effective interventions is made even more poignant.

CHILD SEXUAL ABUSE

Sexual abuse is defined as 'the involvement of dependent developmentally immature children and adolescents in sexual activities that they do not truly comprehend, to which they are unable to give informed consent and that violate the social taboos of family roles' (Kempe & Kempe, 1978). A shorter working definition is 'the exploitation of a child for the sexual gratification of an adult' (Fraser, 1981). Child sexual abuse includes incest and similar intrafamilial abuse of adopted and step-children, but also abuse by strangers. The activity may consist of involvement in pornography, fondling, attempted or actual anal or genital intercourse. It may be homosexual or heterosexual.

In most incidents the child is related to the perpetrator or knows him well as abuse by strangers accounts for only a quarter of cases in most reported series (Mrazek et al, 1981). When the perpetrator is known to the child approximately two-thirds are intrafamilial and in one-third is a family friend or visitor. Intrafamilial sexual abuse is the most common situation then, being usual father–daughter, but the perpetrator may be another sibling, grandparent, uncle, step or adoptive parent. The first three legally constitute incest. Overall the perpetrator is usually male and the victim a girl.

Although overt physical violence constituting rape or assault is not usual (up to 15%) (Holder, 1980, Mrazek et al, 1981), covert violence is common. This may be by coercion, threat, or by the implied threat that a physically larger person (usually male) in a position of authority exerts over his victim over a period of time. De Francis (1969) emphasised the prolonged nature of the abuse, in many cases repeated over months or years. Large family size is associated with an increased incidence of sexual abuse, and the educational achievement of the perpetrators is usually below that expected for an area. However despite these and similar associations with low socio-economic status, overcrowding, parental mental illness and alchoholism, no section of society is immune and no one stereotype is helpful (Brown & Holder, 1980).

Sexual abuse is more common than most people imagine, and it seems that once professionals or the voluntary organisations recognise that such misuse of children is possible, then the recognition of cases increases. In the U.K. an incidence study has been used to give an estimated 1 in 6000 children sexually abused each year (1500 cases over the whole country). This means that 3 in 1000 children are sexually abused in their childhood (Bentovim et al, 1981). Studies of the general population suggest that between a quarter and a third have had some form of sexual experience with an adult during their childhood, ranging from exhibitionism to intercourse (Finkelhor, 1979; DeVine, 1980). It is difficult to determine where abuse begins and ends, but many authorities in the U.S.A. find a rate close to 6% amongst young women, but the true figure, hardly surprisingly, is not known. High rates of sexual abuse have been reported amongst adolescents who run away from home, abuse drugs and other substances, become sexually promiscuous or prostitutes, and self-poison (DeVine, 1980). Sexual abuse accounts for at least 10% of overall child abuse reported in the U.S.A. (Schmitt, 1978).

In the U.S.A. local and national awareness of the problem increased reports of sexual abuse and raised public and professional determination to develop intervention programmes. The U.K. has seen recent reports in newspapers, women's magazines and a television documentary in 1982. The voluntary organisations to support parents, women and rape victims are receiving calls from more and more women who have remained silent until their adult life, and more self-help groups have developed accordingly. Child health professionals have responded more slowly but literature reviews (Mrazek, 1980), study courses and treatment approaches are developing.

Clinically sexually abused children are an older group of children and adolescents than other abused children. The peak age for the presentation of father-daughter incest is 12–17 years (Brown & Holder, 1980), but the Kempes (1978) have evidence to show a recent lowering of this age range in their area.

The younger child may simply tell someone that 'Daddy has been rude to me'. She may tell a teacher, neighbour, family friend or a professional. Sometimes she tells her mother, who may or may not hear what she says. Unfortunately friends and professionals may react alike with revulsion, fear and disbelief. They may even incorrectly quote Freud to bolster up their own denial and mutter about fantasies and obscure wishes. Some children are even scolded and made to feel eternally guilty for uttering such 'disgusting things'. Alternatively the younger child may present incidentally whilst physical abuse or neglect is being investigated: 25% of sexually abused children are neglected and 6% are physically abused (Brown & Holder, 1980). Other presentations at this age include venereal disease, vaginal infections and unexplained genital trauma (Kerns, 1981). The child may become withdrawn, show other behaviour problems, fail at school or develop enuresis, pica or begin inappropriately mouthing objects.

The older child, perhaps adolescent, may tell a best friend or trusted person who may be similarly nonplussed. They may go to the police or a crisis centre. Many studies have indicated that various signs of distress and turmoil may be precipitated by the adolescent's growing intolerance of a secret, which begins to be experienced as wrong and stigmatising. Often sexual abuse is one focus amongst other difficulties and careful prospective and controlled retrospective studies are needed to clarify where exactly help is needed and how it should develop.

The different disciplines who must now evaluate the declared sexual abuse have a responsibility to the child to make the investigation of the incident no more harassing than the assault itself (Giarretto, 1981). Exercising this will depend upon agreed procedures in each area so that social services, police and health services know who to turn to for expert help. In the U.K. the local area review committee on child abuse can address these issues and produce a plan suited to their geographical area.

The child or adolescent commonly ends up with a double burden, that of victim and of being saddled with guilt over the ensuing family breakdown, social decline and perhaps the breadwinner's imprisonment. Many children sense this and keep their secret at all costs until adult life.

To avoid these ill-effects the methods of investigating both alleged perpetrators and victims need to be agreed between social services, medical, police and legal departments. For instance, it is useful to have an agreed procedure whereby the suspected perpetrator is interviewed by plain-clothes police.

The perpetrator and family may be encouraged to clarify what has happened if the professionals realise that a local plan of 2 or 3 years treatment under the supervision of the court is in operation for the majority of cases and that imprisonment is not automatic (Topper & Aldridge, 1981). This serves two important functions—it increases the confession rate (and families are expert at denial), and lessens the burden for the victim, and often her mother, of the inevitable family decline or breakup through criminal proceedings and imprisonment. American experience supports this assertion (Topper & Aldridge, 1981; Giarretto, 1981). Further, the victim needs to be spared repeated interrogation and examination whilst having their safety ensured, making liason between police and social services vital. The child will usually need a safe place to spend the ensuing weeks or months whilst matters are clarified and treatment plans worked out.

Initial assessment is followed by a treatment phase and at present various approaches are used. A whole family perspective to understanding how such a situation came about and was maintained has proved central to many workers and has led to family based treatment (Brown & Holder, 1980; Mrazek et al, 1981; Mrazek & Bentovim, 1981). Notwithstanding the family dysfunction, for practical reasons individual treatment or treatment of relevant pairs within the family usually preceeds family therapy (Giarretto, 1981). Because of lack of research no one yet knows which treatment works best in which situations. The children frequently need help to develop internal controls for their over-solicitous and abnormally sexualised behaviour. This is not easy and whether it is best done in a therapeutic day setting or through family therapy or even both combined is not yet known. Other more withdrawn children may respond to the more familiar psychotherapies which nurture and encourage the children. 'Out of home' care will be required for some children and adolescents and therefore foster parents will need clear explanations of the child's particular problems and they must have opportunities to discuss frankly any difficulties. Over-friendly children are attractive and initially may seem rewarding but the veneer of competence is thin and their difficulties in trusting others shows through. In some areas the partnership between voluntary organised self-help groups which have sprung from the women's and parents anonymous movements, and the local professional services has proved very effective (Giarretto, 1981).

Whilst we do know that improvement of the initial intervention procedures reduces recidivism and lessens the trauma for the victim, we do not know what sort of longer term help influences the eventual outcome for the victim.

The outcome for sexually abused children is not clearly understood, though most studies do show ill-effects especially where the abuse is repeated or violent (See Mrazeks (1981) for a critique of published studies). It is clear that both relatively unscathed survivors and casualities exist but precisely which factors are relevant to the eventual outcome are not known. Many women, sexually abused as children, find to their dismay, great difficulty sustaining warm, loving or committed relationships in adult life with their own children, spouses or friends. It is imperative to find out what factors, including therapies may affect this outcome, which is to some women and men, quite simply, devastating.

REFERENCES

Altemeier W A, O'Connor S, Vietze P M, Sandler H M, Sherrod K B 1982 Antecedents of child abuse. Journal of Paediatrics 100: 823–829

Bentovim A et al 1981 Child sexual abuse. British Association for the study and prevention of Child Abuse and Neglect, Rochdale

Brown L, Holder W M 1980 The nature and extent of sexual abuse in contemporary American society In: Holder W M (ed) Sexual Abuse of Children, Ch 1, pp 1–15. American Humane Association, Englewood

Chase H P, Martin H 1970 Undernutrition and child development. New England Journal of Medicine 282: 491–496

Clarke M G 1980 Psychiatric liason with health visitors. Health Trends 12: 98–100

De Francis V 1969 Protecting the Child Victim of Sex Crimes Committee by Adults. American Humane Association, Colorado

DeVine R A 1980 Sexual abuse of children: an overview of the problem. In: Sexual Abuse of Children: Selected Readings U.S. Department of Health and Human Services: Washington D.C.

Elmer E, Gregg G S, Ellison P 1969 Late results of the failure to thrive syndrome. Clinical Paediatrics 8: 584–589

Finkelhor D 1979 Sexually Victimized Children. Free Press, New York

Finkelhor D 1980 Risk factors in the sexual victimization of children. Child Abuse and Neglect 4: 265–273

Fraser B G 1981 Sexual child abuse: the legislation and the law in the United States. In: Mrazek P B, Kempe C H Sexually Abused Children and their Families, Ch 5, pp 55–74. Pergamon Press, Oxford

Giarretto H 1981 A comprehensive child sexual abuse and treatment program. In: Mrazek P B, Kempe C H Sexually Abused Children and their Families, Ch 14, pp 179–198 Pergamon Press, Oxford

Gray J D, Cutler C A, Dean J G, Kempe C H 1977 Prediction and prevention of child abuse and neglect. Child Abuse and Neglect 1: 45–58

Holder W M (ed) 1980 Sexual Abuse of Children. American Humane Association Englewood

Kempe C H, Siverman F N, Steele B F, Droegemueller W, Silver H K 1962 The battered-child syndrome. Journal of the American Medical Association 181: 17–24

Kempe C H 1978 Child abuse–the paediatrician's role in child advocacy and preventive paediatrics. American Journal of Diseases of Childhood 132: 255–260

Kempe R S, Kempe C H 1978 Child Abuse. Fontana/Open Books, London

Kempe R S, Cutler C, Dean J 1980 The infant with failure to thrive. In: Kempe C H, Helfer R E (eds) The Battered Child, 3rd edn, Ch 10, pp 163–182. University of Chicago, Chicago

Kerns D L 1981 Medical assessment of child sexual abuse. In: Mrazek P B, Kempe C H (eds) Sexually Abused Children and their Families, Ch 10, pp 129–141. Pergamon Press, Oxford

Lynch M A, Roberts J 1977 Predicting Child Abuse: Signs of bonding failure in the maternity hospital. British Medical Journal i: 624–626

Lynch M A 1975 Ill-Health and Child Abuse. Lancet ii: 317–319

Lynch M A, Roberts J C 1982 The Consequences of Child Abuse. Academic Press, London

Money J, Wolff G 1980 Late puberty, retarded growth and reversible hyposomatotropinism (psychological dwarfism) In: Williams G J, Money J (eds) Traumatic Abuse and Neglect of Children at Home, Ch 36, pp 397–407. Johns Hopkins University Press, Baltimore

Mrazek P B 1980 Sexual abuse of children. Journal of Child Psychology and Psychiatry 21: 91–95

Mrazek P B, Bentovim A 1981 Incest and the Dysfunctional Family System. In: Mrazek P B, Kempe C H (eds.) Sexually Abused Children and Their Families, Ch. 13, pp 167–178. Pergamon Press, Oxford.

Mrazek P B, Lynch M A, Bentovim A 1981 Recognition of child sexual abuse in the United Kingdom. In: Mrazek P B, Kempe C H (eds) Sexually Abused Children and their Families, Ch 4, pp 35–50. Pergamon Press, Oxford

Mrazek P B, Mrazek D A 1981 Effects of child sexual abuse: methodological consideration In: Mrazek P B, Kempe C H (eds) Sexually Abused Children and their Families, Ch 18, pp 235–245. Pergamon Press, Oxford

Murphy J F, Jenkins J, Newcombe R G, Sibert J R 1981 Objective birth data and the prediction of child abuse. Archives of Diseases in Childhood 56: 295–297

Ounsted C, Lynch M A 1976 Family pathology as seen in England. In: Helfer R E, Kempe C H (eds) Child Abuse and Neglect, The Family and the Community, Ch 4, pp 75–86. Ballinger, Cambridge

Ounsted C, Roberts J C, Gordon M, Milligan B 1982 Fourth goal of perinatal medicine. British Medical Journal i: 879–882

Roberts J C 1978 Social work and child abuse: the reasons for failure and the way to success. In: Martin J P (ed) Violence and the Family, Ch 10, pp 255–291. John Wiley, Chichester

Roberts J C, Ounsted C 1984 Further goals of perinatal medicine In: Harvey D (ed) Parent Infant Relationships, Ch 7. John Wiley, Chichester

Roberts J C, Beswick K, Leverton B, Lynch M A 1977 Prevention of Child Abuse: Group Therapy for Mothers and Children. Practitioner 219: 111–115

Roberts J C, Dennis J, Jones D P H, Ounsted C 1984 Mother—Infant Relationship Problems Identified in the Maternity Hospital—An 18 Month Follow-Up Study (in preparation)

Schmitt B D 1978 Child Protection Team Handbook. Garland, New York

Stoch M B, Smythe P M, Moodie A D, Bradshaw D 1982 Psychosocial outcome and CT findings after gross undernourishment during infancy: a 20 year developmental study. Developmental Medicine and Child Neurology 24: 419–436

Tanner J M 1978 Physical Growth and Development In: Forfar J O, Arneil G C (eds) Textbook of Paediatrics, 2nd edn, Ch 7, pp 249–303. Churchill Livingstone, Edinburgh

Tanner J M, Whitehouse R H 1973 Height and weight charts from birth to 5 years allowing for length of gestation. Archives of Diseases of Childhood 48: 786–789

Topper A B, Aldridge D J 1981 Incest: intake and investigation. In: Mrazek P B, Kempe C H Sexually Abused Children and their Families, Ch 9, pp 109–127. Pergamon Press, Oxford

Whooping Cough Vaccine Reviewed

INTRODUCTION

At the turn of the century, whooping cough—or by its Latin name pertussis meaning 'intensive cough'—was after measles the commonest fatal, infectious disease of British children under 5. Although the disease remains a common cause of death in many developing countries few children now die from it in the wealthier parts of the world. This reflects the combined effects of high standards of living *and* protection through high immunisation rates. Although some wealthy countries such as Sweden currently do not immunise against pertussis their children are in part protected by the immunisation policies of neighbouring countries. Recent British experience shows that such shelters does not last and a generation of doctors, health visitors and parents suddenly had to learn about a disease that was by the early 1970s nearing extinction in Britain (Christie, 1980).

THE CAUSAL ORGANISM

Although many bacterial and viral pathogens can make children cough, classical whooping cough only follows infection with the bacterial organism *Bordetella pertussis*, which was first grown on culture medium by Jules Bordet and Octave Gengou in 1906 at the Pasteur Institute, Brussels. Although the disease is usually diagnosed on clinical findings there is a strong case for attempting to confirm the diagnosis by culturing the organism so that the epidemiology of the disease can be documented. This must be done by experienced personnel; a special flexible wire swab is passed through the inferior nasal turbinates to the posterior nasal space. The swab must be plated out without delay on to a special medium containing charcoal. Although culture is the only way to confirm the diagnosis, rapid serological and ELISA techniques are becoming available in an increasing number of centres and are likely to be used widely in future.

THE ILLNESS

Pertussis is a highly infectious disease spread by those who are incubating

86

or have the active disease. The disease only affects humans, and there is no firm evidence that symptomless carriers of the disease exist. Following an incubation period of 7–14 days the patient first develops a coryza, with fever and irritability, gradually coughing becomes more marked. Although the disease can occur at any age it is particularly common in infancy and most lethal in the first 6 months of life, when it is less easy to diagnose than in the older child who soon develops the classic whoop. Young infants tend to splutter and choke rather than whoop loudly and are at risk of inhaling vomit, particularly after a paroxysm.

The pathophysiology of pertussis has still not been fully worked out though recent work suggests that the following occurs: those with severe disease get exhausted and this coupled with poor nutrition probably made worse by a tendency to hypoglycaemia due to pancreatic islet hyperstimulation leads to inanition. The debility of whooping cough is due to the production of toxins. Ability to cope with infection is impaired because white cells cannot readily be released from the circulation (hence the presumably useless lymphocytosis characteristic of the disease). It has been suggested that the tendency of the organism to provoke the production of excess adenylate cyclase interferes with the ability of white cells to kill bacteria. At its worst fatal pneumonia results. Fortunately secondary infection can be treated with antibiotics and life maintained with intravenous therapy and ventilation but these are drastic measures. If antibiotics are to be of value in preventing the disease they have to be given in the early coryzal prodromal phase before the cough has developed. Giving them later will not stop the disease. The administration of erythromycin which *in vitro* at least is the most effective antibiotic against the organism in a dose 125 mg in babies, 250 mg over age 2, 6-hourly for a week is commonly advised in cases where an older sibling brings the disease to a house where there is a young unprotected baby. Once the diagnostic cough has presented conventional wisdom is that it is too late to start immunisation; proven contacts should be given erythromycin. One attack of the disease is normally presumed to give life-long immunity, though many cases in adults have occurred in the current epidemic, suggesting that immunity may wane with time.

There is no evidence that whooping cough currently seen in the UK is a milder disease than in the past; the main difference is in availability of better treatment and better general health in childhood. Families are smaller and more widely spaced resulting in fewer young children per household. Infants do not have passively acquired transplacental immunity from their mothers, but there is a possibility that breast feeding might give some temporary protection though so far no specific antibody has been detected in milk.

Official British statistics are derived from notifications by doctors of cases diagnosed in general practice or hospital. Details of every case seen should be notified immediately to the district community physician. This is a statutory duty. However, the incentive to do so is often lacking and many cases go unreported so official figures are greatly underestimated. Deaths are taken

Table 7.1 Deaths by age and case fatality ratios per 100 notifications in England and Wales (1940–1982)

| | Average annual deaths and case fatality ratios | | | | | |
| | All ages | | Age <1 year | | Age >1 year | |
	Deaths	Ratio	Deaths	Ratio	Deaths	Ratio
1940–45	1120	1.20	630	*	489	*
1946–51	639	0.56	411	3.58	228	0.23
1952–57	138	0.13	94	0.96	44	0.04
1958–63	29	0.12	21	0.78	8	0.04
1964–69	23	0.12	19	0.88	4	0.03
1970–75	12	0.11	20	0.73	1	0.01
1976–81	7	0.04	5	0.19	2	0.02
1982	14	0.02	11	0.19	4	0.01

* Not available

Table 7.2 Notification rates by age in England & Wales (1946–1981)

| | Average annual notification rate per 100 000 population | | | |
	<1 year	1–4 years	5–9 years	≥10 years
1946–51	1649	2498	1285	11
1952–57	1417	1963	1101	10
1958–63	439	521	359	5
1964–69	253	310	176	3
1970–75	198	152	92	2
1976–81	460	662	168	4

from death certificates, and presumably are more accurate though they too are also believed to be underestimates (Table 7.1). Fig. 7.1 and Table 7.2 shows the notification rates of the disease and deaths reported since 1940 in England and Wales. The disease has become less common since the war years, tending to occur in 4-yearly epidemics, which were getting smaller every 4 years until 1977. Whilst writing, in late 1982, we are experiencing the greatest weekly notification rates since the 1950s.

Although the number of deaths per 1000 cases notified—the case fatality rate—has dropped markedly, there are no grounds for complacency; pertussis is a preventable disease and the mortality could be zero.

THE NATURE OF PERTUSSIS VACCINE

Attempts to make pertussis vaccines began around 1912. Madsen used one successfully in 1925 in the remote Faroe Isles in the North Sea to quell an epidemic. His account, however, reported two deaths in recently vaccinated infants, thus beginning controversy about the vaccine's safety that has persisted ever since. It must be appreciated that Madsen's vaccine was a

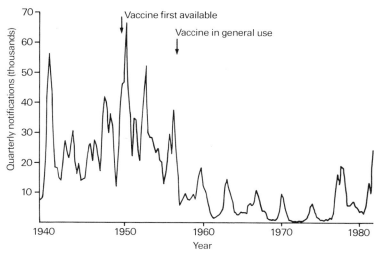

Fig. 7.1 Notifications: England and Wales 1940–82. Whooping cough became notifiable in England and Wales in 1940. There was a peak in 1941 and another more sustained increase between 1948 and 1953 corresponding with the post-war rise in the child population. Notifications fell by more than two-thirds between 1957 and 1961 in the years immediately following the start of widespread immunisation but then declined more slowly with outbreaks every 3–4 years, the smallest in 1974/75

crude product, far removed from present day vaccines and was administered to infants who were already infected.

Pertussis vaccines are now made in most of the larger countries. Basically they consist of a suspension of *B. pertussis* cells derived from the three pathogenic serotypes of the organism that have been killed by exposure to heat or chemicals. Most countries produce the vaccine to specifications laid down by the WHO, though some, notably Denmark, produce a weaker vaccine, whilst that used in the USA contains considerably more cells than the WHO standard. The potency of the vaccine is assessed by a rather crude biological test (Kendrick test) which involves intracerebral injection of virulent strains of *B. pertussis* to unimmunised mice. This test is far removed from human experience but nevertheless the results of this test were found to correlate well with protection in infants in MRC trials of the 1950s.

Unwanted Effects of Pertussis Vaccine

Unlike the biologically much simpler toxoid vaccines used against diphtheria and tetanus, pertussis vaccine contains whole dead bacterial cells. Several theoretically undesirable features can be demonstrated (mainly from animal work). These include an insulin-stimulating factor (though there is no evidence that newly immunised infants actually develop hypoglycaemia), a histamine sensitising factor, and potential haemagglutinins. When large amounts of the vaccine are mixed with brain extract and injected into rats,

Table 7.3 Results of 48-hour follow-up of DTP and DT vaccinees

	DTP (%)	DT (%)
Persistent crying	3.1	0.7
Local redness	37.4	7.6
Local swelling	40.7	7.6
Pain	50.9	9.9
Fever	31.5	14.9
Vomiting	6.2	2.6
Anorexia	20.9	7.0

an auto allergic encephalomyelitis can result. This however is far different from human use and is only of theoretical interest. In practice, pertussis vaccines are more toxic and pyrogenic than those vaccines which only contain toxoids.

In the USA (Cody et al, 1981) DTP vaccine was given to 15 752 children under 6 years whilst a further 784 were given DT vaccine; in order to study sequelae all were followed up, mainly by 'phone for 48 hours afterwards. The results are shown in Table 7.3.

Following DTP immunisation nine developed convulsions and a further nine had brief hyporesponsive episodes but none had any subsequent neurological problems. British experience is that local reactions are less common than this, possibly because British and other vaccines to WHO standard contain rather fewer cells than those used in the USA (Miller et al, 1974).

Is the vaccine effective?

During the 1930s pertussis vaccines were developed in the USA and generally found to be effective but their use in the UK was delayed by the war. During the period from the late 1940s to the mid 1950s, the Medical Research Council made a series of classic field trials of numerous pertussis vaccines supplied by several manufacturers. Some of the vaccines gave excellent protection against naturally-acquired whooping cough, whilst others were useless. One of the good vaccines was selected as being both effective and safe and was subsequently adopted as the British Standard. Later its potency was increased in line with WHO standards. Although the testing was thorough by the standards of the time, much more intensive surveillance is required today before new medical substances can be introduced. Currently there are two British manufacturers, Glaxo and Burroughs Wellcome. They use slightly different manufacturing techniques but no evidence has been produced to show that these vaccines differ for practical purposes. They are supplied in both 'plain' and adsorbed forms. Although the latter is slightly more expensive it is more protective (Griffith, 1978).

The extent to which pertussis vaccines are fully effective has aroused controversy. In the early 1960s three of the four currently used British vaccines were reported to lack the complete range of three agglutinogens which were present in virulent strains of *B. pertussis* isolated in children. This has since been corrected. A series of local studies summarised in a report from the Public Health Laboratory Service (Pollock et al, 1982) has shown that far fewer immunised children than unimmunised have developed pertussis in the recent British epidemic suggesting that the present vaccine has considerable protective activity. Even when cases do occur they are milder than in those unimmunised and hospital admission with serious disease is uncommon. The only contradictory reference came from a small survey from the Shetland Isles (Ditchburn, 1979). No immunising procedure is likely to be 100% protective—sometimes vaccines deteriorate through faulty handling or storage; they may be incorrectly administered—or for unexplained reasons 'not take'. If any vaccine is given to 90% of a child community and is 90% effective, nearly half the cases of the disease that one is trying to prevent will occur in immunised individuals.

VACCINE SAFETY AND VACCINE UPTAKE—THE GREAT DEBATE

Britain has always made pertussis vaccination a matter for parental choice, unlike the Eastern European countries where it is compulsory. In nearly all the states in the USA full vaccination (including DTP) is mandatory before school entry. By 1970 some parts of Britain were using computer based systems for arranging immunisations and achieving up to 90% immunisation rates against pertussis. At the time it seemed that whooping cough might become an extinct disease.

In 1974 a paper from Great Ormond St Hospital, London (Kulenkampff et al, 1974) described 36 children who had been admitted during the previous 11 years with serious neurological disorders which had started within 28 days of immunisation against pertussis. The authors did not claim that these problems had been caused by the immunisation but felt that there was a need for further studies since this immunisation is often followed by fever and irritability. Earlier the British Medical Journal carried an article from Ström (1960) in Sweden entitled 'Is universal immunization against pertussis always justified?'. Ehrengut (1980) from Hamburg had questioned his country's pertussis vaccination policy on the grounds of neurological side-effects and from Paris a further series of children with neurological problems, time associated with pertussis immunisation, was published in 1975 (Aicardi & Chevrie, 1975).

In 1974 the British press and broadcasting media suddenly turned the question of pertussis vaccine safety into red hot news (Clarke, 1980; Griffith, 1981) with the almost nightly spectacle of elderly professors arguing the merits or demerits of the vaccine on television. Wildly extravagant claims against the vaccine started to be made recalling the campaigns against smallpox vaccination nearly two centuries earlier. Not surprisingly the public gained the impression that the vaccine could be very dangerous and demands were made in Parliament for its withdrawal and legal cases for compensation were started. The government decided in the face of much criticism to make *ex-gratia* payments to those who could show that their neurological problems were time associated with immunization (Robinson, 1981). It became clear that the whole situation required intensive review as there was at this time no firm evidence using satisfactory controls, to show whether there really was a case to make against the vaccine or not.

It was against this background that the DHSS agreed to support a scientifically based case-control study into the matter as at the time the case against the vaccine relied solely on testimonial accounts. However, studies of the background incidence of presentation of serious neurological disease in infancy, especially in the age range 6–9 months, show that these conditions are not uncommon and that many are unexplained. Thus, the whole question of vaccine associated brain damage could be explained entirely by coincidence. It was thus necessary to determine the background incidence of the alleged problems and find whether they occurred significantly more often in recently immunised than in non-immunised children. Such problems can be tackled either by the cohort approach where an entire community is studied for a period of time, or a case-control approach where those identified as having a certain disease or condition (in this case serious acute neurological disease) are compared with matched controls. Examples of both types of study have been undertaken recently in the UK.

The Child Health and Education Study (Butler et al, 1982)

Follow-up of the 13 135 survivors of the cohort born in England, Scotland and Wales during the week 5–11 April 1970 through the first 5 years revealed that whilst 4 instead of the expected 1.9 ($P = 0.06$) had a fit within 72 hours of a pertussis immunisation none of the four had any long-term adverse neurological sequelae.

Despite allowance being made in the analysis for social class it was found that children not immunised against pertussis at 5 years were more likely to have had convulsions, be shorter, have speech defects and have poorer educational ratings. The 40 children who had been admitted to hospital with pertussis had particularly low educational test scores at 5.

North West Thames Study (Pollock & Morris, 1983)

Since 1975 the reporting of reactions to all vaccines has been intensified in the North West Thames Region and a special search has been made for instances of serious neurological disease following immunisation.

In one of the seven Areas in the Region (Hertfordshire), 10 000 children given either DTP or DT vaccine have been followed up and the reactions compared.

The NW Thames study embodies a comparison of the relative frequency of reported reactions to DTP and DT, also the relative frequency with which children admitted to hospital with neurological disease have been recently immunised with either vaccine.

The American Collaborative Study (Hirtz et al, 1983)

During the years 1966–74, 54 000 births in eight large American teaching hospitals were intensively studied and followed up with detailed medical surveillance and psychological testing through their first 18 months and again at 7 years. Among these children ten had a seizure within 2 weeks of DTP immunisation but only one had any serious neurological problem when followed up at age 7.

The National Childhood Encephalopathy Study (NCES) (Alderslade et al, 1981)

This study enquired into the serious acute neurological diseases occurring in children aged 2–35 months for a 3-year period starting in July 1976. The aim was to determine whether children with such disorders had a more frequent history of recent immunisation than a group of matched controls. All hospital paediatricians, infectious disease specialists and neurosurgeons in England, Scotland and Wales were asked to notify the study team of any child admitted to their wards with an illness of an encephalopathic type, prolonged fits ($\frac{1}{2}$ hour plus), altered consciousness, or infantile spasms or Reye's syndrome. Those with neurological problems that lasted more than 15 days were visited at home at least twice by a paediatrician member of the study team who undertook a detailed interview with the parents and performed a neurological and developmental examination. Those who were not examined were followed-up by postal enquiries to their doctor.

Each of the 1182 children notified to the study had two controls matched by age, sex and NHS district drawn from the local birth or immunisation register. It was then possible to determine the risk of recent vaccination in the case children and find how this compared to the history in controls by writing to the child's GP and local specialist in community medicine for vaccination histories.

The findings of the Study have been published in medical (Miller et al, 1981), nursing (Miller & Ross, 1981) and health visiting journals (Ross, 1982). Analysis of the first 1000 cases referred to the study showed a slight but significant increase in risk of a child with a serious neurological disease having a pertussis containing vaccine in the 7 days prior to the development of symptoms but no increased risk after this time. The attributable risk— the chance that a reaction occurring in a child following an immunisation is actually due to the immunisation rather than a chance finding—comes out at around one in a third of a million doses given. It must be appreciated that such numerical statements are difficult for the public to comprehend. Whilst 19 children died from pertussis whilst the study was going on and 13 developed encephalitis from pertussis, during the same time 35 children developed a neurological disease within 7 days of a pertussis containing immunisation. One year later 21 of these children were free from neurological deficit, two had died but both had neuropathic virus isolated in the brain at post-mortem. Only six, that is two per year of the study still had serious neurological problems. Even in these children it is still possible that alternative causes for their neurological problems could emerge. Analysis of all 1182 'case' children in the study show that the attributable risk of long term neurological damage is even lower than that reported earlier.

SUDDEN UNEXPECTED INFANT DEATH SYNDROME (SIDS)

About one in 600 children die as 'SIDS' in the UK within the first year. Obviously some of these children will have had recent pertussis immunisation but there is no evidence to show that this occurs more frequently than by chance.

The most thorough enquiries into the question of SIDS and pertussis immunisation come from the USA. In 1978 four cases of SIDS were reported from Tennessee in children who had received DTP vaccine from a single batch within the 24 hours preceeding death. A review was made of the vaccination status of all SIDS children in Tennessee during the 8-month period whilst the suspect vaccine batch was in use. Comparison was made with the equivalent time period in the preceeding year. There was no significant difference in the DTP immunisation rates in the equivalent time periods in the 2 years.

The National Institute of Child Health and Human Development sponsored a multicentre case-control study of SIDS in the USA. Preliminary analysis of data from this study did not show any increased frequency of DTP vaccination among SIDS cases when compared to their matched controls. In fact, there was a lower frequency of DTP vaccination in SIDS cases than in controls.

PERTUSSIS IMMUNISATION IN OTHER COUNTRIES (Miller et al, 1982; Dudgeon & Marshall, 1984)

Although the WHO advises pertussis immunisation and lays down standards for vaccine production there is enormous difference in practice between different countries. In France DT and polio immunisation is obligatory, whilst pertussis immunisation is recommended. In practice about 95% of children receive pertussis vaccine and the clinical disease is rare (Ross & Edouard, 1983). In West Germany practice varies widely; some textbooks strongly advise immunisation but the actual advice given to parents is a matter for individual doctors—probably about 30% of children get the immunisation but it has proved impossible to obtain complete data from German sources. In East Germany and most Eastern block countries pertussis immunisation is compulsory and almost universal. The position in Scandinavia is perverse—Denmark uses a weak vaccine which protects infants but clinical pertussis is occurring in school children, presumably when protection wanes. Sweden gradually reduced the potency of their vaccine during the 1970s, finally abandoning it in 1979. With a population one-sixth that in England and Wales an average 3500 cases of the disease have been confirmed annually by culture of the organism in the period 1977–1981. There have been reports of endemic disease in adults (Trollfors & Rabo, 1981) though there do not appear to have been any infant deaths. The position in neighbouring Norway and Finland is quite different. Both countries widely use a vaccine to WHO standard. Finland (Mertsola et al, 1982) has had no recent epidemic disease though there is some evidence that older children are developing subclinical disease and transmitting clinical infection, presumably due to the locally produced vaccine failing to give long-lasting immunity. Despite careful local study the Finnish authorities are satisfied that their vaccine has not been associated with any neurological sequelae. Unfortunately there is far too little effective international study of pertussis and it is difficult to obtain clear accounts of the position in other countries.

Japanese experience has been very similar to the British (Kanai, 1980). From high immunisation rates after the war and near disappearance of the disease there was a media led campaign against the vaccine in the late 1960s on the grounds of alleged neurotoxicity. Collapse in confidence with the vaccine was followed by epidemic pertussis and a return to higher immunisation rates.

In developing countries uncounted children develop pertussis and the death toll is unknown. The WHO has launched an expanded immunisation programme which includes pertussis immunization to protect children in developing countries. Hopefully this may help to reduce the world's reservoir of the disease.

CURRENT PERTUSSIS IMMUNISATION PRACTICE IN THE UK

Since the use of pertussis vaccine has been so contentious in recent years British doctors are strongly advised to stick to the guidelines advised by the DHSS and published in the National Formulary. These are of course only guidelines, not a legal requirement. They are drawn up by the Joint Committee on Vaccination and Immunization which comprises a group of distinguished clinicians concerned with infections and neurological disease, micro-biology and epidemiology, who advise the DHSS. They meet at regular intervals and monitor the vaccine policy used in this country. The guidelines advise that the vaccine be given as a triple preparation with diphtheria and tetanus toxoids plus oral polio vaccine. This should start at 3 months and two repeat doses given at 6-weekly intervals, when the child is aged 4–6 months. It does not matter if these intervals are extended though makes administration policy inconvenient and delays full protection.

The DHSS guidelines are as follows:

> It is advisable to postpone vaccination if the child is suffering from any acute febrile illness, particularly if it is respiratory, until fully recovered. Minor infections without fever or systemic upset are not regarded as contra-indications. Vaccination should not be carried out in children who have
>
> 1. a history of any severe local or general reaction, *including a neurological reaction*, to a preceding dose: or
> 2. a history of cerebral irritation or damage in the neonatal period, or who have suffered from fits or convulsions.
>
> There are certain groups of children in whom whooping-cough vaccination is not absolutely contra-indicated but who require special consideration as to its advisability. These groups are
>
> 1. children whose parents or siblings have a history of idiopathic epilepsy:
> 2. children with developmental delay thought to be due to a neurological defect: and
> 3. children with neurological disease.
>
> For these groups the risk of vaccination may be higher than in normal children but the effects of whooping-cough may be more severe, so that the benefits of vaccination would also be greater. The balance of risk and benefit should be assessed with special care in each individual case.
>
> Allergy, according to much informed medical opinion, is not a contra-indication to the administration of pertussis vaccine.

Some cynics feel that these guidelines do more to protect doctors from litigation than to protect children. They are not 'tablets of stone' from on high and doctors have to interpret them in the light of the particular child's need. Vaccination schedules and advised contraindications vary greatly and readers outside the UK should ascertain and follow local policy. The number of doses advised varies too: in the USA additional doses are advised at ages 18 months and 5 years. This scheme appears to give very solid protection and may be an additional reason why 4-yearly epidemics of pertussis do not occur there. Many countries, such as France do not impose restrictions and advise antipyretics and anti-convulsants to be given to children with neurological problems prior to immunisation.

Although pertussis immunisation could successfully be given to the newborn, the other components of triple vaccine would not be optimally protective due to the presence of maternal antibody. If there is risk of an infant getting early exposure to pertussis (say proposed admission to a residential nursery) it would be wise to commence vaccination with monovalent pertussis vaccine within the first month of life as it is believed that at least some useful protection begins within 10 days of immunisation. The optimal age to start immunising premature babies with pertussis vaccine has not been determined. If DTP is to be used a reasonable compromise would be to add half the numbers of weeks that the infant is premature to the child's age before starting immunisation; e.g. if a child is 32 weeks gestation, start DTP at 4 instead of at 3 months. The DHSS now advise that those children who were only given DT immunisation in infancy should be offered monovalent pertussis immunisation during their first 6 years (3 doses at 4-weekly intervals). Some doctors advise giving half doses of vaccine with a repeat a week later. There is no documented evidence that this is worth doing and gives twice the work to all concerned.

Practical note

Since vaccines are potent biological substances they should be treated with respect. Children must be seen by doctors prior to immunisation of any type though the actual immunisation can be done by a clinic nurse or health visitor. It is essential that parents are given relevant information about the reasons for vaccination, its benefits and possible risks in a form that they can understand. They should be encouraged to keep the child's immunisation details. It is even more important that an official record is kept. This should include the date, time, maker, doctor involved and the maker's batch number (which are currently needlessly long). This information should be stored indefinitely. Unfortunately much of this vital information has been lost in recent years when computer systems have been changed. This is inexcusable and firm efforts must be taken to prevent this.

Students should be taught to handle immunisation records with the same care given to blood transfusions. Much of the difficulty with pertussis vaccine could have been avoided if proper computerised vaccination data had been available on a national basis.

THE WAY AHEAD

There is now an urgent task to restore a sense of proportion over the safety of pertussis vaccine. Firstly there has to be a mature understanding of the nature of the 'media'. They—newspapers, TV or radio—exist by selling information to the paying public. They stress bad news rather than good and will readily blow a story into a major controversy. It is hard to get a correction or a climb down once a 'scare' has been generated. Those involved in promoting public health should use all appropriate opportunities to give information to the media but must appreciate that misquotation or biased editing often occurs—the golden rule is to get advice from a colleague experienced in this and try to develop mutual trust and understanding with specific people in the media field. The individual, however, has great opportunities for effective health education through patient explanation of facts to colleagues, students and parents. At present many colleagues are confused by the whole matter and until recently felt that withholding pertussis immunisation was the safest course. As the recent return of epidemic disease shows, this position is no longer tenable. Where there is doubt about the wisdom of immunising a particular child, advice should be sought from paediatricians who are known to be experienced in this field. There will continue to be adverse publicity against the vaccine because there are those, mainly in non-clinical positions, who hold strong personal convictions against the vaccine despite the newer evidence. At present intense efforts are being made to develop new, simpler and potentially 'cleaner' pertussis vaccines and one is currently under trial in Japan (extensive study would be needed before it could be cleared for use in the UK). However, for the next few years we are likely to require the present vaccine and therefore there is no logical alternative to encouraging widescale infant pertussis immunisation in the UK. That poses a lot of hard work on all engaged in promoting child health.

Acknowledgements

The author is grateful for the help of many kind colleagues for their advice in the preparation of this chapter.

The opinions expressed are the author's and do not necessarily reflect 'official thinking'.

The author, as a member of the NCES team, would like to thank all readers who so generously provided data or did home visits on behalf of this study. The tables and figure are reproduced (with kind permission) from the weekly Commuriable Disease Report (CDR) of the Public Health Laboratory Service.

REFERENCES

Aicardi J, Chevrie J J 1975 Accidents neurologiques consecutifs a la vaccination contre la coqueluche. Archives Francaise Pediatrie 32: 309–318.
Alderslade R, Bellman M H, Rawson N S B, et al 1981 The national childhood encephalopathy study. In: Department of Health and Social Security. Whooping Cough: reports from the Committee on Safety of Medicines and the Joint Committee on Vaccination and Immunisation. London: HMSO: 79–169
Butler N R, Golding J, Haslum M, Stewart-Brown S 1982, Recent findings from the 1970 child health and education study: preliminary communication. Journal of the Royal Society of Medicine 75: 781–785
Clarke S J 1980 Whooping cough vaccination: some reasons for non completion. Journal of Advanced Nursing 5: 313–319
Cody C L, Baraff L J, Cherry J D, Marcy S M, Manclark C R 1981 Nature and rates of adverse reactions associated with DTP and DT immunizations in infants and children. Pediatrics 68: 650–660
Christie A B 1980 Whooping couch (Pertussis). In: Infectious Diseases, 3rd edn, pp 659–682 Churchill Livingstone, Edinburgh
Ditchburn R K 1979 Whooping cough after stopping pertussis immunisation. British Medical Journal i: 1601–1603
Dudgeon J A, Marshall W 1984 Principles and practices of immunization. Chapman and Hall, London
Ehrengut W 1980 Lässt sich die reserve gegenüber der pertussis-schutzimpgung begründen? Pediatric Praxis 23: 3–13
Griffith A H 1978 Reactions after pertussis vaccine: a manufacturer's experiences and difficulties since 1964. British Medical Journal 33: 107–143

Griffith A H 1981 Medicine and the Media: Vaccination against whooping cough. Journal of Biological Standardisation 9: 475–482

Hirtz D G, Nelson K B, Ellenberg J H 1983 Seizures following childhood immunizations. Journal of Pediatrics 102: 14–18

Kanai K 1980 Japan's experience in pertussis epidemiology and vaccination in the past thirty years. Japanese Journal of Medicine Science and Biology 33: 107–143

Kulenkampff M. Schwartzman J B, Wilson J 1974 Neurological complications of pertussis inoculation. Archives of Diseases in Childhood 49: 46–49

Mertsola J, Viljanen M K, Ruuskanen O 1982 Current status of pertussis and pertussis vaccination in Finland. Annals of Clinical Research 14: 253–259

Miller D L, Ross E M 1981 Whooping cough and brain illness in children. Nursing Times 77: 22 937–939

Miller C L, Pollock T M, Clewer A D E 1974 Whooping cough vaccination: an assessment. Lancet ii: 510–513

Miller D L, Ross E M, Alderslade R, Bellman M H, Rawson N S B 1981 Pertussis immunisation and serious acute neurological illness in children. British Medical Journal ii: 1595–1599

Miller D L, Alderslade R, Ross E M 1982 Whooping cough vaccination: the risks and benefits debate. Epidemiologic Reviews 4: 1–24

Pollock T M, Miller E, Lobb J, Smith G 1982 Efficacy of pertussis vaccination in England. British Medical Journal ii: 357–359

Pollock T M, Morris J 1983 A 7 year survey of disorders attributed to vaccination in North West Thames Region. Lancet i: 753–757

Robinson R 1981 The whooping cough immunization controversy. Archives of Diseases in Childhood 56: 577–579

Ross E M 1982 Pertussis immunization—current knowledge and recommendations. The Health Visitor 12: 648–653

Ross E M, Edouard L J 1983 Whooping cough immunisation: in France and Britain. Journal of the Royal Society of Medicine 76: 374–378

Ström J 1960 Is universal vaccination against pertussis always justified? British Medical Journal ii: 1184–1186

Trollfors B, Rabo E 1981 Whooping cough in adults. British Medical Journal ii: 696–697

Parents' recognition of the ill child

INTRODUCTION

Paediatricians and those professionally involved in the care of ill children have been slow to recognise the obvious—parents, particularly mothers, are the vital link in the care of ill children. If parents fail to recognise or respond appropriately to warning signs of significant illness medical treatment cannot be started. In other words, parental skills are as important to effective treatment of sick infants as medical skills.

Recent interest in the Child Health Services has centred on the quality and quantity of primary and secondary services offered by health professionals. Parents have mainly been considered in terms of the use they make of available services. Their role as *the* primary carers has been minimised and, in some cases, ignored. Even the otherwise far-sighted report 'Fit For The Future' (Committee on Child Health Services, 1976), though paying lip service to the role of parents, concentrates its main recommendations on the organisation of professional services.

This review, starting unashamedly from parents as the main primary carers, looks at the evidence for how much childhood illness is dealt with at home, what skills parents use in recognising and managing their children's illnesses, what advice sources parents use and when do they seek medical advice. Evidence for the breakdown of parental skills and the failure to recognise illness is examined and some ideas advanced for ways of strengthening primary care given by parents.

HOW MUCH CHILDHOOD ILLNESS IS DEALT WITH AT HOME?

It is a commonly held view particularly amongst doctors in primary care that a considerable proportion of their time is spent dealing with trivial symptoms which could have been dealt with at home (Cartwright, 1967: Mechanic, 1974). Parents of small children are regarded as prime 'offenders' consulting unnecessarily for childhood ailments and specific health education initiatives have been undertaken to reduce the frequency of such consultations (Anderson et al, 1980). Though minor symptoms are undoubtedly presented to doctors, there is a large body of evidence suggesting that most symptoms experienced by adults and children are dealt with outside the medical services. What Last (1963) calls the 'Clinical Iceberg' was quantified by Horder & Horder (1954) from a study in their general practice: 75% of patients experiencing symptoms sought no medical advice. More recent studies have shown that the same pattern of self-care occurs for a wide range of problems (Hannay, 1978).

A high percentage of childhood symptoms are also coped with at home. Alpert et al (1967) asked 78 mothers of families with a low income in Boston, USA to keep a diary of their children's symptoms over a 4-week period. For only 10% of symptoms in the 4 weeks did the mothers request medical assistance or advice. Three-quarters of the symptoms needed some action but mothers took action themselves five times as often as they asked for medical assistance. Mothers were most likely to see the doctor when the symptoms were gastro-intestinal.

It could be argued that Alpert et al's (1967) findings merely reflect the financial disincentives for poor families using the health care system in the USA. However, two British studies have produced similar results.

My own study in Nottinghamshire (Spencer, 1980a) in which mothers recorded health problems affecting their infants during a 3-day period showed that medical help (doctor or health visitor) was sought for only 17% of reported symptoms. Mothers reported that they took their children to the doctor not because they thought their symptoms were serious but because the symptoms caused anxiety and might become serious.

In a study of 44 mothers in inner city Newcastle (Pattison et al, 1982) who kept health diaries about their infants for 8 weeks, a doctor or health visitor was consulted on only 6% of days when symptoms were present. Mothers reported that they were making decisions about their baby's health on 75% of the total diary days.

There seems little doubt that the greater part of childhood symtomatology is coped with by parents, particularly mothers, without medical help. Given this situation, what skills do parents use to identify and manage their children's illnesses?

HOW DO PARENTS RECOGNISE AND MANAGE THEIR CHILDREN'S ILLNESSES?

Why, how and when people react to symptoms of illness has been extensively researched under the general heading of 'illness behaviour'. It is accepted that ethnic origin, social class, income and many other factors influence illness behaviour. It is not my intention in this review to examine in any detail these 'external' factors affecting illness behaviour but to concentrate instead on the process of illness recognition and management whilst acknowledging that it is modified by numerous factors. A great deal has been written about the response of adults to their symptoms but there is only a limited literature on the behaviour of parents faced with symptoms in their child. Alpert et al (1967) for instance have the following to say about what they call 'maternal nursing care':

> 'The mother is supposed to assume a complex set of duties that include watching regularly the health of the children, noting any symptoms and complaints, deciding the appropriate action to be taken, administering home-management type of treatments or arranging for medical help.'

These duties comprise observation, recognition, assessment and frequent decisions about appropriate action in response to symptoms. This is not, in any sense, a mechanical passage through the stages of recognition, assessment and action, but is rather, a complex and subtle process requiring frequent reappraisal and reassessment and strongly influenced by other circumstances such as family stress (Roghmann & Haggerty, 1973).

Recognition and assessment

Research into how illness is recognised is fraught with difficulty. Retrospective studies can provide useful insights but rely almost entirely on the respondent's memory of events and their sequence. Diaries and health calenders overcome some of these problems but it remains difficult to be certain firstly that all symptoms recognised are actually recorded and secondly to check that all symptoms have, in fact, been recognised. Thus, the evidence available is limited and incomplete. Notwithstanding these difficulties various studies have thrown useful light on illness recognition. From his detailed examination of a small group of families, Locker (1981), suggests what he calls 'cues' which prompt the recognition of illness. He is concerned with illness recognition by adults in themselves, adults in other adults and adults in children. I have modified the three types of cue identified by Locker (1981) to relate them to parental recognition of illness without altering the sense of Locker's classification. Symptomatological cues are those in which changes in the child's physical or psychological state are observed by the parent; behavioural cues are those in which changes in behaviour or conduct of the child are noted by the parent; communicative cues, which are not applicable to infants, are those in which claims are made by the child to the mother that all is not well.

The changes, forming the substance of the cues, can occur suddenly, as in a previously normal child who starts to convulse, or insidiously, the changes only being fully appreciated some time after their onset. The sudden precipitous event such as a convulsion prompts immediate action from parents (Spencer, 1980a) though their interpretation of the event may be inappropriate (Rutter & Metcalfe, 1978). Insidious change is less easily identified and less easily researched.

The gradual realisation of change in children is beautifully described by Davis (1963) in his study of the parents of 14 children who contracted poliomyelitis. In all cases, the initial symptoms were regarded as commonplace; 'he's got a cold', 'he's got a stomach upset' or 'he's overtired'. Persistence of symptoms beyond the normal period, increasing severity of symptoms and behavioural changes, such as a 6-year-old's inability to fight his 3-year-old brother, obliged parents to rethink their initial assessment and contact the doctor. Davis calls this initial response to symptoms 'normalisation' and there were many examples of the same response amongst the parents I studied in Nottinghamshire. In this extract from one of the diaries kept by mothers to record their infants' symptoms, the baby's mother brings the rash she has observed within a commonplace or know framework.

Diary Extract S14 Day 1

'Small pink spots on face (probably teething) but especially around the eyes. Talked it over with my mother (who lives with me) decided that S. was not his usual self. Decided it was due to either teeth or a slight chill and that the situation needed watching but at this stage no further action needed especially as he had a restful night.'

The spots and the fact that S. was 'not his usual self' are cautiously regarded as due to 'normal' things such as teething or a slight chill but S's. mother is clearly prepared to change her mind in the light of subsequent events.

Field (1976) sums up normalisation as follows: 'This is not simply a case of people failing to recognise that they are 'ill' but is also due to the fact that a great amount of illness is regarded as 'minor' and 'normal'. That is, people may feel that they are 'ill' and accept the need to take some sort of action, e.g. an early night or self-medication, but not define themselves as sufficiently ill to require specialist help.' He is, of course, discussing the response of adults to their symptoms but it would seem to be equally applicable to parents and their children. Specific parental skills seem to be used in the interpretation of cues and when necessary to progress beyond normalisation. In my study I was able to identify a number of skills (see Fig. 8.1) which individually or in combination, as suggested by the theoretical model, serve as pathways to the fundmental decision—is the child ill or not? These skills are best illustrated using my own and others' interview and diary data.

Normal/abnormal judgement

The ability to judge what is normal or abnormal for their own child is a skill which parents alone possess. Its value is illustrated in this diary extract from my study.

Diary Extract S3 Day 1

'R. is an extremely happy and contented baby so although he did not cry a lot, he did cry noticeably more than usual during the afternoon.'

The behavioural cue is picked up by R's. mother and only she or her husband

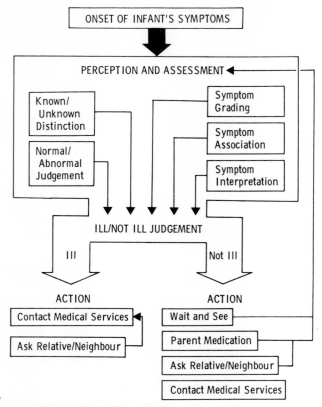

Fig. 8.1 The theoretical model of skills used by parents to determine whether their child is ill

could have been alerted by this because they knew it to be abnormal for their child. An extract from interview transcripts quoted by Locker (1980) shows the same skill.

Interview Extract G15 from Locker, p.91

Interviewer: 'When he was ill with his sickness . . . I mean you said he was sick a lot as a baby.'
Mrs G.:   'Yes but this was violent.'
Interviewer: 'How do you mean?'
Mrs G.:   'Well, you know, he just pumped it all up . . . it wasn't like a normal . . . a sickness where, you know, sort of like wind when the sickness comes up but this was pump, two or three . . . it was all down Roger (her husband), all over the carry cot, Daniel was covered in it as well.'

Mrs G. makes a clear distinction between the 'normal' sickness which she was familiar with in her child and the 'violent' sickness which she is aware is abnormal both for her own child and for others.

Known/unknown distinction

This is closely allied to normal/abnormal judgement but appears to be used to pick out symptoms or changes which are not just abnormal for the child but also outside the parents' experience. A father, interviewed in my study, describes why his boy was admitted to hospital and demonstrates the use of this skill.

Interview Extract S10 Q2

Father: 'He's a happy baby he is . . . he'll sit there and laugh once he's had his fill. He'll sit there and laugh and play contented and that's how he was all the while and then she changed his nappy one day and found this red, you know. We thought it were blood and says we'll take him to doctor's 'cos it worried us a little bit. The doctor says well we'd better take him in.'

The parents' feeling that this unusual symptom must be regarded as serious until proved otherwise, overrides their general assessment of their son as a 'happy and contented' baby and prompts them to consult the doctor.

Symptom grading

Parents in the Nottinghamshire study regarded some symptoms as more important than others: 85% thought that a doctor should be consulted about a baby with a runny nose and a 'chesty' cough whereas only 37% thought a runny nose with a dry cough worthy of medical attention; 75% thought they would contact the doctor if their baby vomited more than twice in 24 hours but only 35% said they would seek medical help if their child had more than two loose green motions in 24 hours. One of the mother quoted by Locker explains how she would grade a cough.

Interview Extract F12 from Locker, p.90.

Mrs F.:   'Well, say it was a cough, it would depend on the cough.'
Interviewer: 'How do you mean, depend on the cough?'
Mrs F.:   'Well, if it was just a normal sort of cough that you've experienced before, fair enough but if it wasn't . . . obviously if you were spitting blood or anything like that then obviously you would go.'

Symptom interpretation

This skill, which I have characterised, is very similar to normalisation discussed above. Many symptoms were attributed to teething as shown by the diary extract below in which the baby's mother is commenting about her nappy rash.

Diary Extract S20 Day 1

'S. has had this nappy rash for a week or two but she has also cut five teeth in the last six weeks which I take to be the cause.'

Symptom Association

The linking of one symptom with another was most frequently used in the Nottinghamshire study in a negative sense: the absence of an expected additional symptom or one perceived as more important served to reassure parents that a 'wait and see' policy was appropriate.

Diary Extract S45 Day 2

'E. was very sick at 9.30 and again at 10.05. Boiled water was given, she had not got a temperature and she slept well the rest of the night.'

E.'s mother recognises, assesses and acts upon her daughter's symptoms but is reassured by the absence of a temperature and by her observation that E. slept well.

Ill/not ill judgement

As postulated by the theoretical model (Fig. 8.1) all the above skills singly or in combination contribute to this judgement which I think is the most decisive. It is this skill which informs the action taken in response to symptoms and determines the urgency of that action. The two interview extracts which follow, the first from Locker's study and the second from my study, show the skilled interpretation of behavioural and symptomatological cues which enables the parents to decide that the threshold between the wellness and illness has been crossed.

Interview Extract G3 from Locker p.51.

Mrs G.: 'The last time I took Daniel to the doctor's he had a really bad, a really high temperature about 5.00 at night. He was sat on my knee, been sort of mouldy all day you know sleeping a lot of the time and he was burning . . . he was just sat on my knee and you could see the glow coming off him it was really bad so I rang the clinic.'

Interview Extract S25 Q2

Interviewer: Had you had a bad night with him before?
Mother: 'Oh yes, yes, yes . . . we'd been up all night hadn't we and we knew that he was bad because he's a baby . . . he's so contented you know from the first day of coming out of hospital he's slept right through you know.
Father: 'We've never lost a night's sleep with him at all.'
Mother: 'Never, never you know he's been so contented even in the daytime hasn't he . . . we knew that there was something wrong with him.'

In both the above extracts, the parents use skilled observations to arrive at their judgement that their child is significantly ill. Mrs G. grades Daniel's temperature as 'really bad, really high' and graphically describes the effect of the temperature on him. She also makes a normal/abnormal judgement when she says that he has 'been sort of mouldy all day you know sleeping a lot of the time.' The parents quoted in the second extract stress the profound change which had occurred in their child's sleeping pattern and the fact that a disturbed night was so unusual for him: again they used a normal/abnormal judgement to arrive at the decision that their child was ill.

WHAT ACTION DO PARENTS TAKE IN RESPONSE TO CHILDREN'S SYMPTOMS AND WHOSE ADVICE DO THEY SEEK?

As discussed earlier in this review, much childhood symptomatology is dealt with at home without medical help. It appears that home management is regarded as appropriate for those symptoms deemed minor, those not apparently affecting the child's well-being and those familiar enough not to cause anxiety. Home management covers a range of possible actions. Alpert et al (1967) found that parents took no action for 25% of the total number of symptoms reported in their children. There was strong anecdotal evidence from my data supporting these findings and indicating that parents frequently adopted a 'wait and see' policy without taking specific action.

Active home management, which Alpert et al (1967) suggest is used for the majority of symptoms handled at home, includes anything from increased emotional support (e.g. extra comforting) through to the use of unprescribed medication. Unprescribed medication given to their children by parents is a widespread practice (Spencer, 1980a; Spencer, 1982). Virtually all the 107 families I studied had unprescribed medication in the house specifically for the baby and a third of the parents reporting problems during the 3-day diary period gave their infants unprescribed drugs. Analgesics, antipyretics, respiratory decongestants and gastrointestinal sedatives formed the bulk of the drugs kept in the home. Other authors (Whyte & Greenan, 1976) have implied that unprescribed medication is used inappropriately by parents but my findings support those of Pedersen (1976) and others (Office of Health Economics, 1968) that parents use familiar drugs for familiar symptoms. Evidence from my study suggests that the use of unprescribed drugs is frequently sanctioned by a doctor or local chemist.

Parents sometimes turn to lay sources for help with their children's symptoms. Grandparents are the most frequent source of help (Holohan, 1978). Their advice was sought on 9% of the days on which symptoms were present in Pattison et al's study in Newcastle (Pattison et al, 1982). Help from other lay sources was sought on 4% of symptom days. It is interesting that lay advice sources were approached almost three times as often as medical sources.

Elliot-Binns (1973) found that 95% of new consulations with a general practice were preceded by lay advice but that much of this advice took the form of 'go and see your doctor'. Parents in my study sometimes sought the 'sanction' of a grandparent or experienced neighbour before contacting the doctor.

The chemist occupies a place between the lay and medical sources of help and tends to be seen as an 'unofficial' easily accessible professional. The chemist's advice is sought on symptoms and he is also asked to 'sanction' visits to the doctor in the same way as grandparents and neighbours.

If parents, using the skills outlined above, conclude that their child is ill then the medical services are contacted either directly or following advice from a lay source. Whether the health visitor, general practitioner or casualty are contacted initially depends mainly on availability and accessibility. My findings indicate that it is not the symptoms themselves, with the exception of fits and other alarming symptoms, but the assessment of the degree of illness that prompts urgent contact with the medical services.

Pattison et al (1982) used stepwise logistic discriminant analysis to select variables which gave the best prediction of whether or not a consultation would take place. They found that the total number of major symptoms (as defined by the authors) in a single illness episode had the greatest predictive value—the more major symptoms present the more likely the consultation. They also found, somewhat to their surprise, that mothers with previous experience with babies were significantly more likely to consult and the authors speculate that this may be related to an increased awareness of the rapidity with which a baby's condition can deteriorate.

Professional advice is sought for symptoms which are not necessarily regarded as serious and for children who are not judged ill at the time. It seems from my findings that consultaions are likely for symptoms causing anxiety or thought to be potentially serious. For example, the parents I studied felt that a 'chesty' cough was potentially serious as this interview extract shows.

Interview Extract S4 Q10 iii

Interviewer: 'What reason would you give for making that distinction between the chesty and the dry cough?'

Mother: 'Well the fact that it was a chesty cough rather than just a dry one . . . with a chesty one it tends to suggest it's more . . .

Father: 'more a guarantee of infection I would have thought.'

There is evidence that factors other than the nature of the symptoms, the anxiety provoked by them or parental judgement of the degree of their child's illness led to consultation: stress increases utilisation of services for children's ailments (Roghmann & Haggerty, 1973) partly as a result of apparent increased vulnerability to infection in the presence of stress (Mayer &

Haggerty, 1963). Mothers may also use relatively insignificant symptoms in their children as a 'screen' behind which to present their own problems to the doctor (Yudkin, 1961).

DO SOME PARENTS FAIL TO RESPOND APPROPRIATELY TO THEIR CHILDREN'S SYMPTOMS AND, IF SO, WHY?

Socio-medical studies of sudden unexpected infant death have consistently demonstrated a small number of infants who die because their parents appear to fail to appreciate the seriousness of their symptoms. Selwyn & Bain (1965) reporting on 184 deaths in Edinburgh designated 23 as preventable of which six were thought to be due to inappropriate parental response. More recent evidence from the D.H.S.S. Multicentre Study of sudden infant death (Stanton et al, 1978) confirms that major symptoms were in some cases either not perceived or inappropriately acted upon by parents. In a retrospective controlled study, McWeeney & Emery (1975) compared the ante-mortem histories of 25 infants dying unexpectedly at home from preventable causes with preadmission histories of 25 infants admitted to hospital with similar conditions who subsequently survived. They found that the parents whose infants died showed a marked reluctance to use the services and a lack of ability to recognise the importance of symptoms compared with the parents of surviving infants.

Little evidence is available as to why these parents fail to develop or use the skills necessary to respond appropriately to their infant's symptoms. However, two large confidential inquiries into infant deaths (Richards & McIntosh; 1972 D.H.S.S., 1970) conclude that poor social conditions, particularly housing, make parents vulnerable. They also found that many of this group of parents were poor users of the services and that there was evidence of parental incompetence and neglect (which terms they do not define) in a percentage of the avoidable deaths.

In the absence of more precise information, it seems reasonable to speculate about those parents most vulnerable to the breakdown of parental skills: young parents because of inexperience or immaturity, socially isolated and disadvantaged parents with little support from family and friends, depressed mothers whose view of the world is distorted, and mothers with a large number of small children. Indirect evidence from various studies (Brown, 1976; Carpenter et al, 1977) lends support to this speculation but more detailed study is required before more accurate characterisation can be made of this group of parents.

The vulnerability of some parents is undoubtedly increased by barriers put up by the services to their proper use. McWeeney & Emery (1975) make the following comment in their paper:

> 'the present organisation of general medical practice services in some areas appears to require too great a degree of drive and persistence on the part of parents to obtain attention.'

Assuming that parents can overcome environmental diffculties such as the absence of functioning telephones in some areas, the urgency of their request for help is often evaluated by an untrained receptionist (Holohan, 1978) and anecdotal evidence from my study illustrates the difficulty parents can experience 'getting past' the receptionist.

Having got to the doctor, parents may not get appropriate treatment for their child and all the infant death studies quoted above reported evidence of inadequate response by doctors as well as parents to infant symptoms. Outright rejection of a mother's assessment of her baby's condition is graphically illustrated in a quote from a young mother in a study of clinic non-users in Rotherham (Hagan, 1981). The mother assessed the baby as 'very ill' and called her doctor apparently only to be told that he would not come out to see the child.

> *Interview Extract from Hagan, p.122*
>
> Mother: 'He said 'I've got better things to do than trail up to (name of area)'. I rang every doctor I could think of, running out of 2ps. in the pouring rain and there weren' one that would come out 'cos I weren't registered under 'em. In the end I got an ambulance and she was in hospital for three weeks with gastric enteritis'.

There is, then, evidence both for a breakdown in parental skills related to environmental factors and factors inherent to the parents themselves and barriers to the use of skills erected by the services. More detailed and extensive research is required to elucidate the relative importance of each factor.

HOW CAN PRIMARY CARE BY PARENTS BE STRENGTHENED?

Parental skills cannot be enhanced unless they are recognised. Increased awareness amongst health professionals of the importance of these skills resulting in greater attention to parents' assessments may lead to prompter action upon life-threatening childhood symptoms. Greater concentration of teaching and research on the parents' role in managing childhood illness would contribute to heightening this awareness.

An essential part of strengthening parental care is acceptance of the parent as a skilled participant in the management and treatment of the child's illness. Many parents do not recognise their own skills and lack confidence in their judgement. If professionals destroy the confidence of parents by ignoring or dismissing their assessments or treating their complaints as time wasting trivia there is the danger of further erosion of already vulnerable skills with potentially disastrous consequences. Parents' judgements do not have to be accepted or agreed with but they should be respected if effective partnership between parent and professional is to develop.

The primary health care services are accepted by most parents as the appropriate source of help with ill children but barriers exist to easy parental access. Urgent attention should be given to reducing these barriers.

Health education directed towards apparently vulnerable parents will strengthen parental care only if it is relevant to the real decisions and judgements parents have to make. 'When to call the doctor' lists take no account of parents' judgements and could be counter-productive if parents, whilst feeling their child to be ill, were discouraged from calling the doctor because their child's symptoms did not appear on the list. Written material is probably of limited value particularly for the most vulnerable parents. Other approaches are likely to be more effective such as mothers groups with more experienced mothers imparting their experience and developing the skills of less experienced mothers (D.H.S.S./Child Poverty Action Group, 1978; Spencer, 1980b).

Lasting improvements in child health demand the strengthening of primary care by both parents and services based on an effective, mutually respecting partnership of parents and professionals. Awareness and respect for parental skills would be a step in the right direction.

REFERENCES

Alpert J J, Kosa J, Haggerty R J, 1967 Medical help and maternal nursing care in the life of low income families. Paediatrics 39: 749–755

Anderson J E, Morrell D C, Avery A J, Watkins C J, 1980 Evaluation of Patient Education Manual. British Medical Journal 281: 924–926

Brown G W, 1976 The social causes of disease. In: Tuckett D. (ed.) An Introduction to Medical Sociology. Tavistock, London

Carpenter R G, Gardner A, McWeeney P M, Emery J L, 1977 Multistage Scoring System for identifying infants at risk of unexpected death. Archives of Disease in Childhood 52: 606–612

Cartwright A, 1967 Patients and their Doctors. Routledge and Keegan Paul, London

Committee on Child Health Services, 1976 Fit for the Future. HMSO, London

Davis F, 1963 Passage through Crisis. Bobbs-Merrill, Indianapolis

DHSS, 1970 Confidential Enquiry into post-neonatal deaths 1964–66. Reports on Public Health and Medical Subjects, No. 125, HMSO, London

DHSS/Child Poverty Action Group, 1978 Reaching the consumer in antenatal and child health services. Report of Conference

Elliott-Binns CP, 1973 An analysis of lay medicine. Journal of the Royal College of General Practitioners 23: 225

Field D, 1976 The social definition of illness. In: Tuckett D. (Ed.) An Introduction to medical sociology. Tavistock, London

Hagan M T, 1981 Positive Pathways—Progress report for the period February, 1980–January, 1981. Department of Health Studies, Sheffield City Polytechnic

Hannay D R, 1978 Symptom prevalence in the community. Journal of the Royal College of General Practitioners 28: 492–99

Holohan A, 1978 The Court Report and acute illness in children in a Northern Town. Health and Social Services Journal, November 10th: 23–28

Horder J, Horder E, 1954 Illness in general practice. Practitioner 173: 177–83

Last J M, 1963 The Iceberg—Completing the clinical picture in general practice. Lancet ii: 28

Locker D, 1981 Symptoms and Illness. Tavistock, London and New York

Mayer R J, Haggerty R J, 1963 Streptococal infections in families. Paediatrics 29: 539–549

McWeeney P M, Emery J L 1975 Unexpected post-neonatal deaths (cot deaths) due to recognizable disease. Archives of Disease in Childhood 50: 191

Mechanic D, 1974 Politics, Medicine and Social Science. Wiley Interscience, New York

Pattison C J, Drinkwater C K, Downham M A P S, 1982. Mothers' appreciation of their children's symptoms. Journal of the Royal College of General Practitioners 32: 149–62

Pedersen P A, 1976 Self treatment by patients prior to consultation with the General Practitioner. Vgeksv. Laeg. 138: 1955–1961

Richards I D G, McIntosh H T, 1972 Confidential Enquiry into 226 consecutive infant deaths. Archives of Disease in Childhood 47: 697

Roghmann K J, Haggerty R J, 1973 Daily Stress, illness and use of health services in young families. Paediatric Research 7: 520–526

Rutter N, Metcalfe D H, 1978 Febrile Convulsions—what do parents do? British Medical Journal, ii: 1345–46

Selwyn S, Bain A D, 1965 Deaths in childhood due to infection. British Journal of Preventive and Social Medicine 19: 123–127

Spencer N J, 1980a The Identification and Management of illness by parents of young children. Unpublished thesis for the degree of Master of Philosophy, Nottingham University

Spencer N J, 1980b Group work with mothers in General Practice: some preliminary observations. Occasional Paper No. 21, Leverhulme Health Education Project, University of Nottingham

Spencer N J, 1983 A Community Survey of Drugs given to infants. Paper presented to British Paediatric Association April 1983.

Stanton A N, Downham M A P S, Oakley J R, Emery J L, Knowelden J, 1978 Terminal symptoms in Children dying suddenly and unexpectedly at home. British Medical Journal, ii: 1249

Whyte J, Greenan E, 1976 Pattern and quality of recording pre-admission drug treatment in paediatric patients. British Medical Journal i: 61–63

Yudkin S, 1961 Six children with coughs: the second diagnosis. Lancet i or ii: 539–549

The myth of bonding

INTRODUCTION

During the last few years a new word has become established in the vocabularies of professionals concerned with neonatal services. The same word has entered the world of popular writing for parents and has been taken up by parents themselves. Many who use this word appear to believe that it has a respectable origin within developmental psychology and that it relates to a theory and a body of experimental evidence that is well established. The word is, of course, 'bonding'. In this chapter I want to suggest that its provenance or, rather, that of the concept it represents, is much more uncertain than some current usage suggests. I shall point out that there may be dangers for parents and children in the well-intentioned but uncritical use of the concept.

Though Donald Winnicott (1958) referred to the relationships between mother* and infant as a 'bond', the term only came into widespread use with the work of the American paediatricians Marshall Klaus and John Kennell (1976). They were concerned about the possible consequences for mothers and babies of the separation that was (and often still is) brought about by the routines of lying-in wards in some maternity hospitals and by the admission of small or sick infants to special care units. They and their collaborators have described a series of studies from which they have concluded that early separation carries the potential risk of damage to the mother-infant relationship. In a mild form this damage might consist of an unusually wide psychological distance between mother and baby while the extreme might include such things as physical abuse, abandonment and 'failure to thrive' in the baby. Klaus and Kennell explained all these effects as the result of a failure of the mother to 'bond' to the baby. They suggested that during the period immediately after the delivery a mother is in a special state (a sensitive

---

* Most of the early work and discussions used the term 'mother' and not 'father' or 'parent'. It is not always clear whether authors are using the term 'mother' interchangeably with 'parent','caretaker' or 'father' or whether they are referring only to the female biological parent. I have tried to be consistent in using the term adopted by other authors when referring to their work and otherwise using 'parent' when I am referring to either or both parents and 'mother' or 'father' when I specifically mean the female or male parent.

period) during which she is more than usually ready to form a bond with her child. If mother and baby are kept separate during this time, which is thought to last from some hours to a day, they argued that bonding would be impaired or even completely prevented. On the other hand they suggested that bonding would be enhanced by particularly close physical contact especially if this is skin to skin ('l'amour c'est le contact de deux epidermes'). Their hypothesis was partly based on an analogy with certain herd-living mammals (e.g. goats) in which post-birth separation can lead to the rejection of an offspring by the mother.

Klaus & Kennell's ideas have received wide publicity and have had profound effects on hospital routines on both sides of the Atlantic. The concept of bonding has provided a readily understandable and acceptable rationale for reducing separation between mothers (and less often fathers) and their babies. In Britain, the biggest changes have occurred in special care baby units. Ten years ago there were few units which offered more than brief visiting times. Today, not only has open visiting become the norm, but visiting often receives positive encouragement, and staff have made great efforts to make parents feel welcome (Brimblecombe et al, 1978; Davis et al, 1983). In some units, as confidence in the more open policies has grown, the circle of relatives and friends who are permitted to visit has been increased and it is not uncommon to see a toddler being lifted up to see a new sibling in an incubator.

Delivery rooms and lying-in wards have changed too. In many hospitals it is now standard practice to hand the baby to the mother at delivery and babies are no longer carried off only to reappear some time later when the mother has been transferred to a ward. On the lying-in wards mothers have much more chance to arrange their day with their baby in the way that they want.

ASSESSING THE EVIDENCE

On the research side Klaus & Kennell's work has been a great stimulus in what was previously a rather neglected field. We now have a considerable number of studies carried out in many different countries and situations which attempt to assess the effects of early separation and there has been a growing theoretical interest in the topic. So how has the original idea of bonding and the sensitive period stood up to this repeated assessment? In making such an evaluation it may be helpful to divide the discussion into two parts:

1. How far has the empirical research supported the idea that early separation disrupts parent-infant relationships?

2. Is there evidence that there is a specific process of bonding which is limited to a sensitive period? Are there other explanations of the data?

In this brief chapter there is not space to review all the studies in detail, so I will provide a bare summary and the reader will need to consult one of the fuller reviews for a more adequate assessment (Richards, 1978, 1979; Campbell & Taylor, 1980; Minde, 1980; Ross, 1980).

Research support for the idea that separation disrupts relationships

Though the earlier studies often suffered from serious methodological weaknesses, their results were at least consistent with the idea that early separation increased the probability of a disturbed parent-infant relationship for some months after birth. In terms of the measures used in the majority of the studies the changes were not profound but they appeared to follow a similar pattern. Today with all the new evidence even such a tentative conclusion is hard to support. These newer studies have embodied better procedures and controls and as this has been done clear evidence of separation effects has become much more elusive.

Typical of the more recent studies is that of Svejda et al, (1980) which compared the behaviour of two groups of normal full-term babies at 36 hours after delivery. Mothers and babies were randomly allocated to an extra contact and normal procedure group. The extra contact group had their babies with them for an hour at delivery (rather than a 'brief contact') and for 90 rather than 30 minutes at each feeding. No consistent differences in behaviour were found in a 25-minute video film including a feed made at 36 hours. The observers who scored the video films did not know which group each mother came from. This desirable control was not included in most early studies. Also, and again unlike the earlier investigations, these researchers made sure that each mother was surrounded by others who were being treated in the same way so that mothers did not feel they were being singled out for special treatment. This answered a criticism of other research which suggested that because extra contact mothers knew they were getting unusual treatment their feeling of 'specialness' rather than the extra contact might make the different.

Studies of separation involving pre-term or sick babies have also produced very mixed and in some cases entirely negative results (e.g. McGurk, 1979). But these studies, because they deal with sick or pre-term babies, face much greater methodological problems and no-one as yet has succeeded in randomising the degree of separation for such groups.

One recent reviewer summarises the situation thus:

> 'There are no data showing that postpartum separation affects interactions between mothers and at-risk infants. Research suggests short-term effects of early and extended contact on maternal behaviour with full-term, healthy babies* . . . and long-lasting effects of early and extended mother-infant contact have not yet been demonstrated.' (Ross, 1980, p. 56)

However, we should be careful not to overstate the negative case. We are

* This conclusion might now be modified in view of the study by Svejda et al, 1980, which appeared after this review by Ross.

dealing with an area of research where our methods are comparatively crude and are only likely to pick up the most gross and obvious differences between the groups. Furthermore, the experimental designs that have been employed cannot cope with the possibility that different mother-baby pairs react to separation in a variety of ways. For instance, there are indications (e.g. Minde, 1980) that some parents react to the birth of a preterm or sick baby by becoming and remaining very anxious. Overfeeding, great concern about trivial events, very high levels of stimulation of the baby and frequent trips to see doctors when the baby is apparently healthy, may all be part of the pattern. Other parents in the same situation may become very withdrawn and distant from their babies at least until they are certain that development will proceed more or less normally. It is not a safe assumption that separation would have the same effects in these two situations. Similarly, with healthy full-term babies there are many individual factors that could lead to widely varying outcomes. For instance, the extent to which parents believe that separation is important (see below) could have a major effect but this and other individual differences await investigation.

Evidence for 'bonding' which is limited to a sensitive period

Insofar as the evidence for an effect of early separation is so confused, our evidence for a process as originally outlined by Klaus & Kennell (1976) must also remain confused. However, there are some theoretical reasons for thinking that their hypothesis is unlikely or, at least, over-simplified.

Their hypothesis is, in essence, a specific event (early separation) specific outcome (damaged parent-child interaction) relationship. Such single factor hypotheses run counter to the widely-held belief that development is well protected from derangement by outside events (see Waddington, 1975). In the usual terminology, the system is well 'buffered' so that a permanent shifting of the course of development is uncommon unless the system is completely overwhelmed. A simple example here is the effect of lack of oxygen for the brain at birth. Given the hazards of the birth process some reduction in the supply of oxygen to the brain of the baby is not uncommon but the brain of the newborn can stand a greater degree of anoxia than that of an adult before obvious damage occurs. In terms of natural selection, it is easy to see that such buffering would likely be of advantage, whereas selection would operate against any single factor having long-term effects especially if that factor is one that is at all likely to occur frequently. Given the likely hazards of a birth for a mother in our evolutionary past, early separation may well have been rather common.

The bonding hypothesis and, especially some of its variants portrayed by popularisers, ignores the general human concern for the meaning and interpretation of events. Separation may well influence a parent in a number of ways depending on the circumstance and interpretation of the separation. Consider two hypothetical mothers: the first has just given birth to a healthy baby. Her labour was relatively easy, the mother had prepared herself well and as she had hoped she was able to avoid all drugs except some gas and oxygen. Immediately the cord was cut, her baby was removed for bathing, weighing etc. because this was the policy of the hospital. Despite the mother's protest, she was not able to see her baby for 40 minutes until they were reunited in the post-natal ward. The reason why this mother had been keen to avoid drugs in labour was because she felt these might blunt her sensations and interfere with the process of bonding with her baby.

Our second mother had a rather different attitude to medical care and she was only too happy to let the doctors and midwives take over and manage her delivery. She was induced and accelerated but despite the oxytocin she had a rather long labour. She was given several doses of Pethidine during labour and had a low forceps delivery. After delivery her baby was removed to a special care baby unit for observation as was the custom in the hospital after a forceps delivery especially when these occurred at night as this one did. The mother was very sleepy and rather confused after the delivery and she was content to sleep having been told that she would see her baby at breakfast time. This mother did not hold her baby for 6 hours after delivery. Would we expect 'separation' to influence these two mothers in similar ways?

It has become clear that we do have to consider the experience of separation as it is perceived by each mother or father. We need to know what their expectations and beliefs are. In particular, we already have some suggestions that the degree to which a parent perceives separation as a threat to, or comment on, their parental abilities may be related to the outcome (see Richards, 1978; Ross, 1980).

We also have to consider how far hospitals may provide a model for some parents of how they should conduct their relations with their babies. In the absence of other information or direct experience parents may believe that hospital routines represent an ideal of good parent-child relations. Thus, if a hospital separates mother and baby for long periods, a mother may believe this is a pattern she should copy when the returns home. Or alternatively, routines can suggest higher than usual levels of contact are desirable. In a recent Swedish study (Rodholm, 1981), fathers of Caesarean delivered babies were given their babies to hold immediately after delivery. When compared with other fathers who were not given their babies at this point those who had had the extra contact were found to show a higher level of involvement with their children several months after delivery.

Finally, another theoretical difficulty of the bonding hypothesis is that there has never been independent evidence for a sensitive period after delivery. No explanation has ever been advanced of the processes that might create such a period or bring it to an end. In fact the concept is one that has been borrowed from the work of animal ethologists who have studied birds like ducks and chickens or mammals such as goats in which the young follow the mother immediately after hatching or birth. It is inherently unlikely that a similar process would be found in species whose parent-child relations are organised in quite another way. In herd-living mammals the young are often very mobile within minutes of birth and there are many reasons why selection pressures will favour processes that foster the individual recognition of offspring by mothers and keep mother and offspring in contact. In our own species infants are immobile for many months and are born into small family groups rather than large moving herds so that there are not the same difficulties in maintaining contact so we might expect parental relations to develop with other patterns.

ARE MYTHS HARMFUL?

Given that most parents appear to want more flexible hospital routines and resent being separated from their newborn babies and there are no substantial arguments that early contact carried risks,* does it matter that changes in policies and routines have been brought about by a hypothesis that appears to be at last over-simplified and at worst plainly wrong? Perhaps the means, in this case, should be justified by the ends? I think not, as there are a number of reasons why the myth of bonding, if it is a myth, could be a dangerous one.

The most obvious danger is that we may create a self-fulfilling prophecy and there are indications that this is already happening. Not only has 'bonding' entered into the policy recommendations of the American Medical Association and the Department of Health and Social Security in Britain, but it is widely discussed in books and on TV programmes intended for parents and at ante-natal classes. It would seem that considerable numbers of parents now believe that early separation may be damaging for them and their children. When such parents are separated their knowledge of the bonding hypothesis is likely to increase their own anxiety and anguish which, in turn, may have consequences for their relationship with their child. Of course, we should strive to reduce early separation to the barest minimum possible. However, so long as birth is primarily a hospital event, and there is centralisation of obstetric services and neonatal paediatric care, some degree of separation is unavoidable.

Because changes in policy have followed the discussions of bonding rather than the requests of parents not to be separated from their babies, there is a danger that we are confirming a system that appears to resist attempts at modification except when there is evidence (or supposed evidence) of long-term damage. The fact that parents and a few professionals have argued that early separation is inhumane, or that it is unnecessary, or simply that they

---

* Fears have been expressed about increased dangers of infection with open visiting in special care baby units. Interestingly, infection rates seem to decrease with increased parental visiting. It is thought that the presence of 'outsiders' may serve to remind staff of the need to maintain the procedures designed to reduce the risks of cross-infection. There is also evidence that contact with newborn preterm infants may increase anxiety. These issues are further discussed in Richards (1978).

do not like it has not been sufficient to change policies. I think there are very good reasons why the system should be responsive to pressures like this.

The example of bonding is not the first one where hospital policies have resisted pressures to change until arguments are used which concern long-term damaging effects. The campaign spear-headed by the National Association for the Welfare of Children in Hospital to give parents free access to their children in paediatric wards began to gain ground when evidence of the long-term consequences of parental deprivation were brought into the argument. Though it was obvious to everyone who saw it that restricted visiting upset both parents and children, at least in the short term, this did not appear to constitute sufficient reason for altering policies. Reliance on the evidence of long-term effects encourages us to avoid taking notice of what users of the health services feel about them. If we are tempted to do this we will fail to make the experience of hospital care satisfying to mothers and their families in the way that Court (1977), for example, has argued we should. In the case of the small and sick babies in special care baby units, the emphasis on bonding may serve to divert attention from other problems. For instance, it is sometimes implied that all the problems of these parents are solved provided that the doors of the unit are constantly open and separation is avoided. Such a view ignores the evidence that a preterm delivery may constitute a severe emotional crisis for parents (e.g. Kaplan & Mason, 1960) or that the 'failure' to visit a baby in special care may be an indication of difficulties in resolving these problems (Minde, 1980). In this kind of situation, early separation may be the effect of a disturbed parent-child relationship. Other evidence suggests that it is not enough to get parents into a special care baby unit as spectators but that they must be given a real share in the care of their own baby (Richards, 1978). This implies changes in the roles of staff: nurses become supporters of parents rather than caretakers of babies and doctors become as much counsellors as neonatal physiologists. Such shifts can be very difficult to achieve but very rewarding for all concerned when they are accomplished successfully. The preoccupation with bonding has led to another important area of research being ignored or at last underplayed. This is the work which demonstrates that preterm babies may have patterns of behaviour that make them unpredictable and unsatisfying partners for parents (e.g. Goldberg, 1978). If this is coupled with emotional problems related to a preterm birth, the social and economic deprivation that is often correlated with prematurity and the anxieties that a sick or damaged infant can engender, then the needs for support may be great. But there has been a tendency not to give these problems the attention they deserve and allow them to become submerged under a concern about early separation.

CONCLUSION

Nothing I have said should be taken as an argument for permitting any avoidable separation of parent and infant. Nor do I feel that it is inappropriate to concentrate a lot of attention on the perinatal period. However, it should be of more than academic concern that the hypotheses that we use to guide action accord with our evidence and theories. Bonding, especially in its popularised forms has failed to meet the necessary tests. We need to develop new hypotheses in this area which attempt to explain the very complex phenomena which recent work has uncovered. Like any parents, those who created the original hypotheses that drew attention to this field should now feel proud as their offspring develops and metamorphoses into new forms that they may barely recognise.

REFERENCES

Brimblecombe F S W, Richards M P M, Roberton N R C 1978 Separation and Special Care Baby Units. Clinics in Developmental Medicine No 68, SIMP/Heinemann Medical Books, London

Campbell S B G, Taylor P M 1980 Bonding and attachment: theoretical issues. In: Taylor P M (ed) Parent-Infant Relationships, Grune & Stratton, New York

Court D 1977 Report of the Committee on Child Health Services, HMSO, London

Davis J A, Richards M P M, Roberton N R C 1983 Parents, Children and Special Care Units. Croom Helm, London

Goldberg S 1978 Prematurity: effects on parent-infant interaction. Paediatric Psychology 3: 137–144

Kaplan D M, Mason E A 1960 Maternal reaction to premature birth viewed as an acute emotional disorder. American Journal of Orthopsychiatry 30: 539–547

Klaus M H, Kennell J H 1976 Maternal-Infant Bonding, C V Mosby, St Louis

McGurk H 1979 Maternal Attachment Behaviour and Infant Development: the Significance of Temporary Separation at Birth. Report prepared for the Department of Health and Social Security, London, unpublished

Minde K K 1980 Bonding of mothers to premature infants: theory and practice. In: Taylor P M (ed) Parent-Infant Relationships. Grune & Stratton, London

Richards M P M 1978 Possible effects of early separation on later development in children. In: Brimblecombe F S W, Richards M P M, Roberton N R C (eds) Early Separation and Special Care Nurseries. Clinics in Developmental Medicine, SIMP/Heinemann Medical Books, London

Richards M P M 1979 Effects on development of medical interventions and the separation of newborns from their parents. In: Shaffer D, Dunn J (eds) The First Year of Life. John Wiley, Chichester

Rodholm M 1981 Effects of father-infant postpartum contact on their interaction 3 months after birth. Early Human Development 5: 1–112

Ross G S 1980 Parental responses to infants in intensive care: the separation issue re-evaluation. Clinics in Perinatology 7: 47–61

Svejda M J, Campos J J, Emde R N 1980 Mother-infant 'bonding': failure to generalize. Child Development 51: 775–779

Waddington C H 1975 The Evolution of an Evolutionist. Edinburgh University Press, Edinburgh

Winnicott D W 1958 Collected Papers. Tavistock, London

Children and divorce

INTRODUCTION

Marital separation or divorce are a commonplace of childhood in Britain today, yet one to which our medical and social services have still to adapt. We have good reasons for thinking that the ending of marital relationships by parents is associated with both mortality and morbidity in children but this fact has almost no impact on our child health policies and seems to be ignored in most encounters between health professionals and children and parents. Antenatal care provides a good example: mothers who describe themselves as divorced or separated are at a high risk of having a child who dies perinatally (Chamberlain et al, 1975). Indeed the correlation between perinatal mortality and marital status is much more impressive than the much more widely discussed relationship with social class. But where is this knowledge used to take preventive action through appropriate antenatal care? In general practice there is the same tendency to miss what could be a very effective form of preventive medicine. Most people visit their general practitioner at the time of a marital separation (Chester, 1971) usually complaining of such things as anxiety, depression and an inability to sleep. Our studies show that these encounters are generally rather brief and usually result in a prescription for Valium or other psychotropic drugs (Richards & Dyson, 1981). Despite our knowledge that children are usually very upset by their parents actions and that many of the parents' anxieties centre on their children, it was rare for a family practitioner to ask parents about their children at these visits or, indeed, to respond to them as parents rather than distressed adults.

The increased rates of divorce have also added to the varieties of parent-child relations. Here the inadequacy of our response is seen in our inability to devise suitable categories to describe the complexities of family life. On many forms we have to decide between 'single', 'married' or 'divorced' but often these terms are less than helpful and do not begin to reflect the kinds of adult-child relations that may be created when parents change their partners.

Of course, one of the main reasons why we have not come to terms with

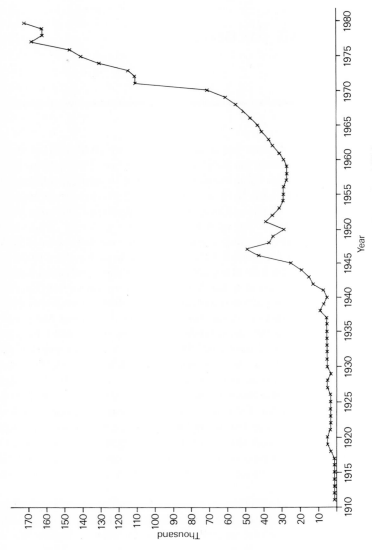

Fig. 10.1 Petitions filed for dissolutions and annulment of marriage in England and Wales for the years 1911–1980 (Source: Office of Population Censuses and Surveys)

living in a high divorce society is that it is only in the last decade or so that Britain could be described in this way. Here, as in most industrialised societies, a dramatic increase in the divorce rate began in the early 1960s and continued until the late 1970s when it levelled off (Fig. 10.1). The rise constituted a more than five-fold increase in the number of divorces to a point where projections suggest that one-third of presently contracted marriages are likely to end in this way. Contrary to popular belief, this increase has little or nothing to do with changes in the legal process, but seems to reflect a profound shift in attitudes towards marriage which has reigned in many parts of the world. It is not that marriage has become less popular—if anything the reverse, as people are tending to do it more than once in a lifetime. Rising divorce rates are paralleled by increasing remarriage rates. One in three marriages now involves at least one partner who has been through it at least once before. Unlike our forebears we do not repent our hasty marriages at leisure but we try again with a new partner. Statistically we are not likely to improve matters, at least if our goal is a persisting marriage, as probability of divorce seems to roughly double at each subsequent marriage. There is a growing concentration of divorce in the early years of marriage (Fig. 10.2). In fact, giving that separation occurs a year or two before a divorce there are now a considerable number of very brief duration marriages. In terms of demography, though not emotionally, children seem to have little bearing on the matter. They do not seem to cement failing marriages and may in fact be associated with increased chances of divorce (Chester, 1980).

A final point worth noting about the divorcing population is that it somewhat over-represents working class couples. But more striking here are the associations with marriage at an early age (also, of course, a tendency more common among working class adults) and occupations with high rates of geographical mobility (hotel and catering trades, the theatre, and hospital medicine, for instance).

About 60% of marriages which end in divorce involve children and a substantial minority of these are under-fives. In considering the nature of the children's responses to these events we need to take into account both the nature of the child and the event. But, of course, though divorce itself may be a single event, the important experience for the child is a long drawn out process that may begin when parents first encounter serious problems and ends perhaps several years later, with the setting up of a new relationship with a step-parent. But the process is variable and can take many forms. It may, for instance, result in a child losing contact with one parent (this seems to happen in about half of all cases (Richards, 1982)), or it may strengthen ties with both parents. The form the process takes is likely to have a great deal to do with the impact for the children. However, this point has been inadequately explored in the research. Too often all the variety is subsumed under the heading of 'divorced' with no account taken of the nature of the child's relationship with the two parents or presence or absence of step-

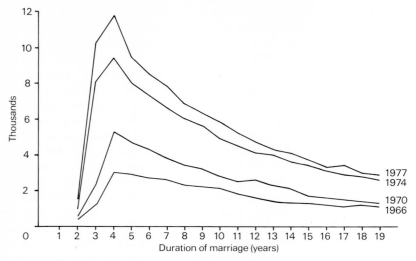

Fig. 10.2 Divorces by duration of marriage for selected years in England and Wales

parent figures. All of this, together with the overall lack of good research, makes it hard to give a very satisfactory general account of how children react to the divorce or separation of their parents. I shall attempt to do this by first describing some of the commonest initial reactions in children and then go on to deal with factors that may modify these. We have recently reviewed the research on this topic and we refer readers to this review for detailed substantiation for the points made here (Richards & Dyson, 1982). I will then briefly deal with longer term effects before concluding with a discussion of some of the help and support that is, or should be, available.

SOME RESPONSES OF CHILDREN

From the point of view of a child, a parental separation may bring for the first time the realisation that social relations are not eternal. If the relationships between their mother and father can end, or at least undergo dramatic modification, it is not surprising that most children begin to question the permanence of their own relationships with their parents. If one parent can leave the home, perhaps the other can too, leaving them alone. Initially, then, fears of separation and abandonment are very frequent. A child may begin to protest at being left at school or nursery. Or they may demand to have a light left on at night or, simply, try never to let the remaining parent out of their sight.

Anger is another common emotion. Most children are angry at their parents for doing something they did not want them to do. Adults may often like to think that children will welcome a separation but in our experience this is very seldom the case and children often retain the fantasy wish of their parents being reunited for the whole of their childhood. They may want the strife and quarrelling to cease if this has preceeded the separation but I have yet to hear a young child describe the separation itself in positive terms. Marital separation demonstrates to children their powerlessness and the fact that their interests and that of their parents may diverge.

It is because their parents are doing things that they do not want to happen that children become angry. The extent to which the anger may be shown directly and overtly varies enormously. Some children are able to tell their parents to their face that they hate them for what they have done (at least, as it seems to the child) while others may feel too insecure and unsure to do this. It may emerge indirectly, perhaps as bedwetting, or is redirected towards a sibling. Usually, the parent with whom the child feels most secure is the butt of the anger. A typical situation is then a mother left on her own with young children, feeling depressed and angry at the departed spouse and unable to cope with all the practical problems of single parenthood. She may blame all that has happened on the husband and his new partner but in the midst of this must face the anger and distress of the children. To make matters worse for her, the children may come to idealise the departed parent and accuse the mother of having driven him away. Sometimes these dynamics may work out in a rather different way. If the mother (and it usually is the mother who is left with the children) expresses a lot of anger about the husband to the children they may become frightened that the anger will be transferred to them. So instead of idealising the departed father, they will run him down to the mother and perhaps refuse to see him in the hope that this will prevent themselves becoming the target of the mother's anger. Much, of course, will depend on the age of the children as well as the particular situation. Adolescents may, in effect, give up on relationships within the family and seek them elsewhere. Earlier heterosexual relationships are associated with parental divorce.

Feelings of the kind I have been describing may spill over from the home into other situations. A child may become very withdrawn and depressed at school or may become unusually involved in activities that take him or her away from home. In the younger age groups a deterioration in peer relationships is not unusual and a child may gain a reputation for being fractious and aggressive which may persist longer than the behaviour itself.

It is commonly believed that children may feel responsible for what has happened to their parents and that they may have done something that has driven one parent away. Such feelings have been recorded (Wallerstein & Kelley, 1980) but they do not seem to be common. I suspect that this is another example of adult projection. It is more comfortable to believe that a child is upset because of supposed guilt at driving a parent out than to accept that the distress arises directly from what the adults have done against the wishes of their children.

Modifying factors

The sorts of behaviour I have been describing may last for a matter of months in an acute phase before gradually retreating. The extent of the reactions and the time that they take to subside vary with the situation. It is rare for a child to exhibit none of the things I have mentioned but on the other hand it is equally unusual for such behaviour still to be prominent after a year.

The most important modifying factor is the quality of the relationships between parents and child after separation. Here the research is quite consistent—children who maintain good relationships with both parents do better. Of course, a bad relationship between the parents often damages the relationship with the children but this is not inevitable and with imagination and ingenuity the two can be kept relatively separate. Interestingly, pre-divorce parent-child relations are not good predictors of what happens afterwards, especially for fathers. Some very involved fathers may disappear completely from the lives of their children (perhaps intermittent relations are too painful) while others who have barely seen their children apart from during brief holidays become devoted and caring part-time parents.

Marital separation can produce quite profound psychological and medical problems for parents which can severely limit their capacity to care for their children. So at a time when children may be particularly demanding and difficult and in need of extra reassurance, parents may be limited in what they can provide and may be more or less completely taken up with their own concerns. A common story is the child who tells of a parent who seldom gets out of bed. Added to the emotional problems may be practical ones. Income almost always drops at a separation and parents may gain their first experience of living on state benefits. A move to a new home is common so children (and adults) may have to face the loss of their friends and a familiar neighbourhood as well as a new school.

The majority of single parent households arise from a marital separation and we have much research that demonstrates that children in such households may be at a disadvantage (e.g. Ferri, 1976). Not least, the children may suffer from having only one parent to cope with all the problems of everyday life and to provide a model of a caring adult. In such situations it is not surprising that the single parent as well as outsiders may see remarriage as the answer to the problem. But the research evidence shows that a new partner can bring problems from the children's point of view (Burgoyne & Clark, 1981) and children who remain with their mothers in single parent households may do better than those whose mothers remarry (Douglas, 1970).

Long-term effects

There has been a good deal of interest among researchers about the effects of parental divorce that might persist into adulthood. All sorts of outcomes have been looked at ranging from various sorts of psychiatric treatment through criminal convictions to divorce itself. Given the complexities of the developmental process it is perhaps hardly surprising that no clear answers have emerged from this work. The usual result is a small increase in the frequency of whatever is being looked at in the group who has experienced a parental divorce in childhood as compared with the group who did not. Such effects are usually more marked in groups where the divorce took place before the age of 5. Where comparisons of groups who have lost a parent through divorce and through death are made, the divorce group usually comes off worst (e.g. Rutter, 1981). However, it should be reiterated that the differences are always small. Another reason for being cautious is that the experience of divorce today when it has become so common is probably rather different for a child than it was a generation ago when it was much rarer. By their nature the longer time follow-up studies are dealing with the history of the last generation and we cannot be sure that the divorces taking place today will have similar effects. It can be argued that the very frequency of divorce makes it less stressful for children and that today when some children are in primary school classes where the non-divorced parental families are in the minority the long-term effects are likely to be minimal.

NEEDS OF DIVORCING PARENTS AND THEIR CHILDREN

In a strict sense, divorce is a legal process. The law has been primarily concerned with the control of entry and exit from the marital state and all that flows from this in terms of such things as property rights and the legitimacy of children and the settlement of disputes that may occur at divorce. Our present law limits divorce for parents to those who can satisfy the court with the arrangements that they have made for the care of their children. However, from the point of view of the welfare of the children, this is little more than an empty gesture and it is very rare for a court not to be satisfied with whatever the parents propose. When disputes arise between parents about children at divorce a court can order a court welfare officer (usually a probation officer) to make a report on the children to help it resolve the matter. In the course of making these reports it is becoming increasingly common for the welfare officers to attempt mediation between the parents and more generally to offer them advice and support in matters related to their children. But despite this, the major role of the courts, in theory or practice, is not a welfare one (Eekelaar, 1978) and courts are very limited in the extent to which they can influence the outcome for children. This has led some people to argue that the law is too blunt an instrument to have the major role in family affairs at such times as divorce and that it should retreat leaving the field to an approach based more on counselling and conciliation. Others point to the symbolic value that the law may have and suggest that we could change the law to use this value more directly in the interests of the children. At divorce, the custody of the children which has been equally shared between the parents during the marriage is usually given to one parent only at divorce. Continuing joint custody is possible but is only used in a tiny minority of cases. The psychological evidence suggests that the best interests of children are usually served if both parental relationships persist and remain intact beyond the divorce. So a major aim of divorce legislation might be to confirm and reinforce the continuing role of both parents. So it might be more appropriate to make joint custody the norm at divorce and only allow departures from this in special cases (Richards, 1982) or in other ways to remove the winner/loser sole custody situation (Maidment, 1982). We are at a point where reform of the divorce law is under wide discussion. It is clear that there is wide dissatisfaction at the present position and there is no doubt that we could improve matters.

A conciliation service working alongside the courts could help to make the pitched court room battles a thing of the past and take the edge from the adversial battles conducted via solicitors, for instance. However, it seems unwise to look to the legal process as the main welfare agency to cope with what is at root a social and psychological process. What most parents and children need is support and the opportunity to talk through their feelings and experiences with a sympathetic person. They may also need access to specific information and advice. Alongside a movement to modify the legal process, we need to think how to provide these. My own feeling is very much against inventing any new profession or service to provide what is needed but rather rely on what we have already in all its variety. As well as the specialised agencies such as the Citizens Advice Bureau and the Marriage Guidance Council, the role that is needed is one that a wide range of professional and lay people could (and do) perform given an appreciation of the need and a minimal amount of information. We could make a very long list of those who might perform this role as well as friends, neighbours, acquaintances, colleagues and relatives. There are health visitors, GPs, paediatricians, vicars, midwives, social workers, psychiatrists, counsellors of all kinds and many others. For the professional groups the need is for them to look at their practice and how it may develop in the future and to see if this does meet the needs of a society in a substantial minority of children will experience at least one major upheaval in their parents' lives during childhood.

REFERENCES

Burgoyne J, Clark D 1981 Parenting in stepfamiles. In: Chester R, Diggory P, Sutherland M B (eds) Changing Patterns of Child Bearing and Child Rearing, Academic Press, London

Eekelaar J 1978 Family Law and Social Policy. Weidenfeld & Nicolson, London

Chamberlain R, Chamberlain G, Howlett B, Claircaux A 1975 British births 1970 Vol 1. The First Week of Life. Heinemann Medical Books, London

Chester R 1971 Health and marriage breakdown: experience of a sample of divorced women. British Journal of Preventive and Social Medicine 25: 231–235

Chester R 1980 A Survey of Recent UK Literature on Marital Problems. Unpublished report prepared for The Home Office Research Unit

Douglas, J W B 1970 Broken families and child behaviour. Journal of the Royal College of
    Physicians 4: 203–210
Ferri E 1976 Growing up in a One-Parent Family. NFER Publishing, Windsor
Maidment S 1982 Law and justice: the care for family law reform. Family Law 12: 229–232
Richards M P M 1982 Post-divorce arrangements for children: a psychological perspective.
    Journal of Social Welfare Law 133–151
Richards M P M, Dyson M 1981 Unpublished observations.
Richards M P M, Dyson M 1982 Separation, Divorce and the Development of Children: a
    Review. Unpublished report for the DHSS, London
Rutter M 1981 Maternal Deprivation Reassessed, 2nd edn. Penguin, London
Wallerstein J S, Kelley J B 1980 Surviving the Breakup. Grant McIntyre, London

Competence and performance of fathers and infants

INTRODUCTION: SOCIOCULTURAL CHANGES

In the past 10 years, investigators have studied the father's role with young infants extensively and suggested the importance of the father-infant relationship (Parke, 1979; Lamb, 1981; Yogman, 1982). This research has important implications for child health and medical care which this and the following chapter will address. At the very least, health professionals caring for children are becoming more aware of the need to obtain clinical data directly from fathers about child health and family adaptation and to include assessments of father as data necessary to good clinical decision making.

Sociocultural changes in Western societies provide the background for understanding why fathers are becoming more involved with their infants. The massive entry of women into the labor force has loosened many of the old sex role stereotypes for men and women and left opportunities for wider variations in the behaviour and roles of the two parents with their infants. In a 1978 U.S. survey, 44% of women between the ages of 18 and 34 with children under the age of 3 were employed (U.S. Bureau of the Census, 1979). Furthermore, the women's work was an economic necessity, since in families where women work full time, they contribute 40% of family income (Kammerman, 1980). When one combines the fact that families move more often and have fewer long-standing neighbourhood friends, the needs for father to share in infant care became clear.

Apart from any response to the women's movement, men are also seeking increased closeness with their infants as part of a men's movement toward a fuller emotional life and a reaction against the alienation and 'burnout' of the purely instrumental role of family provider. While some of the publicity about greater paternal involvement with infants may reflect social acceptability, a 1979 U.S. national survey of father participation in family work does suggest a real increase over the period 1960–1970 (Pleck, 1979).

In addition to changes in parental stereotypes, our views of infant competence have also changed dramatically. The infant now is no longer viewed as passive and limited in social competence but is now seen as an active participant in regulating social interaction (Brazelton et al, 1974), with a wide

130

range of perceptual, cognitive and social competencies (Macfarlane, 1975; Appleton et al, 1975; Meltzoff & Moore, 1977; Lipsitt, 1978). This current view of the competent infant has implied that infants are capable of establishing more than one simultaneous, meaningful relationship and has also provided the opportunity for fathers to be more involved.

These two chapters acknowledge that fathers can and do form a significant relationship with their infants. Therefore, in this chapter, I will briefly review the issue of competence, i.e., what are the capacities of fathers and infants to interact with each other and what are the similarities in behaviour and psychological experience between competent fathers and mothers. I will then address the less well-studied question of father's actual performance with his infant, i.e. what do fathers and infants actually do together, what influences paternal involvement and how does the father's involvement influence the infant's development. In the following chapter, clinical examples will illustrate the importance of father's role in both prevention of and treatment of some clinical disorders of infancy.

COMPETENCE OF FATHERS AND INFANTS

While older theories of child development suggest that parenting is predominantly instinctual, biologically determined, and exclusively maternal, a careful look at cross-species, anthropological and contemporary data in western cultures does not support a view of paternal incompetence with young infants. While primary maternal caregiving is the predominant mode in most animal species, examples of primary paternal caregiving can be found in animals such as the wolf and the stickleback (Tinbergen, 1952; Mitchell, 1969; Redican, 1976; Rypma, 1976) and even in primates such as the marmoset, a new world monkey, and the gibbon (Hampton et al, 1966; Chivers, 1972; Ingram, 1978). Male chimps, baboons and macaques have been found to adopt orphans in the wild (Hrdy, 1976), and even as aggressive a primate species as the rhesus male, when reared in a nuclear family environment in a laboratory, interacts playfully with his infant (Suomi, 1977). Furthermore, hormonal variations in prolactin levels have been related to levels of male caregiving in the marmoset (Dixson & George, 1982) and prolactin responses to tactile stimulation have been demonstrated in the human (Kolodny et al, 1972). The evidence suggests that biological constraints are much less significant determinants of male care of infants than ecological influences such as the modal social structure for each species.

Anthropological data provide further insights into the way social and cultural variables influence paternal care of and involvement with infants. In cultures such as the Arapesh, fathers play an active and joint role with mothers during pregnancy as well as in caring for infants after birth (Howells, 1969). !Kung San (Bushmen) fathers, representative of the earliest hunter-gatherer societies, were found to be affectionate and indulgent, often holding and fondling their infants, although they provided little of the routine care compared with mothers (West & Konner, 1976). Fathers from the Lesu village in Melanesia, who live in monogamous nuclear families and are gardeners, are reported to play with infants for hours.

Analysis of social organisation in different cultures suggests that males have a closer relationship with their infants when families are monogamous, when both parents live together in isolated nuclear families, when women contribute to subsistence by working, and when men are not required to be warriors (West & Konner, 1976; Whiting & Whiting, 1975).

In summary, phylogenetic and anthropological evidence underscores the diversity of the father–infant relationship across species and cultures. Fathers are involved with infants and play a competent role in many species and cultures. Moreover, the conditions of modern Western culture may help explain the current increased involvement and interest by fathers in infant care.

Within contemporary Western society, the evidence that fathers and infants can develop a complex relationship right from birth is impressive. Furthermore, the similarities between the psychological experience of pregnancy and infant care for mothers and fathers are striking. Studies of these similarities can be grouped into four developmental periods (prenatal, perinatal, early infancy (1–6 months) and later infancy (6–24 months)) and a brief discussion of each will illustrate the similarity of maternal and paternal competencies with infants (for a more detailed review see Yogman, 1982). Since most of the studies were conducted in the United States, caution must be exercised in generalising the findings.

During the prenatal period, Bibring (1959) suggests that pregnancy represents a normative psychological crisis for women. Studies by Gurwitt (1976) and Ross (1975) have suggested that during pregnancy men also rework significant relationships and events from early life. This turmoil has been called a crisis of paternal identity (Soule et al, 1979) and involves conflicts of gender, generative and generational identity (Ross, 1975), in which the men's roles as male, son and father become reintegrated.

The occurrence of physical complaints during pregnancy is probably one manifestation of this turmoil and such symptoms are present in men as well as women. Taboos and rituals such as the couvade both restrict and enhance the father's role in many cultures. In the traditional form of the couvade ritual, the father takes to bed during the women's pregnancy, labour and delivery, as a means of sharing in the experience. The remnant of this ritual in modern cultures is evidenced by the couvade syndrome in which men experience psychosomatic symptoms during their wives' pregnancies (Trethowan & Conlon, 1965; Trethowan, 1972).

A recent well-controlled epidemiological survey of patients seen by specialists in internal medicine suggests the clinical importance of couvade symptoms (Lipkin & Lamb, 1982). Almost one-quarter of all men whose wives were pregnant complained of nausea, vomiting, anorexia, abdominal pain or bloating even though a diagnostic evaluation uncovered no objective explanation for these symptoms. These men made twice the number of visits to physicians and received twice the number of medications as their controls, in part because the health provider never asked if the man's wife was pregnant. In other studies, as many as 65% of men complained of physical symptoms which also included backache and weight gain, and described dietary changes and giving up smoking (Liebenberg, 1973).

During the perinatal period, fathers are now almost routinely present during labour and delivery. In fact, Anderson & Stanley (1976) have shown that husband support lessens the degree of maternal distress during this time. In an interview study of fathers of healthy firstborns in London, fathers' descriptions of their feelings after having witnessed the birth were almost identical to those of mothers: extreme elation, relief that the baby is healthy, feelings of pride and increased self esteem and feelings of closeness when the baby opens his eyes (Robson & Moss, 1970; Greenberg & Morris, 1974; Lind, 1974). When fathers are given the opportunity to touch their babies, they do so in the same sequence as mothers: from fingertips to palms, first on the limbs and then on the trunk (Rödholm & Larsson, 1979). While debate goes on about the process by which early contact with newborns influences maternal bonding, similar effects of this intervention have now been shown on the father-infant relationship (Keller et al, 1981; Rödholm, 1981) perhaps mediated by an influence on parental self confidence.

Furthermore, fathers and mothers display similar behaviours when interacting with their newborns. Studies by Parke & Sawin (1975, 1977) of father-newborn interaction in the post partum period suggest that fathers and mothers are equally active and sensitive to newborn cues during the post partum period. In general the conclusions hold for middle-class as well as lower-class families and in both the dyadic (father–infant) and triadic (mother–father–infant) situation. Not only do fathers and mothers share the exhilaration of the perinatal period, but they also share the lows or the normative post partum blues of this period as well. In an interview study of men in the first few weeks post partum, 62% of men reported feelings of sadness and disappointment (Zaslow et al, 1981).

During the first 6 months of life, infants become increasingly social as they begin to smile and vocalise. One might suspect that these socially responsive infants are good elicitors of social interaction with fathers as well as mothers. Since 1974, together with colleagues at Children's Hospital in Boston, I have studied the social interaction of fathers with their infants of 2 weeks to 6 months of age. In contrast to functional tasks such as feeding and diapering, we studied unstructured face-to-face interaction because it placed maximal demands on the social capabilities of the participants. While face-to-face communication may occupy only a small proportion of an infant's day at home, videotaped interactions in the laboratory allowed us to elicit and study in a detailed way brief exchanges of expressive communication that may reflect the developing father–infant relationship. This method of studying early social interaction was developed by Brazelton et al (1975) and has been used to characterise mother–infant interaction as a mutually regulated reciprocal process in which both partners rhythmically cycle to a peak of affective involvement and then withdraw.

We began by demonstrating that infants by 80 days of age and as young as 6 weeks of age would interact differently with their familiar parents than they would with unfamiliar strangers as evidenced by differences in facial expression and limb movements (Dixon et al, 1981; Yogman, 1982).

Infants by 3 months of age successfully interacted with both mothers and fathers with a similar, mutually regulated reciprocal pattern as evidenced by transitions between affective levels that occurred simultaneously for infant and parent (Yogman, 1977; 1982). Mothers and fathers were equally able to engage the infant in games, i.e. episodes of repeated adult behaviour that engaged the infant's attention (Yogman, 1981). Finally, by studying the rhythmicity in an infant's behaviour and heart rate during social interaction with her mother, father, and a stranger, we found that infant and adult behavioural rhythms were synchronous only with father and mother and not with an unfamiliar stranger but that the 3-month-old infant's behaviour and heart rate were synchronised during interaction with all three adults (Yogman et al, 1983). These data suggested that father's and mother's familiarity with their infant enabled them to synchronise their behavioural rhythms with their infant while the stranger did not. In contrast, the relationship between infant measures alone (behaviour and physiology) remained synchronous with all three adults, perhaps reflecting the infant's intactness and organisation. In sum, the studies of fathers and infants in the first 6 months of life supported the hypothesis that fathers are competent and capable of skilled and sensitive social interaction with young infants.

Studies of the father-infant relationship with infants aged 6 to 14 months has focussed primarily on the development of attachment as Bowlby (1969) and Ainsworth (1973) have defined it. These studies have asked questions such as: do infants greet, seek proximity with and protest on separation from fathers as well as mothers? Such studies provide conclusive evidence that infants are attached to fathers as well as to mothers. By 7–8 months of age, when the home environment tends to be relatively low in stress, infants are attached to both mothers and fathers and prefer either parent over a stranger (Lamb, 1975, 1977a, 1978b). During the second year, most studies also show attachment to both mother and father (Kotelchuck, 1976; Lamb, 1977b; Clarke–Stewart, 1978, 1980), although in a more stressful setting in the laboratory, some studies have shown that infants between 12 and 18 months prefer mothers (Ban & Lewis, 1974; Cohen & Campos, 1974; Lamb, 1976). The issue of preference for mother or father depends on what measure is used, but independent estimates by Kotelchuck (1973) in Boston and Schaffer & Emerson (1964) in Scotland are similar: between 12 and 21 months 51–55% of infants show maternal preferences, 19–25% show paternal preferences, and 16–20% show joint preferences. Lamb's data (1978a, 1979) suggest that it is mainly boys who prefer their fathers because fathers engage them more actively.

Not only are infants attached to fathers, but the study of qualitative aspects of infant attachment to mothers and fathers using Ainsworth's 'Strange Situation' has suggested that infants could develop a secure attachment with the father in spite of an insecure attachment with the mother (Lamb, 1978b; Main &Weston, 1981). In sum, studies of the father–infant relationship in each of these developmental epochs (the prenatal, perinatal, early and later infancy periods) demonstrate both the similarity of the father–infant and mother–infant relationship and the capacities of fathers and infants to interact successfully.

PERFORMANCE OF FATHERS AND INFANTS

Regardless of these capacities, what fathers and infants actually do together seems increasingly variable and diverse as stereotypes for the male role shift. In general, however, fathers spend much less time with their infants than mothers do. The specific role fathers play and activities they engage in seems highly dependent on the surrounding context.

In natural observations, the mother is clearly the predominant partner (Clarke–Stewart, 1980). Reports of father involvement vary from a mean of 8 hours per week spent playing with, and 26 hours per week available at home with awake 9-month-old babies (Pedersen & Robson, 1969) to 3.2 hours per day (1/3 that of mother) spent with the infant (Kotelchuck, 1976), or 30 minutes per day spent alone with the infant (1/2 that of mother) (Pedersen et al, 1979). When one looks at specific activities (feeding, cleaning, play), fathers also spend much less time in these activities than mothers do, although a greater proportion of fathers' time with the baby is spent specifically in play (37.5% vs. 25.8%) (Kotelchuck, 1975). With toddlers (20 months of age), fathers are reported to spend an average of 3 hours/day playing with their infants although the variability was extensive (Easterbrooks, 1982). Even though fathers do not spend as much time with their babies as mothers do, at least 25–50% of fathers are involved in some caretaking responsibilities, as shown by surveys from the U.S., England and Ireland (Newson & Newson, 1963; Kotelchuck, 1975; Richards et al, 1977; Nugent et al, 1982). Almost 90% of fathers played with their infants and while fathers would sometimes feed their infants, they were less likely to change diapers (nappies) and bathe the baby (Newson & Newson, 1963; Kotelchuck, 1975; Richards et al, 1977). The degree to which fathers participate in caregiving and in play with their infant has been related to their sex role classification: increased participation has been associated with androgynous sex roles (Russell, 1978). Finally, one must remember that the actual time parent and infant spend interacting may be substantially less than simply the total amount of time they spend engaged in any of these specific activities. Differences in the time mothers and fathers spend interacting with their infants may be less than they first appear.

Father–infant play

Regardless of the amount of time fathers spend with their infants they are more likely to be the infant's play partner than the mother, and father's play tends to be more stimulating, vigorous, arousing and state disruptive for the infant. In our studies of infant games during the first 6 months of life, fathers engaged their infants in tactile and limb movement games in which their behaviour attempted to arouse the infant. Mothers more commonly played visual games in which they displayed distal motor movements that were observed by the infant and appeared to be attempts to maintain visual attention (Yogman, 1981).

The visual games most often played by mothers may represent a more distal attention-maintaining form of interactive play than the more proximal, idiosyncratic limb movement games played more often by fathers. Studies of the games parents play with 8-month-old infants show similar findings: mothers played more distal games, while fathers engaged in more physical games (Power & Parke, 1979). Stern (1974) has suggested that the goal of such games is to facilitate an optimal level of arousal in the infant in order to foster attention to social signals. The more proximal games of infants and fathers may serve to modulate the infant's attention and arousal in a more accentuated fashion than occurs during the distal games of infants and mothers. These findings are surprisingly robust in that they have been replicated with different age infants in different situations. Fathers of newborns, while similar to mothers in most behaviours, tended to hold and rock their newborns more (Parke et al, 1972). In interviews conducted after holding their newborns, fathers emphasised the physical contact, the feeling of the baby 'moving up against them' (Greenberg & Morris, 1974). Differences in interaction between mothers and fathers and their older infants all involve play: fathers engage in more play than caretaking activities with 6-month-olds (Rendina & Dickersheid, 1976) and more often pick up their infants (8 months) to play physical, idiosyncratic, rough-and-tumble games. By comparison, mothers are likely to hold infants, engage in caregiving tasks, and either play with toys or use conventional games such as peek-a-boo (Lamb, 1977a). By age $2\frac{1}{2}$ when parents were asked to engage the child in specific play activities, fathers were better able to engage the child in play. Father's play with his child was likely to be proximal (as was described for younger infants), physical, and arousing, and fathers reported that they enjoyed it more than mothers (Clarke–Stewart, 1978, 1980). Infants at 8 months responded more positively to play with fathers than mothers (Lamb, 1977a) and by age $2\frac{1}{2}$ not only preferred to play with fathers but were judged to be more involved and excited with them (Clarke–Stewart, 1978). It is fascinating to note that fathers' physical play with their infants correlates most highly with mothers' verbal stimulation (0.89) and toy play (0.96) (Clarke–Stewart, 1980). These are maternal behaviours found in other studies to be part of a pattern of 'optimal maternal care' (Clarke–Stewart, 1973).

These differences in play and quality of vigorous stimulation are quite robust and persist even in studies of primary caregiver fathers in the U.S. (Field, 1978; Yogman, 1982) and in studies of non-traditional fathers taking advantage of paternity leave in Sweden (Frodi et al, 1982; Lamb et al, 1982). It is interesting to speculate that these play differences may become less tied to gender as socialisation of young children changes. It is important to note that in contrast to these play differences the performance of caregiving tasks seems easily modifiable and closer in its relationship to role rather than to gender.

Influence on paternal involvement

The father's involvement with his infant is influenced by a number of inter-personal, intrapersonal, social, cultural and economic variables. One of the major influences on father's involvement is the marital relationship. High marital satisfaction has been associated with the quality of both parents' relationship with the baby. Heightened paternal feelings of competition with his spouse have been shown to occur after the birth of an infant, particularly if the father has a close relationship with the baby and the mother is nursing. Husbands of nursing mothers described feelings of inadequacy, envy, and exclusion, and the competition may actually undermine the mother's attempts at breast-feeding unless these feelings are addressed (Lerner, 1979; Waletzky, 1979).

The importance of the family context for understanding the father's role has been illustrated by studies that suggest that the mother–infant relationship is typically dyadic while the father-infant relationship typically is triadic and involves the mother (Pedersen et al, 1980). In families in which the mother is at work all day she actually spends more time with the infant in the evening and this is associated with lower levels of father-infant interaction (Pedersen et al, 1982). The mother seems to function much as a gatekeeper, regulating the father's involvement with the infant. The mother's feelings about father's involvement become one determinant of this gatekeeper function and they are influenced by her relationship with her own father. Mothers who perceive their own fathers as having had a minimal role, tend to be married to men who are highly involved in childcare (Radin, 1981). The mother continues to influence a father's relationship with his infant even when he is not home, since mother conveys a representation of father in his absence (Atkins, 1981) that influences the father-infant relationship after father's return.

Father's relationship with his own father has also been associated with his high involvement in infant care (Cordell et al, 1980) and conversely, father's negative self esteem was associated with less involvement (Gamble & Belsky, 1982). The most satisfied fathers were those who were more strongly identified with the parenting role than the average person (Dickie et al, 1981).

Cultural practices, economic constraints and employment policies such as paternity leave and flexible work schedules all have major influences on paternal involvement. Stresses such as job loss may be associated with paternal depression and although this may result in additional free time for these men, they are less likely to assume infant care responsibilities (Cordell et al, 1980). Further, paternal unemployment may have adverse influences on both behavioural disorders in children and on the incidence of minor infectious illnesses (Margolis, 1982a, b).

Changes in hospital policies and simple interventions may have dramatic influences on paternal involvement in childbirth. The changes in obstetric and neonatal services which encourage the father's presence during labour and delivery and in the nurseries have gone far toward reversing the separation and exclusion of fathers from their infants. Postpartum support groups for fathers described by Rizzuto (1978) document father's unmet needs for discussing their concerns and fears without being labelled aberrant. Several educational programmes have shown that brief interventions with fathers in the perinatal period could influence their attitudes, caregiving skills, and knowledge of infant capabilities for as long as 3 months (Parke et al, 1980). In Sweden, fathers who received simple instructions on bathing, changing, and feeding in the perinatal period were found to have higher degrees of infant caretaking activity as recorded on a maternal questionnaire 6 weeks after discharge (Johannesson, 1969). Demonstrations of neonatal behaviour to fathers in the newborn period has been shown to influence paternal involvement for as long as 6 months. In Australia, fathers of full term and preterm newborns administered and scored a behavioural assessment of their baby and discussed a videotape of their baby. Compared to an intervention control group, fathers of the term infants engaged in more face-to-face play at 6 months and fathers of both full term and preterm infants provided more stimulation in a home observation (Dolby et al, 1982). In the USA, a similar study showed an increase in paternal caregiving at 4 weeks of age (Myers, 1982). Simple interventions with fathers of older children (instructing them to play with their 12 month-old sons 50 minutes a day) were also effective. One month later, infants in the intervention group showed greater degrees of proximity-seeking to their fathers in a free play context than fathers in the non-intervention group (Zelazo et al, 1977). More prolonged interventions have been shown to improve the infant's competence as well (Dickie & Carnahan, 1979). Changing our stereotypes about the relationship of fathers and infants probably requires educating children and adolescents about infants as part of a school curriculum in parenting education.

Paternal influences on infant development

The influence of the father–infant relationship on later cognitive, social, and emotional development of the infant has not been well studied. In a prenatal and postpartum interview study of the influence of maternal and paternal expectations and roles, Fein (1976) suggests that the most effective male post-partum adjustment was related not simply to high or low paternal involvement but rather to a coherent role that met both the needs of the father himself, the mother, and the baby.

The influence of the father-infant relationship on the infant during these early months is suggested by the report that, at least for boys, increased father involvement at home is associated with greater infant social responsiveness at 5 months of age during a Bayley test (Pedersen et al, 1979). Infants whose fathers participate highly in caregiving show less separation protest and cry less with a stranger than infants whose fathers are less involved (Spelke et al, 1973; Kotelchuck, 1975). The amount of time father spends alone with his 20 month-old infant directly predicted 23% of the variance of the infant's affect during a task with the mother and 10% of the variance of the infant's task orientation and concentration (Easterbrooks, 1982). In our own longitudinal study of healthy full term infants in Boston, paternal involvement defined by the sum of measures of prenatal and peri-natal involvement and caregiving was correlated (r = 0.39) with infant Mental Developmental Index (MDI) scores on the Bayley test at 9 months. A similar measure of the involvement of young fathers living in Dublin also correlated with 12-month Bayley MDI scores and, when combined with measures of parental social class, neonatal behaviour and maternal socialisation goals in a multiple regression analysis, 57% of the variance in Bayley MDI scores at 12 months was accounted for (Nugent et al, 1982). Concurrent predictions of infant Bayley scores at 16 and 22 months were related to the father's positive perceptions of the child and his ability to engage the child in play and to anticipate independence on the part of the child. Predictions of concurrent social competence were related to the father's verbal and playful behaviour and for girls, his expectation of independence (Clarke-Stewart, 1978, 1980). Boys in particular have been found to be more autonomous when both parents are warm and affectionate (Baumrind & Black, 1967). While causation cannot be inferred from correlational studies, Clarke-Stewart (1980) suggested that the mother's warmth, verbal stimulation, and play with toys with infants at 15 months of age was related to higher infant Bayley scores at 30 months which, in turn, influenced fathers to engage in play more often, to expect more independence, and to perceive their children more positively.

Most attempts to assess the impact of the father infant relationship on later development have looked at father-absent families and the relationship to sex role identification. Father-absence, particularly prior to age five (Mischel, 1970) has been shown to influence masculine sex role adoption and cognitive style among boys (Carlsmith, 1964; Hetherington, 1966; Biller, 1970; 1976) and heterosexual roles among girls (Johnson, 1963). Since these studies have been criticised for combining very different underlying reasons for the father's absence and for confounding the direct effects on the infant with indirect effects mediated through the mother (Herzog & Sudia, 1973), the focus has shifted to understanding the differential relationship of fathers with sons and daughters during infancy. These studies show that not only do fathers vocalise and play more with sons than daughters but that this is especially true for first-born sons (Parke & O'Leary, 1976; Parke & Sawin, 1975; 1977; Parke et al, 1979). The preference seems true not only in the United States but in Israel (Gerwirtz & Gerwirtz, 1980) and among the Kung San bushmen (West & Konner, 1976). Studies of infant preferences show that 1-year-old male infants look more at fathers than at mothers during free play in the laboratory (Ban & Lewis, 1974), remain closer and vocalise more to fathers than to mothers during a more stressful laboratory procedure (Spelke et al, 1973), and that by 20 months of age, male infants show specific play preferences for fathers (Clarke–Stewart, 1980). Belsky (1979) attempted to determine the direction of this preference in home observations and attributes the preferences of male 15-month-olds for their fathers primarily to the behaviour of their fathers.

CONCLUSION

In conclusion, these studies of fathers and infants are beginning to form a basis for theorising about the influences of paternal involvement on infant personality development.

First of all, studies of father-infant interaction suggest that fathers can have a meaningful and direct relationship with their infants right from birth and that the pregnancy experience is a time of developmental transition for fathers as well as mothers.

In spite of different research strategies and samples, the studies have shown considerable consistency in describing the nature of father-infant interaction. In the newborn period fathers held and rocked their babies more than mothers and were more stimulating (Parke & Sawin, 1975). By 3 months of age, fathers and infants in our studies engaged in more proximal, arousing, idiosyncratic games, whereas mothers and infants were more likely to engage in smoothly modulated, soothing distal games, especially verbal ones. Others have found that fathers are more likely to play physical, arousing idiosyncratic games with their infants at 1 and 2 years of age while mothers are more likely to play conventional games (Lamb, 1977a; Clarke-Stewart, 1980). Furthermore, infants respond to their fathers with more excitement. In sum, while fathers have been shown to be sensitive to infant cues (Parke & Sawin, 1975, 1977) and skilled interactants with young infants (Yogman, 1977), consistent and rather stable differences in the quality of behavioural regulation have been demonstrated between father-infant and mother-infant interaction. Fathers seem more likely to develop a heightened, arousing, and playful relationship with their infants (Parke, 1979; Clarke-Stewart, 1980; Yogman, 1982) and to provide a more novel and complex environment (Pedersen et al, 1979).

Acknowledgements

The research in this and the following chapter was supported by the National Foundation March of Dimes, with additional assistance from NICHD Grant No. 10889, NIMH Grant No. TO1MH14887–06, MCH Grant No. MGR-250460, the Robert Wood Johnson Foundation, and the Carnegie Corporation of New York. I also wish to thank my colleageues Suzanne Dixon, Edward Tronick, Barry Lester, Joel Hoffman, Diana Dill, Nancy Jordan and to thank T. Berry Brazelton for his support and encouragement in this research.

REFERENCES

Ainsworth M D S 1973 The development of infant–mother attachment. In: Caldwell B and Ricciuti, H (eds) Review of Child Development Research, Vol. 3. University of Chicago Press, Chicago

Anderson B J, Standley K 1976 A methodology for observation of the childbirth environment Paper presented to the American Psychological Association Washington, DC

Appleton T, Clifton R, Goldberg S 1975 The development of behavioural competence in infancy. In: Horowitz F (ed) Review of Child Development Research, Vol. 4. University of Chicago Press, Chicago

Atkins R 1981 Discovering daddy: the mother's contributions to father-representations. Paper presented to American Psychiatric Association, New Orleans

Ban P L, Lewis M 1974 Mothers and fathers, girls and boys: attachment behaviour in the one-year-old. Merrill-Palmer Quarterly 20: 195–204

Baumrind D, Black A E 1967 Socialization practices associated with dimensions of competence in preschool boys and girls. Child Development 38: 291–327

Belsky J 1979 Mother–father infant interaction: a naturalistic observational study. Developmental Psychology 15: 601–607

Bibring G 1959 Some considerations of the psychological processes in pregnancy. Psychoanalytic Study of the Child 14: 113

Biller H 1970 Father absence and the personality development of the male child. Developmental Psychology 2: 181–201

Biller H B 1976 The father and personality development: paternal deprivation and sex-role development. In: Lamb M (ed) The Role of the Father in Child Development. Wiley, New York

Bowlby J 1969 Attachment and Loss Vol. 1. Basic Books, New York

Brazelton T B, Koslowski B, Main M 1974 The origins of reciprocity. In: Lewis M, Rosenblum L A (eds) The Effect of the Infant on its Caregiver. Wiley, New York

Brazelton T B, Tronick E, Adamson L, Als H, Wise S 1975 Early mother infant reciprocity. In: Hinde R (ed) Parent-Infant Interaction. Ciba Foundation Symposium No. 33. Elsevier, Amsterdam

Carlsmith L 1964 Effects of early father absence on scholastic aptitude. Harvard Education Review 34: 3–21

Chivers D J 1972 The Siamang and the Gibbon in the Malay Peninsula. Gibbon and Siamang 1: 103–135

Clarke-Stewart K A 1973 Interactions between mothers and their young children. Monographs of the Society for Research in Child Development 38

Clarke-Stewart K A 1978 And daddy makes three: the father's impact on mother and child. Child Development 49: 466–478

Clarke-Stewart K A 1980 The father's contribution to children's cognitive and social development in early childhood. In: Pedersen F A (ed) The Father-Infant Relationship: Observational Studies in a Family Setting. Holt, Rinehart and Winston, New York

Cohen L J and Campos J J 1974 Father, mother and stranger as elicitors of attachment behaviours in infancy. Developmental Psychology 10: 146–154

Cordell A S, Parke R D, Sawin D B 1980 Father's views on fatherhood with special reference to infancy. Family Relations 29: 331–338

Dickie J, Carnahan S 1979 Training in social competence: The effect on mothers, fathers and infants. Paper presented at the biennial meeting of the Society for Research in Child Development, San Francisco

Dickie J, VanGent R, Hoogerwerf E, Martinez I and Dieterman B 1981 Mother-father-infant triad: who affects whose satisfaction. Paper presented to Biennial Meeting of SRCD, Boston, MA

Dixon S, Yogman M W, Tronick E, Als H, Adamson L, Brazelton T B 1981 Early social interaction of infants with parents and strangers. Journal of the American Academy of Child Psychiatry 20: 32–52

Dixson A F, George L 1982 Prolactin and parental behaviour in a male New World primate. Nature: 551–553

Dolby R, English B, Warren B 1982 Brazelton demonstrations for mothers and fathers. Paper presented to International Conference on Infant Studies, Austin Texas

Easterbrooks M A 1982 Father involvement, parenting characteristics and toddler development. Paper presented to International Conference on Infant Studies, Austin, Texas

Fein R A 1976 Men's entrance to parenthood. Family Coordinator 25: 341–351

Field T M 1978 Interaction behaviours of primary versus secondary caretaker fathers. Developmental Psychology 14: 183–184

Field T M 1979a Interaction patterns of preterm and fullterm infants. In: Field T M (ed) Infants Born at Risk: Behaviour and Development. SP Medical and Scientific Books, New York

Frodi A, Lamb M, Hwang C, Frodi M 1982 Increased paternal involvement and family relationships. Paper presented to International Conference on Infant Studies, Austin, Texas

Gamble W C, Belsky J 1982 The determinants of parenting within a family context: a preliminary analysis. Paper presented to International Conference on Infant Studies, Austin, Texas

Gerwirtz H R, Gerwirtz J L 1968 Visiting and caretaking patterns for kibbutz infants. American Journal of Orthopsychiatry 38: 427–443

Greenberg M, Morris N 1974 Engrossment: the newborn's impact upon the father. American Journal of Orthopsychiatry 44: 520–531

Gurwitt A R 1976 Aspects of prospective fatherhood. Psychoanalytic Study of the Child 31: 237–271

Hampton J K, Hampton S H, Landwehr B T 1966 Observations on a successful breeding colony of the marmoset. Oedipomidas Oedipus. Folia Primatologica 4: 265–287

Herzog E, Sudia C E 1973 Children in fatherless families. In: Caldwell B M, Ricciuti H N (eds) Review of Child Development Research, Vol. 3. University of Chicago Press, Chicago

Hetherington E M 1966 Effect of paternal absence on sex-typed behaviours in negro and white preadolescent males. Journal of Personality and Social Psychology 4: 87–91

Howells J G 1969 Fathering. In: Howells J G (ed) Modern Perspectives in International Child Psychiatry. Oliver and Boyd, Edinburgh

Hrdy Sarah B L 1976 Care and exploitation of nonhuman primate infants by conspecifics other than mothers. In: Rosenblatt J R, Hinde R A, Shaw E, Beer C (eds) Advances in the Study of Behaviour, Vol. 6, pp 101–158. Academic Press, New York

Ingram J C 1978 Social interactions within marmoset family groups. In Chivers D, Herbert J (eds) Recent Advances in Primatology, Vol. 1. Academic Press, New York

Johannesson, Patricia 1969 Instruction in child care for fathers. Dissertation at University of Stockholm

Johnson, M M 1963 Sex role learning in the nuclear family. Child Development 34: 315–333

Kammerman S 1980 Maternity and Parental Benefits and Leaves. Impact on Policy Series, Monograph No. 1, p. 8. Columbia University Press, New York

Keller W D, Hildenbrandt K A, Richardson M E 1981 Effects of extended father-infant contact during the newborn period. Paper presented to Biennial Meeting of SRCD, Boston

Kolodny R C, Jacobs L S, Daughaday W H 1972 Mammary stimulation causes prolactin secretion in non-lactating women. Nature 238: 286–286

Kotelchuck M 1973 The nature of the infant's tie to his father. Paper presented to Society for Research in Child Development, Philadelphia

Kotelchuck M 1975 Father-caretaking characteristics and their influence on infant–father interaction. Paper presented to American Psychological Association, Chicago

Kotelchuck M 1976 The infant's relationship to the father: experimental evidence. In: Lamb M (ed) The Role of the Father in Child Development. John Wiley, New York

Lamb M E 1975 Fathers: forgotten contributors to child development Human Development 18: 245–266

Lamb M E 1976 Twelve-month-olds and their parents: interaction in a laboratory playroom. Developmental Psychology 12: 237–244

Lamb M E 1977a Father–infant and mother–infant interaction in the first year of life. Child Development 48: 167–181

Lamb M E 1977b The development of mother-infant and father-infant attachments in the second year of life. Developmental Psychology 13: 637–648

Lamb M E 1978a The father's role in the infant's social world. In: Stevens J E Jr, Mathews M (eds) Mother/Child, Father/Child Relationships. National Association for the Education of Young Children

Lamb M E 1978b Qualitative aspects of mother- and father–infant attachments. Infant Behaviour and Development 1: 265–275

Lamb M E 1979 Paternal influences and the father's role: a personal perspective. American Psychologist 34: 938–943

Lamb M E (ed) 1981 The Role of the Father in Child Development. John Wiley, New York

Lamb M, Frodi A, Hwang C, Frodi M, Steinberg J 1982 Mother and father-infant interaction involving play and holding in traditional and nontraditional Swedish families. Developmental Psychology 18: 215–221

Lerner H 1979 Effects of the nursing mother-infant dyad on the family. American Journal of Orthopsychiatry 49: 339–348

Liebenberg B 1973 Expectant fathers. In: Shereshfsky P, Yarrow L (eds) Psychological Aspects of a First Pregnancy and Early Postnatal Adaptation. Raven Press, New York

Lind J 1974 Observations after delivery of communication between mother–infant–father. Paper presented at International Congress of Pediatrics, Buenos Aires

Lipkin M, Lamb G S 1982 The couvade syndrome: an epidemiologic study. Annals of Internal Medicine 96: 509–511

Lipsitt L 1978 Developmental Psychobiology: The Significance of Infancy. Lawrence Erlbaum, Hillsdale, NJ

Macfarlane A 1975 Olfaction in the development of social preferences in the human neonate. In: Hinde R (ed) Parent–Infant Interaction (Ciba Foundation Symposium No. 33). Elsevier, Amsterdam

Main M, Weston D R 1981 The quality of the toddler's relationship to mother and to father. Child Development 52: 932–940

Margolis L 1982a Work in progress at University of North Carolina School of Public Health. Personal communication

Margolis L 1982b Help wanted. Pediatrics 69: 816

Meltzoff A N, Moore M K 1977 Imitation of facial and manual gestures by human neonates. Science 198: 75–78

Mischel W 1970 Sex typing and socialization. In: Mussen P (ed) Carmichael's Manual of Child Psychology. John Wiley, New York

Mitchell G D 1969 Paternalistic behaviour in primates Psychological Bulletin 721: 399–419

Myers B J 1982 Early intervention using Brazelton training with middle class mothers and fathers of newborns. Child Development 53: 462–471

Newson J, Newson E 1963 Patterns of Infant Care in an Urban Community. Penguin, Harmondsworth

Nugent J K, Yogman M W, Lester B M, Hoffman J 1982 The father's impact on infant development in Ireland in the first year of life. Paper presented to Tenth International Congress for Child and Adolescent Psychiatry and Allied Professions, Dublin, Ireland

Parke R 1979 Perspectives on father-infant interaction. In: Osofsky J D (ed) Handbook of Infancy. John Wiley, New York

Parke R D, O'Leary S 1976 Father-mother-infant interaction in the newborn period. In:
    Riegel K, Meacham J (eds) The Developing Individual in a Changing World, Vol. 2.
    Mouton, The Hague
Parke R, Sawin D 1975 Infant characteristics and behaviour as elicitors of maternal and
    paternal responsibility in the newborn period. Paper presented to Society for Research in
    Child Development, Denver
Parke R, Sawin, D 1977 The family in early infancy: social interactional and attitudinal
    analyses. Paper presented to Society for Research in Child Development, New Orleans
Parke R, Hymel S, Power T, Tinsley B 1980 Fathers and risk: a hospital based model of
    intervention. To appear in: Sawin D B, Hawkes R C, Walker L O, Penticuff J H (eds)
    Psychosocial Risks in Infant Environment Transactions, Vol. 4. Bruner Mazel, New York
Parke, R D, O'Leary S E, West S 1972 Mother-infant-newborn interaction: effects of
    maternal medication, labor, and sex of infant. Proceedings of the American Psychological
    Association, pp 85-86
Parke R D, Power T G, Tinsley B, Hymel S 1979 The father's role in the family system.
    Seminars in Perinatology 3: 25-34
Pedersen F A, Robson K S 1969 Father participation in infancy. American Journal of
    Orthopsychiatry 39: 466-472
Pedersen F, Rubinstein J, Yarrow C T 1979 Infant development in father-absent families.
    Journal of Genetic Psychology 135: 51-61
Pedersen F, Yarrow C J, Anderson B J, Cain R L 1979 Conceptualization of father
    influences in the infancy period. In: Lewis M, Rosenblum L (eds) The Child and Its
    Family. Plenum Press, New York
Pedersen F, Anderson B, Cain R L 1980 Parent-infant and husband-wife interactions
    observed at age 5 months. In: Pedersen F A (ed) The Father-Infant Relationship,
    pp 71-86. Praeger, New York
Pedersen F, Zaslow M, Suwalsky J, Cain R 1982 Infant experience in traditional and dual
    wage-earner families. Paper presented to International Conference on Infant Studies,
    Austin, Texas
Pleck J 1979 Men's family work: three perspectives and some new data. Family Coordinator
    28: 481-488
Power T G, Parke R D 1979 Toward a taxonomy of father-infant and mother-infant play
    patterns. Paper presented to the Society for Research in Child Development, San Francisco
Radin N 1981 Child rearing in intact families I. Merrill Palmer Quarterly 27: 489-514
Redican W K 1976 Adult male-infant interactions in nonhuman primates. In: Lamb M E
    (ed) The Role of the Father in Child Development. John Wiley, New York
Rendina I, Dickerscheid J D 1976 Father involvement with first-born infants. Family
    Coordinator 25: 373-379
Richards M P M, Dunn J F, Antonis B 1977 Caretaking in the first year of life: the role of
    fathers' and mothers' social isolation. Child Care, Health and Development 3: 23-26
Rizzuto A 1978 Intervention with fathers in the perinatal period: fathers' support group.
    Paper presented at the Annual Meeting of the Seminar in the Development of Infants and
    Parents
Robson K, Moss H 1970 Patterns and determinants of maternal attachment. Journal of
    Pediatrics 77 976-985
Rödholm M, Larsson K 1979 Father-infant interaction at the first contact after delivery.
    Early Human Development 3: 21-27
Rödholm M 1981 Effects of father-infant post partum contact on their interaction 3 months
    after birth. Early Human Development 5: 79-85
Ross J M 1975 The development of paternal identity: a critical review of the literature on
    nurturance and generativity in boys and men. Journal of American Psychoanalytic
    Association 23: 783-817
Russell, G 1978 The father role and its relation to masculinity, femininity, and androgyny.
    Child Development 49: 1174-1181
Rypma C B 1976 The biological bases of the paternal responses. Family Coordinator
    25: 335-341
Schaffer H R, Emerson P E 1964 The development of social attachments in infancy.
    Monograph of the Society for Research in Child Development 29
Soule B, Standley K, Copans S 1979 Father identity. Psychiatry 42: 255-263

Spelke E, Zelazo P, Kagan J, Kotelchuck M 1973 Father interaction and separation protest. Developmental Psychology 9: 83–90

Stern D 1974 The goal and structure of mother-infant play. Journal of American Academy of Child Psychiatry 13: 402

Suomi S 1977 Adult male-infant interactions among monkeys living in nuclear families. Child Development 48: 1215–1270

Tinbergen N 1952 The behaviour of the stickleback. Scientific American 187: 28–38

Trethowan W H 1972 The couvade syndrome. In: Howells J (eds) Modern Perspectives in Psycho-obstetrics. Oliver and Boyd, Edinburgh

Trethowan W and Conlon M F 1965 The couvade syndrome. British Journal of Psychiatry 111: 57

U.S. Bureau of the Census 1979 Current Population Reports, Series P-20, No. 341 'Fertility of American Women: June 1978' Washington, DC U.S. Government Printing Office

Waletzky L 1979 Husband's problems with breast-feeding. American Journal of Orthopsychiatry 49: 349–352

West M M, Konner M J 1976 The role of the father: an anthropological perspective. I: Lamb M E (ed) The Role of the Father in Child Development. John Wiley, New York

Whiting B, Whiting J 1975 Children of Six Cultures. Harvard University Press, Cambridge

Yogman M W 1977 The goals and structure of face-to-face interaction between infants and fathers. Paper presented to the Society for Research in Child Development, New Orleans

Yogman M W 1981 Games fathers and mothers play with their infants. Infant Mental Health Journal 2: 241–248

Yogman M W 1982 Development of the father–infant relationship. In: Fitzgerald H, Lester B, Yogman M W (eds) Theory and Research in Behavioural Pediatrics, Vol. I, pp 221–279. Plenum Press, New York

Yogman M, Lester B, Hoffman J 1983 Behavioural and cardiac rhythmicity during mother–father–stranger–infant social interaction. Pediatric Research 17: No. 10

Zaslow M, Pedersen R, Kramer E, Cain R, Suwalsky J, Fivel M 1981 Depressed mood in new fathers. Paper presented to Biennial Meeting of SRCD, Boston

Zelazo P R, Kotelchuck M, Barber L, David J 1977 Fathers and sons: an experimental facilitation of attachment behaviours. Paper presented to the Society for Research in Child Development, New Orleans

The father's influence on infant health

INTRODUCTION

Given the paucity, until recently, of any theoretical or empirical guide to understanding a father's role in early infancy, it is hardly surprising that fathers have been excluded, ignored and patronised in both health promotion and medical management of clinical disorders of infancy. The father's role in the family and with his infant represents important clinical data which should prove essential in promoting child health. While other family members may often be used to describe the father's contributions, in most cases data obtained directly from the father will be more valid. By discussing some general aspects of involving the father in health maintenance visits and a few specific clinical disorders, I hope to illustrate the effects of systematically including fathers in paediatric care on improved health outcomes.

Including fathers as well as mothers in prenatal visits is an effective way of initiating contact directly with the father and establishing trust. However, in this situation we may have to actively engage the father in the interview by posing questions directly to him. If a prenatal visit is not feasible, visits in the newborn nursery become a second opportunity to establish direct contact with the father. Interventions with fathers during this period involving demonstrations of neonatal behaviour (Dolby et al, 1982; Myers, 1982) or demonstrations of caregiving (Johannesson, 1969; Parke et al, 1980) have substantially increased paternal involvement with their infants in the first few months. Given what is known about learning from role models, demonstrations of caregiving by males would be likely to have a greater effect.

Once a trusting relationship has been established with a father, specific problems can sometimes be handled on the telephone and fathers can be offered a specific call hour to use for their questions. For fathers whose work schedule conflicts with office (surgery) hours, evening hours may offer an efficient solution. For each of the health maintenance visits, knowledge of the developmental stage of the father-infant as well as the mother-infant relationship may help one to understand the questions the parents bring to the office visit (Mandell & Yogman, 1982).

146

INFANTS AT BIOLOGICAL RISK

The birth of a high risk infant confronts fathers as well as mothers with a major stress. This may have a direct effect on the father-infant relationship, but it may also have an indirect effect on the infant mediated through the father's support of the mother. The utilisation of supports becomes a major coping mechanism for dealing with stress and the father is the most readily available source of support within the family. Preterm birth is a good example of a major stress.

Following a preterm birth, both mothers and fathers reported more depression, anxiety, emotional turmoil and difficulty caring for the baby than a matched group of parents of full term infants (Jeffcoate et al, 1979). Initially, fathers are often required to play a primary role in decision-making either because the infant has been transferred to a different hospital or because of the physical incapacity of the mother. In a study done in Canada, of preterm infants weighing less than 1500 grams, fathers were first to visit their newborns though subsequently mothers and fathers developed similar visiting patterns. Nursery observations suggest that parents display fairly similar behaviour toward their neonates during these visits (except that fathers were more responsive to newborn limb movements and mothers talked more) (Marton, et al, 1981; Parke & Tinsley, 1982).

Fathers who visit the nursery are likely to be committed to learning about their baby and to participate in caregiving. In one study in progress, the father's behaviour at this initial visit appears to be associated with their behaviour at subsequent contacts during the first month. Fathers who touched and talked to their newborns and visited longer than 15 minutes were more likely to call and visit more frequently during the subsequent 4 weeks (Johnson & Gaiter, 1980). In the context of a longitudinal study of 20 preterm infants, we offered the fathers as well as mothers the opportunity to observe an assessment of their neonate's behaviour (Brazelton, 1973). Half of the fathers participated. These participating fathers were younger and more likely to be having their first baby than non-participants. There was no association between neonatal medical complications and father participation. Compared to the fathers who did not observe this demonstration of neonatal behaviour, the fathers who participated had made more nursery visits in the subsequent month and both they and their wives reported that they were doing more caregiving tasks after the infant was home for 1 month.

Studies of paternal interaction with older preterm infants have produced conflicting findings, in part because the infants are often quite heterogeneous in their medical complications and behavioural difficulties and parental reactions are also variable. In two studies of preterm infants at 3 months post-term, their face-to-face play with fathers and mothers was similar (Marton et al, 1981; Parke & Tinsley, 1982) except for more maternal touching. A study at 4 months post-term found that fathers played more games than mothers with their preterm infants, although less than with full-term infants (Field, 1979b).

We recently completed a longitudinal study of preterm infants over the first 18 months of life in which we looked at how the father's involvement with his infant influenced outcome. First, many of the fathers responded to this stress by providing extensive support to their spouses, both emotional support and physical support by helping with caregiving tasks. While fathers still did far less caregiving than mothers, fathers of the preterm infants reported doing more of the caregiving tasks at 1, 5, and 18 months post term than a comparison group of fathers of fullterm infants. While all fathers helped with diapering, the preterm fathers were more likely to get up at night to console their infant, to bathe the child and to take the infant to a physician. There was some association between obstetric complications and paternal involvement in caregiving so that fathers of newborns with more complications were more involved in caregiving.

Interestingly, there was little relationship between paternal involvement in caregiving and father-infant games seen during a face-to-face play session at 5 months post-term. In this setting, fathers of preterm infants played both fewer and shorter games and fewer arousing games, in particular, than did fathers of full-term infants. Tactile games were the most common games played by fathers of preterm infants. Fathers played fewer games with their preterm infants than mothers did although this is probably the effect of infant fatigue since fathers always interacted with their infants after 9 minutes of mother-infant interaction.

One suggested explanation of these findings is that we are seeing a strong influence of the infant's behaviour on the parent so that in a stressed high risk infant, hypersensitive to stimulation and arousal, father's arousing stimulation drops out while the father attempts to adapt to the individual behaviour of his infant. Given the difficulties of social interaction with a premature infant whose state and motor organisation may be labile (Goldberg, 1978; Field, 1979a) and whose cry seems more aversive to father and mother (Frodi et al, 1978), the tendency of many fathers to excite, play with, and vigorously stimulate their infant may stress an already vulnerable infant, interfere with social interaction, and lead a father to withdraw. Describing the baby's cues (particularly when they are poorly readable) may be of great help to a father in this situation and may offer him a more adaptive alternative to complete withdrawal. Unfortunately, most intervention programmes for high-risk infants do not specifically address the father's role with these infants (Bricker & Bricker, 1976). The expectation that most fathers will not participate quickly becomes a self-fulfilling prophecy unless the father's participation is actively encouraged.

A case example from our longitudinal study should illustrate the difficulties faced by some fathers in making this adjustment:

> 'This male infant is the first infant born to parents in their early thirties, delivered prematurely after a 29-week pregnancy and weighing 1080 grams at

birth. After a prolonged neonatal hospitalisation complicated by respiratory problems, the infant was discharged home at 36 weeks of age weighing 1500 grams to his mother and father. He had considerable problems with sleep, feeding, and crying in the first few weeks at home. Both parents worked at a local TV/radio station and were isolated from their extended families. Father became very involved with the infant, helping with a substantial portion of the caregiving. When the family was seen for the 5 month face-to-face play session, the father interacted with the baby with continual tapping and shaking the infant's limbs in spite of the fact that the infant spent much of the interaction looking away from his father, squirming and finally fussing and crying.'

On the basis of a few families referred for psychiatric help, Herzog (1979) has expressed concern about early increased paternal involvement with the infant at the expense of maternal attachment. Fathers may need permission to express their feelings of fear and grief during the perinatal period even if it violates the stereotype of masculinity. Zilboorg (1931) has examined the interaction between psychodynamic and sociocultural influences on post-partum reactions in men and women and suggests that men are more likely than women to develop symptoms of extreme regression, psychosis, or paranoia because depression is a socially unacceptable symptom in males. According to Zilboorg, society instructs men to view symptoms such as passivity, impotence, and crying as a threat to their self-image. Therefore, professionals working with fathers in a premature nursery may need to view bizarre and regressive behaviour as less pathological than in other situations and as analogous to maternal depression.

Despite the low frequency of games fathers play with preterm infants, we found a significant association between the father's ability to engage his preterm infant in play in the 5 month sessions and the infant's developmental outcome at 9 and 18 months post-term on a Bayley Test. The total number of games played by father ($r = 0.79$) (as well as by both parents combined $r = 0.77$), were significantly correlated ($P < 0.05$) with the Mental Development Index (MDI) at 18 months. The total duration of all games played with both parents was also significantly correlated with MDI scores at 9 and 18 months and with the Psychomotor Index (PDI) at 18 months, while the duration of nonarousing games with both parents was correlated with the MDI at 9 months and the PDI at 18 months. Perhaps this association reflects the infant's behavioural robustness and capacity to engage in play since measures of paternal caregiving involvement and support which were associated with outcome in a fullterm comparison group (see p. 139 in previous chapter) were not associated with outcome in this preterm group. Conceivably, some fathers may react to the stress of a preterm birth by withdrawing and others may become more supportive so that overall support is not associated with outcome. These measures of social interaction were significantly correlated with outcome even though measures of obstetric and paediatric complications and a neonatal neurological exam showed no significant correlations. Beckwith & Cohen (1980) have reported similar findings for social interaction with mothers of preterm infants: infants with higher scores on reciprocal social interaction and severe medical complications performed better at 2 years of age than infants with lower scores on reciprocal social interaction and milder perinatal complications.

CHILD ABUSE AND FAILURE TO THRIVE

The clinical importance of the father's role with young infants is perhaps best illustrated by the literature on child abuse. Green (1979) and Green et al (1974), on the basis of studies of a cohort of 60 abused children in New York, reported that 43% of the children were abused by their fathers or father surrogates and 14% were jointly abused by mothers and fathers. Gil (1970) concurs, reporting that when fathers were present in the home, they were involved in two-thirds of the abusive incidents. He suggests that personality disorders of parent, environmental stresses, and child character-istics are all potentiating factors, just as with abusing mothers (Newberger et al, 1977). Other reviews (Rigler & Spinetta, 1972) suggest that substitute or social fathers (in most cases, a boyfriend) more commonly abuse children conceived from a prior relationship of the mother than biological fathers abuse their own children.

Infants who are failing to thrive suffer from a complex mix of caloric deprivation, behavioural vulnerability and interactive failure with their parents. While neither maternal nor paternal deprivation (Green & Beall, 1962) accurately describe the parenting contributions (which reflect inap-propriate interactions rather than absent interactions), a case example may illustrate the dynamics of the father's contribution to his infant's failure to thrive:

> 'A 12-month-old white male presents with a 4-month history of poor weight gain (failure to thrive), a history of spitting up since early infancy, and two episodes of diarrhoea, one with dehydration requiring a hospital admission. The family consists of mother, a 28-year-old of French Canadian extraction whose extended family now lives nearby; a 3-year-old female sibling; and father, a 28-year-old truck driver of Portuguese ancestry from a very deprived background. The parents had labelled their infant as medically ill and vulner-able. Mother was quite depressed and one of her major symptoms was with-holding food from her hungry infant whenever he developed a minor illness in the hope of protecting him from a medical complication. Father was frequently away for long periods up to a week at a time for his job as a long distance driver. When he was home, he spent a great deal of time interacting with his son but his interactions with his son went beyond the vigorous, arousing play of a typical father. He would abruptly withdraw from the inter-action in a teasing fashion without any effort to prepare his infant or to modulate his aggression and anger.'

In this case, father's deprived background and resultant anger became a major determinant of marital conflict, mother's depression and interactive failure with his infant. Obviously, adequate management of such an infant requires direct intervention with father as well as mother.

PATERNAL GRIEF: SUDDEN INFANT DEATH

Paternal responses to sudden unexplained infant death are another instance in which health professionals must be sensitive to the father's grief reaction as well as to the mother's. (The term 'health professionals' is used to cover all those concerned with child health including paediatrician, general practitioner, health visitor, paediatric nurse, etc.) In a study of 46 such families (Mandell et al, 1980), in which both parents were interviewed, several identifiable mourning patterns seemed more characteristic of men: (1) the necessity to keep busy with extra jobs or increased work loads; (2) a feeling of diminished self-worth; (3) self-blame because of lack of 'care' involvement; and (4) a marked inability to ask for help. Health care providers often seemed unwittingly to promote masculine stoicism and managerial functions which may serve to obstruct the full expression of grief. While mothers often request help, their presenting problems were often their concerns about the fathers who would not ask for help. On the basis of these interviews, the authors suggest that if fathers are given an opportunity to express feelings and a validation of their feelings, they will constructively utilise support. The task for the health professional is to respond to masculine expressions of distress as well as to the more overt feminine ones.

A case example best illustrates the way the father's responses become crucial to managing the problems of the older sibling:

> 'Mother comes to your office for follow-up 3 months after having lost an infant from SIDS. Father is 28 and has just taken on a second job because he says they need the income. When you ask, she admits that her husband seems irritable and angry, but when she tries to discuss the baby, he says he'd rather not talk about it or think about it. Meanwhile, he is spending much less time with their 8-year-old daughter who now has asleep disturbance and for the first time, has failed a subject in school in which she previously did well.'

This case exemplifies the importance of having established a direct relationship with the father prior to this tragedy so that one can help this father to move beyond his defensive withdrawal and allow himself to grieve and express his feelings. Grief reactions associated with any loss (parent, or even more rarely a spouse) may have a major impact on any subsequent pregnancy as well.

HANDICAPPED INFANTS

The paternal response to the birth of a retarded or defective infant is similar in some ways to his response to the sudden loss of a child. When informed, fathers are less emotional and expressive than mothers and ask questions about future problems (Price-Bonham & Addison, 1978). Gath's (Gath, 1974) case control study of families experiencing the birth of an infant with Down's syndrome suggests that the birth resulted in severe degrees of marital tension and strain during the subsequent 18 months. The study also

suggested that the source of marital tension was commonly sexual dissatisfaction, which may have been a reflection of the fact that the father needs
to mourn just as the mother needs to after having produced a defective
offspring.

These fathers are often expected by extended family members to be strong
and invincible and moreover to rectify the situation and make the child well
again regardless of how unrealistic that may be. The communication of
complex information by medical professionals to these families makes it
imperative that fathers be present, since otherwise mother is put in the
awkward position of translating information from physician to father.
Fathers as well as mothers of these infants must grapple with the issue of
focussing on the normal developmental strengths as well as the handicaps of
these infants so that they are not being over-protective and treating the
infants as excessively vulnerable.

BEHAVIOURAL PROBLEMS OF INFANTS AND TODDLERS

When a health professional is asked for help with the behavioural problems
of infants and toddlers, meeting with the father as well as the mother may
be essential to understanding these problems and helping the family find
solutions. For example, helping a family whose baby is persistently fussy
may require establishing a strong alliance between the parents that supports
them both and avoids placing responsibility or blame on either. Sleep problems are another example. Difficulties in bedtime settling may be exacerbated
if the father arrives home just before bedtime, elicits the predictable excited
reaction from the baby, and then attempts to convince the baby to go to
sleep. Night terrors in infants between 15 and 30 months have been related
to the loss, either partial or complete, of the father at this time (Herzog,
1980). Persistent waking at night can create substantial marital tension.
Issues such as who goes to the baby, do the parents take the baby into bed,
and the impact of sleep loss on the parent's job may become major sources
of conflict between parents and result in a fixed symptom for the infant. By
directly talking with fathers as well as mothers about these problems, the
health professional can diffuse some of the tension while remaining the
child's advocate.

Although scheduling office visits when working parents can come is often
difficult, it is surprising how willing fathers are to modify their own schedules
in order to come to see a health professional when they are concerned about
their infant and when they believe that the health professional is really willing
to listen to them. When parents are having difficulties with their child's
negativism or with discipline and control during the second year, discussions
with the father as well as the mother may be crucial. Toddlers are unusually
capable of highlighting any inconsistencies between mothers and fathers in
discipline and limit-setting. Unless parents have an opportunity to discuss

their feelings about the child's behaviour and with each other, they may find themselves competing for the child's favor and exacerbating the problems. By discussing the situation with fathers and mothers together in a few extended counseling visits, the health professional can be very helpful in either alleviating the problems or helping the parents to accept a referral for more intensive therapy.

ADOLESCENT FATHERS

Given the current concern about teenage pregnancy, the needs of the adolescent father must also be addressed. Recent US reviews suggest that one teenage boy in 10–20 will father a premarital pregnancy and that 20% of all births to teenage girls are fathered by adolescent males (Elster and Panzarine, 1981). These fathers have an established relationship with their girlfriends when conception occurs, and usually maintain it following delivery (Platts, 1968; Ewer & Gibbs, 1975). Almost 2/3 of teenage mothers get some financial help from the father.

While these fathers often remain involved with their infants, they may have little or no knowledge of infant development and have unrealistic expectations. Some of these boys are also depressed (Elster & Panzarine, 1980) and themselves need both educational and psychological services. Even when matched for social class, they are less likely to graduate from high school (Elster & Panzarine, 1981).

It is obviously difficult to reach the adolescent father but enlisting the support of the girlfriend, seeing the couple together and creating a role for the father at the visit has been suggested. The father's initial reaction to the pregnancy, in particular the presence of depressive symptoms, has been found to be a good screen for the male's later adaptation to fatherhood (Elster & Panzarine, 1981). Information on his supports, future plans for the relationship with the mother, and for his education and vocation can also be obtained.

Many of these fathers sustain an investment in their infant long after their emotional relationship with the baby's mother has ended. In fact, the father's parents often play an active role as substitute caregivers or even primary caregivers if the mother gives the child up. Health professionals may find themselves in the middle of this complex web if the mother begins to amplify symptoms or illnesses in the baby as a way of maintaining a relationship with the father. An optimal role for the professional in this situation must be to remain the advocate for the child, and I believe that this often requires direct communication with the father as well as the mother. Unfortunately, such contact is often difficult to arrange, a problem very few programmes have addressed. Given the continuing involvement of these fathers with their infants, our exclusion of fathers and our failure to provide educational and social support for paternal roles leaves fathers uninformed about infant care, infant competencies, and infant needs. To be truly effective in reaching adolescent males, such education should be offered as part of a school curriculum (Sawin & Parke, 1976).

CUSTODY ISSUES IN INFANCY

The more active role in child-rearing played by fathers has begun to influence child custody decisions in divorce cases. Courts have begun to award contested custody to fathers (10% of cases in one U.S. study) (Weitzman & Dixon, 1979), and joint custody arrangements are becoming more common. I believe that health professionals must become forceful advocates for the child's interests in these situations and must make this role explicit to the parents. The difficulty often lies in coordinating the child's needs for consistent, stable, secure caregiving with the needs to maintain the already established relationship with both parents. Whenever possible, parental counselling and mediation serve the child's interests more than a contested court struggle.

In the few limited follow-up studies comparing the effects of different custody arrangements on older children, parental cooperation appears to be more highly related to outcome than is any specific custody arrangement (Abarbanel, 1979; Warshak & Santrock, 1979). Thompson (1983) suggests that better long-term adaptations are helped by minimizing the transitions for the infant in the first year after divorce. Others have suggested that children do better with the same sex parent (Santrock & Warshak, 1979) but the real debate is whether the courts are equipped to decide which is the 'psychological parent' who can meet the 'best interests' of the child (Goldstein et al, 1973).

Single parents, both mothers and fathers, are increasingly common in the United States, and the demands on them to play dual roles often require that the health professional be a supportive listener, educator, and at times, interpreter for the child. Not only are fathers becoming single parents as a result of divorce or the death of a spouse, but single males are becoming adoptive parents as well (Levine, 1976). In the United States census, 324 000 males were single parents. Although it is estimated that only 1% of children are reared by primary caretaker fathers in this country, more than 15% of children under age 14 are cared for by fathers while the mothers work, and health professionals must increasingly deal with the concerns of these fathers as well.

In summary, these are just a few examples of the importance of understanding the father-infant relationship for more effective management of child health problems.

CONCLUSION

In spite of all that has been written about the father-infant relationship, new questions have replaced the old ones. The competence of fathers and infants to develop a significant and successful relationship is well established. While the fathers' role as play partner for the infant has been a consistent finding, the robustness of this finding remains to be seen. Our understanding of the influence of context on what the father actually does with his infant is just beginning but is likely to have important clinical implications.

In the meantime, the major clinical application of this research is that it emphasises the importance of getting to know fathers and of understanding their relationship with their infants in order to play the most effective role in promoting child health. Only when we begin systematically to include fathers in our preventive work and in our diagnostic assessments and treatments will we be facilitating the father-infant relationship. Finally, given our limited knowledge, any efforts to change clinical care or hospital policy toward fathers should aim to increase the options available to fathers as well as mothers rather than promoting specific alternative prescriptions.

REFERENCES

Abarbanel A 1979 Shared parenting after separation and divorce: a study of joint custody. American Journal of Orthopsychiatry 49: 320–328

Beckwith L, Cohen S E 1980 Interactions of preterm infants with their caregivers and test performance at age 2. In: Field T (ed) High Risk Infants and Children, pp. 155–178. Academic Press, New York

Brazelton T B 1973 Neonatal Behavioral Assessment Scale. J B. Lippincott Co, Philadelphia

Bricker W A, Bricker D A 1976 The infant, toddler, and preschool research and intervention project. In: Tjossem T D Intervention Strategies for High Risk Infants and Young Children. University Park Press, Baltimore

Dolby R, English B, Warren B 1982 Brazelton demonstrations for mothers and fathers. Paper presented to International Conference on Infant Studies, Austin, Texas.

Elster A B, Panzarine S 1980 Unwed teenage fathers. Journal of Adolescent Health Care 1: 116–120

Elster A, Panzarine S 1981 The adolescent father. Seminars in Perinatology 5: 29–51

Ewer P, Gibbs J 1975 Relationship with putative father and use of contraception in a population of Black ghetto addolescent mothers. Public Health Reports 90: 417

Field T M 1979a Interaction patterns of preterm and full-term infants. In: Field T M (ed) Infants Born at Risk: Behavior and Development. SP Medical and Scientific Books, New York

Field T 1979b Games parents play with normal and high-risk infants. Child Psychiatry and Human Development 10: 41–48

Frodi A, Lamb M, Leavitt L, Donovan W, Neff C, Sherry D 1978 Fathers' and mothers' responses to the faces and cries of normal and premature infants. Developmental Psychology 14: 490–498

Gath A 1974 The impact of an abnormal child upon the parents. British Journal of Psychiatry 125: 568

Gil D 1970 Violence Against Children. Harvard University Press, Cambridge

Goldberg S 1978 Prematurity: effects on parent-infant interaction. Journal of Pediatric Psychology 3: 137–144

Goldstein J, Freud A, Solnit A 1973 Beyond the Best Interests of the Child. The Free Press, New York

Green A H 1979 Child-abusing fathers. Journal of the American Academy of Child Psychiatry 18: 270–282

Green A H, Gaines R, Sandgrund A 1974 Child abuse. American Journal of Psychiatry 131: 882–886

Green M, Beall P 1962 Paternal deprivation—a disturbance in fathering—a report of nineteen cases. Pediatrics 30: 91–99

Herzog J 1979 Disturbances in parenting high-risk infants: Clinical impressions and hypotheses. In: Field T M (ed) Infants Born at Risk. Spectrum Publications, New York
Herzog J M 1980 Sleep disturbance and father hunger in 18-to-28 month-old boys. Psychoanalytic Study of the Child 35: 219–233
Jeffcoate J A, Humphrey M E, Lloyd J K 1979 Role perception and response to stress in fathers and mothers following pre-term delivery. Social Science and Medicine 1304: 139–145
Johannesson, Patricia 1969 Instruction in child care for fathers. Dissertation at University of Stockholm
Johnson A, Gaiter J L 1980 Father-infant bonding in the intensive care nursery. Work in progress, Children's Hospital National Medical Center
Levine J A 1976 Who will raise the children? New options for fathers. J J Lippincott, Philadelphia
Mandell F, McAnulty E, Reece R 1980 Observations of paternal response to sudden unexplained infant death. Pediatrics 65: 221–225
Mandell F, Yogman M W 1982 The use of child development during well child visits. Journal of Developmental and Behavioral Pediatrics 3: 118–122
Marton P, Minde K, Perrotta M 1981 The role of the father for the infant at risk. American Journal of Orthopsychiatry. 51: 672–679
Myers B J 1982 Early intervention using Brazelton training with middle class mothers and fathers of newborns. Child Development 53: 462–471
Newberger E, Reed R B, Daniel J H, Hyde J, Kotelchuck M 1977 Pediatric social illness: toward an etiologic classification. Pediatrics 60: 178–185
Parke R, Hymel S, Power T, Tinsley B 1980 Fathers and risk: a hospital based model of intervention. In: Sawin D B, Hawkes R C, Walker L O, Penticuff J H (eds) Psychosocial Risks in Infant Environment Transactions, Vol. 4. Bruner Mazel, New York
Parke R D, Tinsley B 1982 The early environment of the at risk infant. In: Bricker D D (ed) Intervention with At-Risk and Handicapped Infants, pp 153–177. University Park Press, Baltimore
Platts K 1968 A public agency's approach to the natural father. Child Welfare 47: 530
Price-Bonham S and Addison S 1978 Families and mentally retarded children: emphasis on the father. The Family Coordinator 27: 221–230
Rigler D, Spinetta J 1972 The child-abusing parent: a psychological review. Psychological Bulletin 77: 296
Santrock J W, Warshak R A 1979 Father custody and social development in boys and girls. Journal of Social Issues 35: 112–125
Sawin D, Parke R 1976 Adolescent fathers: Some implications from recent research on paternal roles. Educational Horizons 55: 38–43
Thompson R 1983 The father's case in child custody disputes. In: Lamb M E, Sagi A (eds) Fatherhood and Social Policy. Erlbaum, Hillsdale
Warshak R, Santrock J W 1979 The effects of father and mother custody on children's social development. Paper presented to the Society for Research in Child Development, San Francisco
Weitzman L J, Dixon R B 1979 Child custody awards: legal standards and empirical patterns for child custody, support and visitation after divorce. University of California Davis Law Review 12: 472–521
Zilboorg G 1931 Depressive reactions to parenthood. American Journal of Psychiatry 10: 927

Language development in the young child

INTRODUCTION

The sophistication of human communication which not only allows us to talk to each other now, but also to remember information from the past is fundamental to the success of the human species. Given this, it is surprising how little attention the early students of human behaviour paid to trying to understand the problem of language development. Freud, for example, stressed during the second year of life not the blossoming of language, but the achievement of bowel control. The early psychologists such as Watson and Skinner, who saw most learning as a mechanical process, regarded language as something which was simply learnt by imitation of adults and failed to stress its importance in relation to understanding the way people think and children develop.

All this changed about 25 years ago and one can pick out two seminal workers who have led to today's enormous expansion in our knowledge and understanding of language development. The first was Professor Brown at Harvard University who started collecting detailed information on tape of a child's language development. He soon recognised what a wealth of data such studies generated and began the struggle with the methological problems of how one should understand the data one acquires. Second was the work of the flamboyant Professor Chomsky who startled the psychological world with his suggestion that the brain contained some essential pre-programmed part—a language learning device with grammar already embedded which was really responsible for the child acquiring language and that the fundamental issue in understanding language development was to look therefore at brain mechanisms rather than emphasize the importance of incoming stimuli. The provocative nature of his ideas together with the steady analytical work of Brown and others has lead to a huge expansion of work by psychologists and linguists into the nature of language development and the field is now such a vast one that the simple clinician trying to apply some of the new information to understanding the children who are brought to see him can reasonably feel bewildered as to where to begin. In this paper I am going to try and summarise some of the more recent findings which have clear implications for children whose speech and language development is delayed.

PRE-NATAL DEVELOPMENT

Unlike virtually every other part of the body, the middle ear with its ear ossicles and the cochlea are initially laid down at their full adult size. This is essential because if the three ear ossicles grew throughout childhood they would not deliver a consistent vibration to the inner ear and the child would have the confusion of changing signals reaching his brain at different ages. In consequence the system is capable of receiving sounds from an early stage and there is no question that the fetus responds to sounds *in utero* probably from mid-term onwards. Mothers will report that her fetus kicks her if a loud noise is transmitted to the baby and all sorts of claims have been made for the importance of the sounds that a child receives *in utero*, in terms of later development. What in fact is the childs hearing? If, by way of the cervix, you place a microphone into the uterus of a human, or more readily into that of an animal and measure the level of sound reaching the fetus's ear, it is surprisingly high—something in the order of 70 to 90 decibels—a noise level which adults find almost intolerable. These sounds are caused by movement of air around the intestines and movement of blood through the placenta and uterine wall. It seems likely that the infant can also hear her mother's voice and it has been suggested that the fetus gets accustomed to its sound before she is born and indeed the mother's voice is almost certainly transmitted to the child.

A much more important task that the infant probably learns at this time is the ability to ignore certain sounds: this subsequently leads her onto selective attention—deciding what she will listen to—not the background noise of the car in the street but the voice of the person who is speaking to her. Thus a new born baby will happily sleep in her pram near a main road but may wake up when her mother speaks to her.

On the output side the child has in time first to learn to control and integrate the activities of the lungs working, as it were, as a pair of bellows to deliver air streams through the vocal apparatus to make sound—modified by integrated movements of tongue, lips, pharynx and larynx. Movements of these parts of the body can be observed *in utero*, using radio opaque dye injected into the amniotic cavity, which is then swallowed. Thus the fetus possibly 'practices' making the appropriate movements which subsequently allow her to use the system for meaningful communication as soon as she is born. While we do not yet fully understand the way these different mechanisms develop *in utero*, as soon as the baby is born we can identify a very effective communications system.

THE NEWBORN BABY

Shortly after birth, the baby can hear sounds throughout the whole human voice range and her ability to locate them is quite good (Turner & Macfarlane, 1978). Indeed it seems better at this time than it is at the age of 2 or

3 months. She tends to respond most to sounds made in the human voice range and turns more to the human voice sounds than pure tones. This is explicable on the basis of earlier myelination of some fibres of the auditory nerve than others. Later, at around 10 days, it is possible to demonstrate that the baby is able to discriminate between the sounds of her own mother's voice from other sounds in general and the sound of other adult women in particular. Such directed head-turning can of course only occur when she is in a position to make it and given her problem with head control it is best to carry out such testing when the child is lying in a cot or even better with her head supported in some sort of cradle.

The response is not stereotyped and the clinician may find it quite difficult to elicit it at the specific time when he/she sees the baby. The baby must also be in the 'alert awake' state (not crying) for a response to be seen.

On the output side the child is born with a sophisticated signalling system to indicate her wants. Scandinavian workers (Wasz-Hockert et al, 1968) have demonstrated that there are different qualities to the cry and although this signal rapidly turns into a generalised distress signal mothers are able to distinguish between the 'hunger' cry of a baby and the 'pain' cry even though they are often unaware of the part it plays in their assessment of the child's wants. The cry is a most powerful biological sign. It arouses enormous emotion in the mother as she first hears it and for both parents it is a signal that is hard to ignore—it is an expression of need, the child wants something and when it cannot be interpreted, parents can become distressed.

The fact that the baby seems programmed to focus her attention on her mother, and the sounds she makes to her, and the mother equally responds to the child is an essential prerequisite on which language can be built.

PHONETICS AND PHONOLOGY

One of the first tasks the child has to achieve before she can use speech as a method of language communication is to develop a full range of sounds. The human speech sounds vary from language to language, some languages such as Chinese involve the use of different qualities to those that are used in English. When born, the baby clearly has the potential to acquire any language but as everyone knows as she becomes older it becomes increasingly difficult to acquire the skill to make the sounds of another language. Apart from the cry, the first sounds the baby makes are largely vowel sounds and guttural noises at the back of the throat.

As she begins to sit up more she makes clicking and blowing noises at the front of her mouth and around about 5 months or so the first consonatal sound. Any consonantal structure involves complicated movements of the lips against the palate and teeth and subtle control of the air stream; blending the two together is clearly a highly complicated activity.

The first consonantal sounds heard in English children are often a G or a D sound, with others following rapidly—though there is much individual

Table 13.1 Most frequently mispronounced, substituted or omitted sounds in 80 children with specific developmental speech disorders and 112 normal children

Sounds	% with defective sounds	
	Group 1	Group 2
r	78	37
S (sh)	74	15
o (thing)	66	31
s	63	5
l	62	1
k	36	12
tS (church)	34	13
d₃ (hedge)	34	13
g	26	9
f	20	6
v	17	—
p	17	1
b	17	—

Group 1: 80 children with specific developmental speech disorders
Group 2: sample group of 112 unselected children aged 3½ years (Morley, 1957)

variation in the way consonants are developed. During the second year the child becomes able to make enough consonantal sounds to be fully understood, although some sounds go on being acquired throughout the pre-school years. The 5-years-old child still has difficulty with sounds like the voiced 'Th', and may still have one or two other problems and if she has three or more consonantal substitutions her speech should be reviewed (See Table 13.1).

Apart from the issue of single sounds, the babbling 3-month-old is putting chains of noises together which develop increasing complexity until, around the 8-month stage, it begins to be possible to identify sounds associated with different languages. The production of this babble is at least in part generated within the central nervous system independent of input because congenitally deaf babies will also babble. The presence therefore of sound making is not good evidence of intact hearing. However, around the age of 7 or 8 months the babble of the deaf baby begins to diminish unless vigorous steps are made to sustain it.

What is the deaf child missing? As mentioned the system by which a received sound is converted into a nervous impulse is normally fully functional at birth. Signals are transmitted by the auditory nerve to the auditory cortex. How does the brain go about making sense of them. The visual cortex recognises certain patterns (e.g. obliques as against verticals) and probably the auditory cortex has a similar mechanism for recognising certain segments of sound.

The incoming signal is decoded and in the adult recognised as a meaningful signal. In order to do this the system must *selectively* attend to certain sounds, and decode those which are parts of language. In other words extraneous sounds (such as street noises) are largely ignored while the child concentrates on listening to and decoding the sounds which it *chooses* to hear. In certain children it is possible to demonstrate that although sounds reach the auditory cortex they are subsequently ignored; such children are spoken of as being centrally deaf.

When a foreign language which we do not understand is spoken, we *hear* it (it is transmitted to the auditory cortex) we *listen* to it (we recognise its segmental qualities and think this person is communicating to us) but we are unable to *decode* it. The decoding process is thus clearly a very complex one especially for the child and she likes to be close to the speaker often using the additional visual cue of lip reading to help her in the process. The visual aspect of this communication is easily observed as the 8-month-old baby converses with her mothers, staring intently at her face.

(Phonetics studies the sound system of speech and phonology is concerned with meaningful sound system which are appropriate to the language being spoken. A phonological error therefore would involve the child consistently mispronouncing a sound within a language. The most famous example of this of course is the biblical one of a *s*ibboleth and *sh*ibboleth).

DEVELOPMENT OF IDEAS OF SELF AND TURN TAKING

A prerequisite for communication is that the child should recognise herself as an individual and then be interested in interacting in a systematic way with other people. There is not space to review the enormous amount of work which has been done in the last two or three decades on attachment behaviour between the infant and those around him but simply to stress here that by the time the child is 5 or 6 months old he knows clearly his immediate adults and becomes distressed if they leave him.

That is to say she has identified her mother and father as distinct and separate individuals in contrast to other human beings. Round about this time she also achieves the notion that objects (including people) exist when they are not in her immediate presence. She looks for objects that are missing and begins to show such behaviour as looking towards the door to see whether her father is arriving home. In recognising that there are other people in the world she must begin to have some concept of herself as an individual, separate from the rest of the world and able therefore to receive and initiate communications. Initially we see this communication going on in the form of games; the child at the age of around 8 or 9 months sitting in a chair will, with delight, throw objects onto the floor—wait until they have been picked up again and then repeat the game. An older brother or sister is an ideal playmate for this type of repetitive activity but it does involve turn taking which is of course the essential basis for conversation. We see at this time therefore delight by the child in 'conversation' with her mother: that is to say she makes a string of babbling noises and she responds to them while the child listens and then makes a further contribution. This 'turn taking' may be observed in 'babbling' play with her mother under six months of age.

As her manipulative skills develop and she is able to make hand gestures she begins to use these to make demands and the vigorous 10- to 12-month-old child who points at things is in the process of developing her communication system. She learns the very favourite gesture of waving good-bye and again this becomes a turn taking game. Gesture has been developed by deaf people so that they communicate through a sign system. Such sign systems are now also used with handicapped people. Evidence suggests that far from inhibiting speech development signing helps communication. Signing and speech are both *mediums* for expressing *language* and are usually used simultaneously. Language is hard to define but put at its simplest it is the inner symbolisation of thought and the world around us.

It is interesting to note that sign systems while probably rarely achieving the complexity of the spoken language are easier to learn than the spoken system so that children of deaf parents acquire their first (signed) words earlier than ordinary children. Also mentally handicapped children seem to find signing easier than speech.

The inflexion in the child's voice begins to assume different qualities under different circumstances—an enquiring grunt when she is simply pointing at something to draw your attention to it or the more frustrated or angry grunt when she is demanding to be given food or something that she desperately wants. The prosodic or inflexional qualities of speech remain important throughout life—the enormous range of meaning we can give to the word 'yes' reflect this. Prosodic elements in vocalisation—rising falling melody forms—in sounds like 'da da' become apparent during the second half of the first year.

It is difficult to be certain of the significance of the very first words when these emerge. They are usually naming words for members of her family and possibly for animals and they seem to many observers to have different qualities to the words which emerge later on in the second year around about the 15–17 month period. Certainly sounds are beginning to be blended into shapes; Crystal and his colleagues at Reading, back-tracking to earlier tapes that they had made of a particular baby, found that they were picking out the sounds which became a distinctive word at 15 or 16 months, in the first year of life, given they knew the form in which the word eventually emerged. It is impossible to say whether these sounds really have meaning for the child in the sense that words do later, 'ad' or 'da' is seen sometimes to the parents to be used appropriately for father but disconcertingly the baby may suddenly start pointing at many other individuals using the same label. While these processes are going on it is extremely difficult to identify what precise role the adults (usually parents) around the child are playing.

Without them the child would not learn to talk, but attempts to 'teach' a child particular words often leave them frustrated (e.g. the child who says Dad before Mum). Later on perhaps it is easier to see the adult's role as correction and example, restricting the use of an individual word to its precise meaning. But during the first year and early part of the second year what we observe is the parent initiating 'games of communication' rather than succeeding in initiating particular vocalisations, although paradoxically we can also often observe a great deal of imitation of sounds.

INTO LANGUAGE

What are the processes which allow the child to use words with meaning? One suggestion has been that the child has a mechanism which allows him to recognise appropriate segments of sounds. These exists in all languages and are the basis for the analysis that all children must make of the incoming sound to make sense of it. Thus, if you listen to a foreign language, while its meaning may not be understandable to everybody, most people seem to be able to separate it into appropriate structures. They recognise qualities of speech even though they don't know the meaning. At the same time the child is certainly blending his own sound system into discreet outputs which of course eventually form intelligible words to the observer. On the cognitive side, the child is recognising that objects have characteristics that distinguish the one from another. They have different shapes, textures, weight consistencies by which she identifies them as she explores with her hands and prehensile fingers. Can she associate 'differences' with labels—labels emitted as words? Language is a system of classifying the world and often therefore the first words are labelling words such as 'car', 'doggie' and so on. Equally the child wants to use words which effect the world like 'up' 'want' 'more'. These expressive words may communicate not only wants but feelings— 'naughty' is another early word. These early words of course get generalised to a very much larger range of objects than is appropriate, for example, the child will initially use the word 'doggie' to apply to all four legged animals e.g. cows and cats.

What is quite striking however is how quickly she begins to correct this and makes sophisticated distinction; for example, she begins to learn the doglike features of dogs despite their enormous ranges of shape and size whereby she distinguishes them from sheep and cats. How these distinctions are made is often surprising. For example, I once showed a group of 3-year-olds from the Isle of Wight a picture of a double decker bus and was startled that unlike London children quite a number of them referred to it as a car or a lorry. These children saw double decker buses in their own environment but they were green not *red* as in my picture.

The number of words that a child learns varies greatly but the average two-year-old has a vocabulary of 200 words (although it is extremely time consuming and difficult to find out what words they do know). One has to distinguish words whose meaning they understand, so that if you ask the child to find you a fork she will pick it up but if you hold a fork up to her in the air she may refer to it as 'spoon'. This distinction between receptive language — words which she understands, and expressive language — words which she speaks, is obviously an important one.

FIRST SENTENCES

If the understanding of the way in which single words emerge is still ill understood the development of grammar and sentence structure is equally if not more difficult to comprehend. Various chimpanzees have been taught to 'sign' up to 50 single 'words' but they never go on to develop sentence structures and the fact that they can label various 'wants' such as a banana, does not mean that they are capable of developing the sophisticated type of communication system that we identify as human. The development of grammar is essential to develop communication beyond the labelling stage. Thus, 'cat chase dog' means the opposite to 'dog chase cat' and even single word order alone is essential to the meaning. It certainly seems likely that there are innate brain mechanisms which underlie sentence development. One feature of the early sentence a child has is that they are not copies of the sentences which adults are using around him but they are instead particular to children.

These are sometimes referred to as 'telegrammatic speech'; they follow a consistent pattern and they indicate that the child has a grammar system or rule system which he is clearly using. Although two word utterances begin to be used around the age of 2, various studies suggest that about 65% of utterances at 2 years are still single word utterances. One assessment of the developing complexity of speech is measurement of minimum length of utterance by simply counting the number of words which occur in the child's sentences; this development is quite slow during the period between 2 and 3. By $4\frac{1}{2}$ the mean length of a sentence is coming up about five words but many are shorter. Beyond this simple count, the analysis of early sentence structures becomes complex and is a matter of considerable debate among linguists who find it difficult to produce even simple rules to describe their structures. One can however note certain features; for example, that the child may either correctly identify the position of the word or not, so she might use a sentence like 'all gone car' or 'car all gone' where only the two words 'all gone' are consistently used in their correct place relative to another. Prosodic information (i.e. emphasis on words like 'doggie hurt' which could mean according to the child's intonation 'Is the dog hurt?' or 'the dog has hurt me!') are other important elements in early language and indeed persist throughout life. But the reader who wishes to become involved in understanding some of these issues must refer to more extensive texts such as Fletcher & Garman (1979).

NEUROPHYSIOLOGICAL CONSIDERATIONS

The task of relating some of the findings above to possible morphological features of the central nervous system is a difficult one but it is worth examining some of the relevant information which comes from looking at adults with aphasia. These findings relate to the notions which have been outlined above; for example, the separation between 'vocabulary'and the construction of sentences. Thus in Broca's aphasia, speech is poorly articulated and effortful, and tends to be dramatically impoverished, whereas in Wernick's aphasia the patient is fluent and articulates normally but the production is devoid of content and prone to error (a very useful review of these issues is by Saffron (1982) from which I quote). Anomic aphasia is actually a difficulty of word finding and this may be very specific (i.e. in relation to proper names only). Quite clearly this information ought to help us to have ideas about how language is developing and which parts of the brain is being used and such theoretical juxtapositions are clearly going to become more important in the future.

One other group of patients who have excited some interest are those who have a deficit of short-term memory. It is clear that in order to comprehend a sentence one must retain the earlier parts of a sentence while listening and absorbing the latter parts, for the utterance to make sense. Certain patients have been described who have problems of short-term memory (such as a shortened digit span) and have displayed curious problems with language. Thus Saffron and Merin (reviewed in Saffron, 1982) report a patient who when asked to repeat the following sentence 'the residence was located in a peaceful neighbourhood' produced 'the residence was situated in a quiet district', a suggestion that while the conceptual basis of what was going on was being absorbed, perhaps into the permanent memory store, the lexical and semantic aspects of the sentence was not being stored. Saffron makes a distinction between firstly a conceptual system which is described as a general purpose system of the representation of knowledge, inferential processes etc, and secondly a lexical semantic system—a system of units each of which corresponds to a word in the language and each unit incorporating the definition of a word in the form of instructions for projection onto units in the conceptual system. She also derives from this lexical semantics system what she calls an 'output logogen' system in which each word in the language is represented in the form of a phonological code that can be utilised by the speech production system. Each of these systems must be represented in the brain.

THE CLINICAL PROBLEM

The perplexities at all levels in our understanding of how language is acquired and the implication that the process is indeed a complex one make it hardly surprising to find that delayed speech and language development is the most common developmental disorder in childhood. The clinician faced with a child who has such problems has to be aware that the problem may arise at many different levels: in the external environment (in terms of the stimulus that the child is receiving), at a simple level on the input side— be it a problem at the conductive level to the inner ear or a simple relay of the signal to the auditory cortex (a nerve deafness), within the process of decoding the signal and presumably supplying it to the conceptual system, in handling it conceptually—deciding to make a response and then in constructing a response first at a conceptual level, then at the lexical semantic system and then in the form of phonological code that can be utilised for speech production. Even after this the speech apparatus itself might have a defect in it which might itself be at a neurological level such as the interference with the breathing mechanism or actually be at a mechanical level as say in a cleft palate. I have not in this chapter said anything about speech and language disorders but I simply stress here the importance of normal development. A first essential in helping children with a disorder is adequate diagnostic work, based on this understanding and this has been so rudimentary in the past that it is perhaps not surprising that attempts at evaluating therapy have been few. The iconoclast derides a successful diagnostic process as a time wasting procedure when there is no appropriate therapy. But without adequate understanding of the nature of a childhood language it is difficult to see how effective therapy for language disorders can be devised.

REFERENCES

Crystal D, Fletcher P, Garman M 1976 The Grammatical Analysis of language Disability. Edward Arnold, London.
Fletcher P and Garman M 1979 Language Acquisition. Cambridge University Press, Cambridge
Morley M E 1961 The Development and Disorders of speech in Childhood. E & S Livingstone, Edinburgh
Saffron E M 1982 Neuro-psychological approaches to the study of Language. British Journal of Psychology 73: 317–337
Turner S and Macfarlane A 1978 Localisation of human speech by the Newborn Baby and the Effects of Pethidine ('Mereridine'). Development Medicine and Child Neurology. 20. 727–734
Wasz-Hockert O, Lind J, Vuorenkoski V, Partanen T, Volanne E 1968 The Infant Cry—A Spectographic and Auditory Analysis. S.I.M.P/Heineman, London.

FURTHER READING

Bullowa (Ed). 1979 Before speech: The beginning of Interpersonel Communication. Cambridge University Press, Cambridge
Elliot A J 1981 Child Language. Cambridge University Press, Cambridge
Fry D B 1979 The Physics of Speech. Cambridge University Press, Cambridge
Olson D R (Ed) 1980 The social Foundation of Language and Thought. W. W. Norton and Company, New York
Snow C, Furguson C (Eds) 1977. Talking to Children: Language Input and Acquisition. Cambridge University Press, Cambridge
de Villiers P A, de Villiers J G 1979 Early Language 'da-da'. Fontana/Open Books, London

Socio-economic factors related to child health

INTRODUCTION

This chapter examines the way in which the social environment of Britain in the 1980s makes its mark upon the health of its children.* The examination is based on an obvious and deceptively simple fact. The majority of Britain's children grow up in families: less than 1% are cared for in residential institutions like long stay hospitals and local authority homes. Child health is first and foremost a family responsibility. It is thus dependent upon the capacity of parents, and mothers in particular, to secure the resources known to be necessary for sound physical and mental development. Specifically, the welfare of children is determined by the capacity of parents to provide safe accommodation, a reasonable diet and access to good quality health care and to protect their children against physical and emotional trauma. This simple fact opens up two areas for the chapter to explore; areas, however, in which the issues are complex and, as yet, only partially understood.

Firstly, since children are cared for in families, their health is closely tied to the distribution of resources *between* families. We know that health-promoting resources are not randomly distributed across the population. Instead, children who benefit from one such resource—a safe home for example—are likely to enjoy the benefits of good food and good health care as well. Material deprivations of various kinds are similarly related: children in poor health tend to suffer from a cluster of such deprivations. Because of the dependency of children upon the economic position of their parents, the patterns of child health follow the contours of social class. In fact, it is in the patterns of childhood morbidity and mortality that the reality of class inequality is most sharply and cruelly depicted (Fig. 14.1). The infant mortality rate of children born into families of unskilled manual workers (social class V) is twice that of children born into professional families (social class I): the chances of being killed by a motor vehicle is five times greater for the child pedestrian of the unskilled worker (OPCS, 1978).

It is not only the social and economic deprivations associated with social class that have an adverse effect on child health. The ethnic origin, marital

* This paper draws from the arguments developed in Stacey (1980).

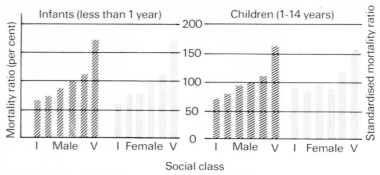

Fig. 14.1 Mortality by occupational class: infants and children (Source: Occupational Mortality 1970–72, HMSO, 1978, p. 196)

status and regional background of Britain's parents are also related to the quantity and quality of health-resources available to their children. In consequence, there is a greater than average incidence of ill-health and premature death among children in black communities, in single parent families and in the less prosperous northern regions of the country (Hart, 1978; Townsend, 1979; Rathwell 1981). However, it is in the relation between social class and child health that the importance of socio-economic factors is most apparent—if only, as Townsend & Davidson (1982) point out, because there is more data to work on. For this reason, it is social class which is the subject of the second section below.

Understanding more about the socio-economic influences on child health involves not only an appreciation of the distribution of resources *between* families. It involves, secondly, an appreciation of the organisation of resources *within* families. For it is within families that the work of making and keeping children healthy takes place. It is here that the impact of material deprivation is felt, as parents endeavour to meet the health needs of their children with the limited (and often insufficient) resources at their disposal. This unenviable task typically falls on 'the woman of the house'. It is the wife-mother who takes responsibility for health, often making up for deficiencies by going short herself (Land, 1977). It is the mother, too, who mediates with the professional carers in the health service. Research confirms everday observations: it is mothers who make and maintain contact with GPs; dentists, health visitors and social workers (Litman, 1974; Carpenter, 1980).

Through this labour of love, mothers, and not infrequently fathers, have acquired a deep understanding of their children's health. The research of Spencer indicates that parents, and especially mothers, are sensitive to changes in their children and are quick to appreciate the significance of symptoms. However, while knowledgeable, parents often doubt their competence as carers. A recurrent theme in studies of childrearing is the anxiety which accompanies responsibility, and the guilt mothers experience when their children's needs are neglected (Stacey et al, 1970; Hall & Stacey, 1979, Graham,

1979, Burghes, 1980). It is this perspective of the patients which is explored in the third section of the chapter.

The final section considers the present and future role of the professional in child health. It highlights two areas in which an appreciation of social class and family life have resulted in an re-evaluation of professional practice. Firstly, it has stimulated a wide-ranging critique of the way in which our maternal and child health services are delivered to patients (Hall & Stacey, 1979; Graham & Oakley, 1981). The traditional roles of 'providers' and 'consumers' are being challenged, and alternative models of care, like the Tyneside project are being developed. Central to these developments, is the philosophy of a 'child and family-centred health service' described by Donald Court (DHSS, 1976), in which professionals 'should see themselves as partners with parents', pooling their knowledge and sharing their skills. Secondly, it has been persuasively argued by a number of researchers that if the determinants of child health lie in the social and physical environment into which the child is born, then health policy can no longer be defined narrowly in terms of the provision of medical care (Draper et al, 1978; Stacey, 1979; Townsend & Davidson, 1982). Those members of the medical profession convinced by such arguments clearly have an important part to play in bringing their professional influence to bear on the centres of political power where our welfare policies are formulated.

SOCIAL CLASS & CHILD HEALTH: THE DISTRIBUTION OF RESOURCES BETWEEN FAMILIES

The pervasive influence of occupation and income on child health has been recorded since the collection of statistics on infant mortality by Farr & Chadwick in the nineteenth century. As Fig. 14.1 indicates even before children are old enough to earn their 'own' social class by entering the world of paid employment, the experience of class inequality is real enough (Hart, 1978). Wilson et al (1978), in their study of inner city families, record the way in which the multiple deprivations of poverty, overcrowding and urban decay are etched into the health of children. Most, they state, 'have first-hand knowledge of illness, disability, accidents and mental stress experienced in a variety of symptoms. They must learn, in growing, to come to terms with or to contain situations of stress to which they are subjected day by day. The draining of human energy and potential is the element that outweighs all others and has an overpowering effect on the growth of children that no other element can counterbalance'.

It is important to note that it is not only those children at the bottom of the class structure who are disadvantaged. There are marked differences in life expectancy and health experiences between each social class, and even between social class I and II. As the Black report on *Inequalities in Health* observes, the poor health status of working class children cannot be explained in terms of the irresponsible or incautious behaviour of those 'deprived' communities (Townsend & Davidson, 1982). It is not, as Preston (1979) concludes from her analysis of mortality data, 'just a question of the unsatisfactory life-styles of "problem families"'.

If the forces which fuel these continuing inequalities are not those of individual improvidence and irresponsibility, where do they originate? A powerful factor, undoubtedly, is poverty—in plain terms, a shortage of cash. In the classic studies of Booth & Rowntree in the nineteenth century, as in the collection of statistics today, poverty is defined in terms of a level of income insufficient to meet the health needs of oneself and one's children. Poverty, by definition, is therefore incompatible with good health. The standard measure of poverty is the current rate of supplementary benefit. However, the stringency of the rates has led social researchers to include among the poor those whose incomes are up to 40% above the level of supplementary benefit (often identified as 'on the margins of poverty'). Over the last twenty years, the proportion of the population in poverty or on the margins of poverty has increased substantially from 14% in 1960 to 27% in 1977 (Townsend 1981). The most up-to-date figures, for 1979, reveal that 2¼ million children are in or on the margins of poverty, about 18% of all children in Great Britain (Burghes, 1982). Since 1979, of course, unemployment has risen significantly, and the level of earnings and benefits among the low paid has failed to keep pace with inflation. These figures are therefore likely to underestimate the numbers of children whose health is threatened by poverty.

Of the mechanisms through which poverty operates, particular emphasis has been placed on diet (Table 14.1). Studies have highlighted the way in which maternal nutrition is related to reproductive outcome: to birthweight, handicap and stillbirth. (Baird, 1974; Wynn & Wynn, 1981). The introduction of food rationing and welfare foods in Great Britain in the second world war demonstrated what social policy could achieve to equalise the distribution of food across the social classes, and underlined the importance of nutrition in childhood in improving the health of working class children (DHSS, 1978). Recent research by the Child Poverty Action Group sets these findings in a contemporary context. It is known, for example, that families

Table 14.1 Household consumption of certain food items by social class (ozs per person per week)

Social Class	Potatoes	White Bread	Sugar and preserves	Fruit	Cheese	Meat (excluding meat products)
1	36	12	10	44	5	34
2	33	15	12	37	5	31
3A	34	14	11	39	5	32
3B	37	21	11	29	4	27
4	45	24	13	24	4	27
5	49	27	14	20	3	25

Source: adapted from *Household Food Consumption & Expenditure: 1980*, the Annual Report of the National Food Survey Committee, Ministry of Agriculture Fisheries and Food, HMSO, 1982, pp. 105–6 in poverty try and make ends meet by reducing their expenditure on food. Of all the basic necessities—fuel, housing, clothing—it is spending on food which can be most easily reduced. A survey of families on supplementary benefit (Burghes, 1980) records that one-third of families occasionally or never bought fresh vegetables, fresh fruit, fresh meat, fresh fish or cheese. Poverty determined not only the quality but the quantity of the diet. As Burghes observes, 'having too little money for food also means that, in many families, parents and their children go without meals. In eight out of 10 families, adults frequently missed meals and, in four out of 10 families, children did' (Burghes, 1980).

Research by Piachaud (1979, 1981) confirms that it is the level of benefit and not the standard of housekeeping that is the problem. He calculated the minimum expenditure necessary to keep a child 'in health'. Food emerged as the largest item of expenditure: according to Piachaud's calculations the minimum expenditure on food for an 8-year-old (at 1981 prices) would consume all but 24p of the supplementary benefit awarded to the child (£7.06 for food out of a benefit of £7.30). Not surprisingly, Piachaud (1981) concludes that the benefit rates for children, rates designed to keep children out of poverty and ill-health, are 'below—for some substantially below—the estimated cost of modern minimum requirements for young children'.

The effects of poverty are mediated through environmental as well as nutritional deprivation. Environmental deprivation manifests itself in damp, overcrowded houses lacking in basic amenities in which it is estimated that 18% of pre-school children live (Bone, 1977). It manifests itself in neighbourhoods with no safe play space and which are 'disliked by most who have to live in them' (Wilson et al, 1978). Townsend's (1979) national survey of poverty indicated that one third of children aged 1–10 had no safe place to play, with the proportion rising to 44% in social classes IV and V. The impact of such deprivation is baldly demonstrated in the rates of fatalities among children from accidents and infectious diseases: the causes of death in infancy which exhibit the steepest class gradients. Concluding its review of the evidence, the Black report on *Inequalities in Health* suggests that, 'the important causal variables are contained within the socio-economic environment' (Townsend & Davidson, 1982). They continue, in a passage which comes close to explaining the relationship between social class and child health:

> 'any factors which increase the parental capacity to provide adequate care for an infant will, when present, increase the chance of survival, while their absence will increase the risk of premature death. The most obvious of such factors fall within the sphere of material resources: sufficient household income, a safe, unpolluted home, warmth and hygiene, a means of rapid communication with the outside world, for example, a telephone or car and an adequate level of manpower—or woman power (two parents would normally provide more continuous care and protection than one). In addition to these basic material needs must be added other cognitive and motivational factors which are not independent of the distribution of material advantage . . . knowledge, skill in verbal communication . . . motivation.'

Recognition of these social and economic factors is not, of course, limited to social scientists. Professional health workers, too, have highlighted the way in which the British class structure places the health of its citizens at risk (Tudor Hart, 1971; DHSS, 1976). However, the policy response has been disappointing. The Black report failed to win Government approval because the financial and political costs of attacking class inequality were regarded as too high. Instead, while acknowledging that child health is determined by forces deeply-rooted in our social structure, recent governments have favoured so-called 'low-cost solutions' which emphasise the personal (and parental) sources of ill-health. Preventive health is welcomed, and lines of responsibility are identified, but the arena is that of the family and not the society. The model of prevention emphasises individual effort; it is not a model which highlights the more urgent need for a government initiative, backed by decisive and comprehensive social policies, to eliminate poverty in childhood.

The case for such policies is re-examined in the final section. Meanwhile, it is time to turn to the arena in which government programmes of prevention are currently focussed: that of family life.

FAMILY LIFE AND CHILD HEALTH: THE ORGANISATION OF HEALTH RESOURCES WITHIN FAMILIES

An appreciation of class inequality can only take us so far in our understanding of child health. It can tell us about the distribution of resources between families, but not that which occurs within families. It can tell us about the material pre-conditions for child health—adequate income, housing, play space—but not about the human pre-conditions: the labour and the love necessary to marshall these things for healthy children. To understand more about the care which creates health, we need to learn more about the sexual division of labour. We need to inquire more deeply into the organisation of work within the home which leaves men responsible for making money and women responsible for keeping the house in good shape and the children in good health.

This time-honoured division is linked to child health in obvious, but nonetheless important, ways. Firstly, it means that when we talk about 'improving child health' we are talking about altering the shape or the pace of women's work. Empirical investigations have noted repeatedly 'the pervasive role played by the wife-mother in the health and health care of the family' (Litman, 1974). It is the wife-mother who takes responsibility for the day-to-day management of child health; a responsibility which commits her, along with her sisters in Europe and America, to a 77-hour week of housework and child care (Oakley, 1974). It is she too, who typically makes decisions about the involvement of professionals: she is the one to accompany children to the doctor and dentist and it is she who receives and attempts to implement medical advice (Carpenter, 1980). It is thus the wife-mother who is most directly implicated in the current emphasis on parents 'carrying out their responsibilities for the promotion of their children's physical and mental health' (DHSS, 1980).

Policies of prevention and community care inevitably add to the already heavy burdens which women carry as the principal care-takers of family health (Graham, 1979; Finch & Groves, 1980). In so doing, they tend to exacerbate rather than relieve the pressures which force mothers to adopt habits and patterns of behaviour which are detrimental to their children. Rather than solving the problem, these policies are likely to fuel it. To understand this paradox, we need to introduce a second important dimension of the sexual division of labour. While women take responsibility for health, few have the resources to do their job effectively. Few mothers have control over the family purse, and housekeeping money has been found to be particularly unresponsive to inflation (Pahl, 1980). Only a small proportion of mothers have access to a reasonable and efficient means of transport which, with the increasing distance they need to travel to hospitals, clinics, health centres and supermarkets, is now an essential prerequisite for effective child care. While, according to the 1980 General Household Survey, nearly 60% of households have a car, it tends to be 'Daddy's car'. A government survey indicates that, among car-owing families, one-third of mothers had the use of the car more than once a week (Bone, 1977). Another study in inner London found that only 7% of mothers got to drive 'the family car' during the week (Bax, 1979).

It is not just the necessary material resources of money and transport which are in short supply, the all-important human resources of energy and strength are equally stretched. Tiredness, poor health and lack of sleep are constant themes in studies of caring (Hughes, 1980). In situations where demand exceeds supply, compromises must be made. Caring inevitably involves difficult decisions in which some needs are sacrificed in order to promote others. Activities which benefit one child are all-too-often measured in costs for another. Breast feeding a new baby means less time and attention for another; avoiding the early introduction of solids in the interests of the baby's health involves disturbed nights for the rest of the family—and less energy for the carer to devote to their health needs the following day (Graham, 1979). The costs are likely to be particularly high when the carer is involved in activities outside the house: going to the clinic and the doctor, travelling to a source of cheap, nutritious food or a safe play ground. As Perkins (1980) reports in her study of ante-natal classes:

> 'attending classes will involve mothers with children under five in making arrangements for their care, which may be difficult, time-consuming and, in the case of a clinging toddler, emotionally exhausting. The uncertain benefits of attending classes may be outweighed by the costs in the family disturbance'

This opportunity-costing is even more critical in families at breaking point, the very families most in need of the support that the professional services can provide. According to Wilson et al (1978), in such families 'the objective is survival . . . Decisions were made at family level . . . the needs of individuals must take second place.'

Cost-cutting and compromises leave a legacy of anxiety and guilt, however. A number of studies highlight the sense of inadequacy among those who fail to breast feed successfully, to feed their children adequately and to have the time and energy to be constantly responsive to their children's needs (Graham, 1979, 1980; Hughes, 1980; Burghes, 1980). Health professionals are well-placed to understand the emotional burden of being the one ultimately responsible for a child's life. It is something many of them have experienced first hand. Yet mothers report that the professional carers are not sympathetic to their position and perspective. They do not listen; they do not encourage mothers to ask questions; they do not offer realistic advice which takes account of the physical and emotional demands of caring (Perkins, 1978; Oakley, 1979; Graham & McKee, 1980). In so doing, professionals clearly lose the opportunity of becoming more effective health workers themselves. As Spencer's research suggests, while professionals can learn from parents, mothers often have difficulty convincing doctors that 'mother knows best'—or even that mother knows anything at all.

As in the case of class inequalities, governments seem aware of the problems faced by those who care for children. Court, as noted earlier, spoke emphatically of the need for a partnership in child health. However again, the change of direction appears to be superficial. 'Partnership', rather than transcending the traditional division of labour between the 'skilled' professional and the 'unskilled' parent, often involves formalising it. It now appears that the drift to prevention and community care has meant an intensification of the work-load of women in the home, while professionals are encouraged to devote more time to assessment and surveillance (as outlined, for example, in *Prevention in the Child Health Services*, DHSS, 1980). With the present reduction in services, this division is likely to be sharpened, with the rhetoric of partnership becoming increasingly at odds with reality. Faced with the prospect of a further deterioration in the position of the child and the family, the medical profession is beginning to play a more positive and forceful role in the formulation of Britain's health policies. It is to the nature and direction of this professional intervention that we now turn.

THE ROLE OF THE PROFESSIONAL IN CHILD HEALTH

It is not only children (and their parents) who draw their strength and vitality from their environment. The health of the national health service depends, too, upon the social and economic context in which it operates. For the last decade, the NHS has been operating in a distinctly hostile economic environment (Draper et al, 1978). In this climate of cut backs and claw backs, it is particularly important that the services which professionals provide for children are as effective as possible. Noting the way in which the structure of social class and family life determines the health experiences of children, how can effectiveness in our child health services be achieved?

Recent debates have highlighted two directions for professional intervention. Firstly it is argued that professional health workers should play a more active part in developing and delivering a new kind of service which would facilitate the involvement of patients and their families. We know that the health services are a lifeline—metaphorically and literally—for many families. Yet barriers exist between professional and parent. Services are designed to maximise the flow of information and expertise from doctor to patient. Other inputs typically flow the other way: it is parents who travel, it is parents who sit and wait, and it is parents who return home, confused and demoralised by the encounter (Hall & Stacey, 1979; Oakley, 1979; Graham & McKee, 1980).

The concept of partnership implies a radical restructuring of this relationship, and recent initiatives reflect the attempt to build a service in which care becomes a two-way process. Much has been written about the need for a more equal relationship between professional and parent in the 'in-house' services: in the ante-natal and child health clinic, in the paediatric wards and in the surgery (DHSS 1976; Hall & Stacey, 1979; Perkins, 1980).

Attention has for some years been drawn to the importance of 'outreach' services (Brotherston, 1976) and recently more attention has been given to these ideas (Rosenthal, 1980; Smith, 1982). These efforts are not merely a question of taking services to the women and children but also of involving them themselves in the service provision. Mother and baby clubs, started perhaps by health visitors who quickly cede the running to the mothers, have proved of great benefit to isolated and possibly depressed mothers. Such clubs can make a contribution to child health above and beyond that possible for professionals working on their own. Furthermore, such groups need not only be composed of adults. A simple and direct medium for skill-sharing is a children's health club. The St Thomas' Health Club in South London, for example, is run by children, with sessions on those issues crucially related to their health: nutrition, pollution and smoking.

A second arena for professional intervention is more ambitious in scope. It has been cogently argued by the Black report, by Draper and others, that, since health is a measure of our collective social life, health policies should be policies about the structure of our society (Draper et al, 1978; Townsend & Davidson, 1982). Health policy, it is argued, cannot be limited to the provision of medical services; it must encompass areas not traditionally the preserve of the Minister of Health. Policies for health, and child health in particular, must inevitably cover social security and education, industry and employment, housing and environmental planning. To answer those who believe such policies to be utopian, the Black report on *Inequalities in Health* translated them into a package of practical and carefully-costed proposals (Townsend & Davidson, 1982). They calculated the cost (at 1980 prices) at £1500m a year, under 2% of Britain's total annual public expenditure.

Such a broad strategy for the improvement of child health implies activities which most doctors involved in clinical practice in child health, whether predominantly from a curative or a preventive point of view, have not taken to be their own. Their attention and their prime responsibility is correctly directed to the delivery of personal health care to individual mothers and their children. The broad strategy is aimed at creating an environment in which 'healthier choices' are 'easier choices' (Draper et al, 1978). In the context of child health, this is its major appeal. For many parents, particularly those on low incomes, 'choosing' health is not in reality an available option. Whatever their commitment to their children, the structure of their lives forces choices on them in which the health of their family is put at risk. Making health choices easier choices involves improvements in the financial position of families, in the design and location of medical services, in the production and distribution of nutritious food, in public health, in domestic architecture and urban planning. While within limits practitioners can make their services and the way they run their clinics more acceptable and accessible to mothers, many of the implications of the policy outlined fall outside those which most medical practitioners take to be their own.

It is they, however, who see the consequences of failed social and economic policies in the health of the children whom they are surveilling or treating. Constituencies of support, both public and political are needed, to attain the larger goals which will improve the life chances of children and reduce the health inequalities so apparent today. The political dimension cannot be avoided. The medical profession is in a unique and powerful position to inform and guide such constituencies. The profession, like the parents, has an obligation, as Court reminds us, to ensure that 'the child's right to continuing and positive health care is upheld' (DHSS, 1976). Unlike parents, the medical profession has ways of speaking collectively through its professional organisations. These ways have in recent years been used to good effect in issues such as the adverse consequences of cigarette smoking. We know from such activities and from other facets of the history of the organisation of the NHS itself, that the medical profession is one which can make its voice heard. Its voice could well be raised in the present day in the interests of these broader aspects of child health.

REFERENCES

Baird D 1974 The epidemiology of low birth weight: changes in incidence in Aberdeen, 1948–1972. Journal of Biosocial Science 6: 323

Bax M, Moss P, Plewis I 1979 Pre-School Families & Services, unpublished report. Thomas Coram Research Unit, London University Institute of Education

Bone M 1977 Pre-School children and their need for day care. HMSO, London

Brotherston J 1976 The Galton Lecture, 1975: Inequality, is it Inevitable? In: Carter C O Peel J (eds) Equalities and Inequalities in Health. Academic Press, London

Burghes L 1980 Living from Hand to Mouth: a study of 65 families on supplementary benefit. Poverty Pamphlet, 50 Family Service Units/Child Poverty Action Group, London

Burghes L 1982 Facts and Figures Poverty, 52: 28–33

Carpenter E 1980 Children's health care & the changing role of woman Medical Care 12: 1208–1218

Department of Health & Social Security 1976 Fit for the Future: the Report of the Committee on Child Health Services. Cmnd 6684, HMSO, London (The Court Report)

Department of Health & Social Security 1978 Eating for Health HMSO, London

Department of Health & Social Security 1980 Prevention in Child Health Services. DHSS, London.

Draper P, Dennis J, Best G, Popay J, Patridge J, Griffiths J 1978 The NHS in the next 30 years: a new perspective on the health of the British, Unit for the Study of Health Policy, Guys Hospital Medical School, London

Finch J, Groves D 1980 Community Care & the family: a case for equal opportunities. Journal of Social Policy 4: 437–451

Graham H 1979 'Prevention & Health: every mothers' business: a comment on child health policies in the seventies, in Harris, C. (Ed.) The Sociology of the Family: New Directions for Britain Sociological Review Monograph 28, University of Keele

Graham H 1980 Family influences in early years on the eating habits of children. In: Turner M. (Ed.) Nutrition and Lifestyles, Applied Science Publishers, London

Graham H, McKee L 1980 The First Months of Motherhood Monograph No. 3, The Health Education Council, London

Graham H, Oakley A 1981 Competing ideologies of reproduction: medical & maternal perspectives on pregnancy. In Roberts H (Ed.) Women, Health and Reproduction. Routledge & Kegan Paul, London

Hall D, Stacey M (Eds.) 1979 Beyond Separation: Further Studies of Children in Hospital. Routledge & Kegan Paul, London

Hart N 1978 Health and Inequality University of Essex

Hughes M, Mayall B, Moss P, Perry J, Petrie P, Pinkerton G 1980 Nurseries Now: A Fair Deal for Parents and Children, Penguin, Harmondsworth, Middlesex

Land H 1977 Inequalities in Large Families: More of the same or different In: Chester R, Peel J (Eds.) Equalities and Inequalities in Family Life, Academic Press, London

Litman T 1974 The Family as a Basic Unit in Health and Medical Care: a socio behavioural overview Social Science and Medicine 8: 495–519

Oakley A 1974 The Sociology of Housework Martin Robertson, Oxford

Oakley A 1979 Becoming a Mother Martin Robertson, Oxford

Office of Population, Censuses & Surveys 1978 Occupational Mortality 1970–1972, Decennial Supplement. HMSO, London

Pahl J 1980 Patterns of money management within marriage Journal of Social Policy 9, 3: 313–35

Perkins E 1978 Having a Baby: an Educational Experience? Leverhulme Health Education Project, Occasional Paper 6, University of Nottingham

Perkins E 1980 The pattern of women's attendance at ante-natal care: is this good enough? Health Education Journal, 39 1: 39

Piachaud D 1979 The Cost of a Child, Poverty Pamphlet 43, Child Poverty Action Group, London

Piachaud D 1981 Children & Poverty, Poverty Research Series 9, Child Poverty Action Group, London

Preston B 1979 Further studies of inequality Sociological Review 27: 343–50

Rathwell T 1981 Meeting needs—health planning for ethnic minorities Medicine in Society 7: 14–15

Rosenthal H 1980 Health & Community Work, KF80/117 King Edward's Hospital Fund for London, London

Smith C 1982 Community Based Health Initiatives: a Handbook for Voluntary Groups National Council for Voluntary Organisations, London

Stacey M 1979 New perspectives in clinical medicine: the sociologist Journal of the Royal College of Physicians of London 13: 123–9

Stacey M 1980 Realities for change in Child Health care: existing patterns and future possibilities. British Medical Journal 281, 6238: 493–495

Stacey M, Dearden R, Robinson D, Pill R 1970 Hospitals, Children & their Families. Routledge & Kegan Paul, London

Townsend P 1979 Poverty in the United Kingdom Penguin, Harmondsworth, Middlesex

Townsend P 1981 Toward Equality in Health through Social Policy International Journal of Health Services 11: 63–75

Townsend P, Davidson N 1982 Inequalities in Health Penguin, Harmondsworth, Middlesex (The Black Report)

Tudor Hart J 1971 The inverse care law Lancet 1: 405–412

Wilson H, Herbert G, Wislon J 1978 Parents & Children in the Inner City Routledge & Kegan Paul, London

Wynn M, Wynn A 1981 Historical associations of congenital malformations International Journal of Environmental Studies 7: 7–12

Britain's National Cohort Studies

INTRODUCTION

The quotation 'the child is the father of the man' is intuitively recognised as valid. Biographers and autobiographers generally start their story with the birth of the subject and his early development. Although forming an important background in individual cases, it is not easy to generalise from an interesting story to the population in general. For example, on the basis of the circumstances of Sir Winston Churchill's birth it would be dangerous to say that infants born very pre-term are likely to exhibit impressive qualities of leadership; nor should one extrapolate from the death of Bertrand Russell's parents early in his life to say there are major intellectual advantages in being brought up by a grandmother. It is only by looking at truly representative samples of the population, with relatively large numbers, that one may be able to identify factors that will predict an increased likelihood of advantageous or deleterious outcome in the child.

Collection of information is possible in two different ways. One could start with a population of adults and interview them or one could start with a population of infants and follow them throughout their lives. The difficulties in the retrospective questioning of adults about their childhood lies in the fact that the most valuable information is usually that not known to the adults themselves (it may be more apposite to question their mothers, but even this would be fraught with difficulty in view of the long period of time that had transpired between the events and interview); in addition, the recall of events will be subject to the biases inherent in any situation where the outcome is known. In comparison, information collected at intervals throughout the individual's life has the advantage of being much more accurate.

Any study of long-term associations has the disadvantage that there is often a long period of time before the results are available. Thus, if a new obstetric regime is instituted which has a long-term adverse effect on the infant, it may be anything from 20 years onwards before it is discovered. A dramatic example of this, of course, lay in the use of diethyl stilboestrol in pregnancy subsequently found to be associated with an increased risk of vaginal carcinoma in young women (Herbst et al. 1971).

Longitudinal studies of small sub-populations have been undertaken in many countries. Britain is unique, however, in that there have been three national longitudinal studies which have followed nationally representative samples of children from birth throughout their lives. The first of these was initiated in 1946, the second in 1958 and the third in 1970. None of these surveys was started as a longitudinal study. Rather, they were all started as studies of the circumstances surrounding birth. All three then became longitudinal studies, with albeit slightly different designs and somewhat different aims.

THE NATIONAL SURVEY OF HEALTH AND DEVELOPMENT (1946 COHORT)

As already mentioned, this cohort grew out of a birth survey carried out at the end of the last war with the aims of determining the state of the maternity services. The study was carried out under the joint auspices of the Royal College of Obstetricians and Gynaecologists and the Population Investigation Committee. An attempt was made to identify and survey all births occurring in England, Scotland and Wales in the week 3–9 March 1946. Health visitors were asked to interview the mother and fill in structured questionnaires some 6 weeks after delivery. A total of 13 687 questionnaires were completed. The aims of the study were to examine the availability and effectiveness of the ante-natal and maternity services. Analysis of the results produced a fascinating glimpse of the child-bearing scene at that time—with recommendations for future improvement that included the possibility of taking antenatal care into the community, reducing waiting times in antenatal clinics and providing facilities in clinics for older children to play (Smith, 1948). The report ended with the statement: 'The present inquiry has been limited to a study of pregnancy, labour and the first 2 months of puerperium; but in order to make a complete assessment of the achievements of the maternity services it would be necessary to observe the health of mothers and infants over a much longer period.' This was to herald the start of a longitudinal study that is still proceeding.

When the children were aged 2 a follow-up was planned but, for financial reasons, only a sub-sample of the original 13 687 infants in the birth survey was selected. Selection was stratified, and all illegitimate and multiple births were excluded. The remainder, however, contained substantially more children of manual than non-manual workers (Atkins et al, 1981), so for follow-up, only a 1 in 4 sample was taken of the manual workers, but all children of all non-manual workers were included as were all children of agricultural workers (a group of special interest at that time). In all there were 5362 children in this sample—and information has been collected on each child at ages 2, 4, 6, 7, 8, 9, 10, 11, 13, 15 and every year thereafter until aged 26. James Douglas remained Director of the Study throughout this period. They are currently being contacted again at the age of 36. At the same time a study is being made of the children born to this cohort, and inter-generational studies are also being carried out.

The social and educational implications have been profound, but from the health point of view perhaps the most interesting findings from the first years of the study fall into three groups: social class differences, disadvantages in low birthweight and the advantages of breast feeding. In 1951, Douglas (1951a,b) showed that children in the 'lower' social classes not only had a higher mortality rate in the first years of life but they also had a greater risk of upper and lower respiratory tract infection. Interestingly, he also showed that the infants in the lowest classes were not only more likely to fall ill in this way, they were more likely actually to get the illness at an earlier age. In contrast there was no social class association with discharging ears, whooping cough or mumps and only a slight trend with the proportion of children who had had measles in the pre-school period (Douglas & Blomfield, 1958). There was a reverse social class trend, however, in the likelihood of the child having had a tonsillectomy or, if a boy, circumcision (MacCarthy et al, 1952).

Unlike the findings in later cohorts, it was the norm in 1946 to breast feed: 76% of mothers did so for at least 2 weeks and 53% breast fed for over 2 months. There was no social class variation in the likelihood of breast feeding, but the subsequent health of the breast fed baby differed markedly (Douglas, 1950). Those children who had never been breast fed were more likely to have had diarrhoea in the first 4 months of life (though there was no difference thereafter). Bottle fed babies were also slightly more likely to have had a lower respiratory infection during the first 9 months of life, and more likely to have had measles. Developmentally, Douglas (1950) showed that the longer the child had been fed by the breast the earlier he walked. A later study on the cohort by Rodgers (1978) indicated that breast feeding was associated with a slightly higher score on intellectual testing—and following the cohort into adulthood, Marmot et al (1980) found some indication that serum cholesterol was lower in men who had been breastfed.

All these studies took into account the fact that children of low birthweight were less likely to have been breast fed. Not only were low birthweight children more likely to die during the neonatal period, and the rest of the first year but they were also twice as likely to have died during the second, or even third year of life (Douglas & Mogford, 1953). In addition, they were over 4 times as likely to have been admitted to hospital with bronchitis or pneumonia during the first 2 years of their lives. This was not due to differential admissions policies for low birthweight infants since these children also had more episodes of lower respiratory tract infection that were treated at home.

That bronchitis and pneumonia in infancy have a long-term adverse effect was demonstrated when the cohort was followed up at ages 20 and 25. The adults who as infants had had such a history were much more likely to have chronic coughs than were those adults without such a history (Kiernan et al,

1976). Long-term effects were also shown among children who had had repeated or prolonged hospital admission during their pre-school years. They were shown to be at increased risk of later troublesome behaviour at school, poor reading ability, unstable employment patterns and delinquency (Douglas, 1975).

THE NATIONAL CHILD DEVELOPMENT STUDY (1958 COHORT)

The second national cohort again started as a birth survey. This time it was the National Birthday Trust Fund in association with the Royal College of Obstetricians and Gynaecologists who sponsored the study which was under the direction of Professor Neville Butler. The survey was specifically designed to look at causes of perinatal death at a time when the perinatal death rate had remained static for some years. To this end, pathologists all over the country arranged to carry out detailed post-mortems on stillbirths and neonatal deaths occurring in the 3-month period: March–May 1958. In order to compare the clinical and social backgrounds of the deaths with those of the background population, a sample of surviving births was selected, i.e. all infants born in one week of March (3–9), 1958. Questionnaires on the 7117 deaths and on the week's 16 994 births were filled in shortly after delivery by midwives. In the event, some 95% of all stillbirths and neonatal deaths were included, and able to be compared with the 98% of all births occuring in one week. From this survey, much was learnt about the clinical and pathological causes of stillbirth and neonatal death (Butler & Alberman, 1969; Butler & Bonham, 1963). Analysis of the information collected in the one week was valuable in assessing various factors contributing to low birthweight or pre-term gestation; these included the contributions of maternal smoking, pre-eclampsia, age, parity and social class. The data were analysed to assess the optimum interval between pregnancies (Fedrick & Adelstein, 1973), and the possible consequences of maternal infection during pregnancy (Fedrick & Alberman, 1972).

Follow-up of these children was long delayed, compared with the previous cohort. Finally, after representation from various sources it was decided to mount a comprehensive survey when the children were 7 years old with the primary aims of: (a) gathering normative data on the educational, behavioural, social, medical and physical development of the children, documenting the inter-relationships between them and delineating the incidence of handicap; and (b) evaluating the long-term relationships between aspects of pregnancy, delivery and the neonatal period with the medical and educational development of the children. Subsequent follow-ups have been carried out at the ages of 11, 16 and 23 (Fogelman & Wedge, 1981).

For the first three of these follow-ups, the children received medical examinations by clinical medical officers, the local health visitor took a complete medical and social history from the parents, the teacher filled in a questionnaire on the child and the children completed a number of educational tests. Analyses of the results at 7 showed the dramatic associations of social disadvantage with poor intellectual ability, even as early as 7 years of age (Davie et al, 1972). They showed, too, that children who were socially disadvantaged were the least likely to take up primary health care facilities, their dental health was poor and their physical coordination, speech and bladder control were less well developed. From a study of the longitudinal data it was shown that smoking in pregnancy did appear to have a long-term effect on the child, over and above that associated with low birthweight: children of mothers who smoked were, in general shorter at the age of 7 than those of non-smokers (Butler & Goldstein, 1973). This association remained even when other factors known to be associated with the child's height were included, such as maternal height, birth order and social class.

The data collected in this cohort have been valuable in estimating the prevalence of various potentially handicapping conditions, with the documentation of their long-term effects. For example, Sheridan and Peckham (1978) examined the results at follow-up of 215 children with normal hearing but whose speech was rated as unintelligible at 7. By the age of 16, 51% still had speech problems. Less than a fifth (40 children) were classified as educationally subnormal (ESN), but with few exceptions the rest had done badly at school. Among those not classified as ESN, there was also an increased incidence of both visual impairment and clumsiness.

Examination of the audiometric results as the children grew older showed that, on average, hearing acuity had declined significantly between the ages of 11 and 16. Richardson and his colleagues (1977) also showed that the decrease was greatest among children in the manual social classes and suggested that the results were a function of increased exposure to highly amplified 'pop' music.

THE CHILD HEALTH AND EDUCATION STUDY (1970 COHORT)

Once again this started as a national birth survey, and included all births in a given week (4–11 April 1970). The information differed somewhat from that collected in the preceding studies in that, for the first time, Northern Ireland was included. The study was known as the British Births Survey and was again sponsored by the National Birthday Trust Fund in association with the Royal College of Obstetricians and Gynaecologists. It's major aim was concerned with the quality of life in the first week after birth. Information was again collected by midwives during the first week postpartum. This included details of the social background of the mother, her past obstetric history, the history of the pregnancy, labour, delivery and the postpartum period.

The results of this survey (Chamberlain et al, 1975, 1978) showed once again the disadvantage to the fetus in having a mother who smoked, as well as the increased risk of perinatal death when there had been a history of bleeding in pregnancy or if severe pre-eclampsia had developed. The survey also showed the variation in obstetric practice with social class and parity. Comparison of information from the 1958 and 1970 birth surveys (Peters et al, 1983) has shown that whereas the perinatal death rate had fallen dramatically the proportion of infants born of low birthweight had increased rather than decreased. Further analysis showed that part of this increase was related to an increase in maternal smoking rates. Interestingly in both surveys, although there was *prima facie* evidence for the prevalence of low birthweight increasing in the lower social classes, this could be entirely explained by the fact that women in the lower social classes are shorter and more likely to smoke.

A study was undertaken on sub-populations of the infants in the British Births Study at the ages of 22 months and 42 months, to assess the effects of fetal malnutrition on the subsequent mental and physical progress of the babies. To this end three groups were selected: those born at, or after 42 weeks gestation, those with birthweight below the 5th percentile for their gestational age, sex and parity, and all multiple births (twins and triplets). These were compared with a random sample of 1 in 10 of the original study. Children whose mothers were single, widowed, divorced or separated from their husbands at the time of birth were excluded.

Analysis of the random sample (Chamberlain & Simpson, 1979) showed that; (a) although children in large families were most likely to contract infectious diseases, they were the least likely to be vaccinated; (b) the most significant association with lower respiratory tract infection in infancy was maternal smoking; (c) there was an increased risk of accidents to children of working mothers; and (d) sudden unexpected infant death was more likely if the mother had smoked during pregnancy.

At the age of 5, an attempt was made to trace the whole cohort of children born in the survey week and resident in Great Britain (Northern Ireland was omitted for political and technical reasons). Health visitors went to the homes of the children, interviewed the mothers, measured the height and head circumference of the children and administered simple intellectual tests. Subsequently the children have been traced at 10, medically examined and given a barrage of educational tests. At both ages a full social and medical history was taken from the mother.

Among important findings has been a detailed analysis of smoking in pregnancy. Not only have the 1958 cohort results been replicated, with a demonstrable reduction in the child's height associated with maternal smoking, it has also been shown that there is an increased prevalence of various types of behaviour problems and a reduction in intellectual performance at 5 (Rush, 1982) among this group. The 1946 cohort finding of better intellectual performance in children who had been breast fed was also replicated (Taylor et al, 1983) but there was no longer evidence for a protective effect of breast feeding in relation to lower respiratory tract infection or gastroenteritis (Taylor et al, 1982).

Social differences remained important in conditions such as bronchitis and pneumonia, behaviour problems and intellectual outcome, but there were no social class differences in the overall prevalence of accidents or convulsions (Golding & Butler, 1984). The children from the upper social classes were more likely to have had eczema, to suck their thumbs or bite their nails. These socially advantaged children were also more likely to have been breast fed, to live in well-to-do urban areas and come from small families.

One of the ways in which the data have been analysed concerned possible adverse reactions to pertussis vaccination. Studies had already shown that there was a small but statistically significant risk of encephalopathy occurring within 48 hours of pertussis immunisation (Miller et al, 1981). The cohort data were used to assess whether there were other adverse effects, of less acute onset. We, therefore, compared the intellectual ability of the children who had received immunisations with those who had not. We found that far from there being evidence for an adverse effect of immunisation, the reverse was true: children who had been immunised were performing substantially better than those who had not (Butler et al, 1982). This was true even after standardisation for various social factors as well as for indications for withholding the immunisation. In contrast, children who had actually had pertussis itself early in infancy were at increased risk of mental subnormality.

The major aim of the 10 year follow-up of this cohort has been to study the prevalence and antecedents of handicap and disability. The longitudinal data will shortly be ready for analysis and should provide fascinating evidence on a number of points. Already it has become apparent that diabetes, for example, is increasing markedly in prevalence. In the 1946 cohort, only 1 of the 5362 children had developed diabetes by the age of 10 giving a rate of 0.2 per 1000, in the 1958 cohort there were 10 out of 15 500, giving a rate of 0.6 per 1000 (Calnan & Peckham, 1977) and in the 1970 cohort 18 of 13 823 children had diabetes at the age of 10 (rate of 1.3)—this implies a 7-fold increase in the 24 years between the cohorts (Stewart-Brown et al, 1983).

CONCLUSIONS

In this chapter it has been possible only to sketch in a few details of the methodology and findings of our unique resource—the national longitudinal studies. There have always been antagonists and protagonists of this method of study. The antagonists will suggest that smaller surveys in more depth would be preferable; they point out, too, that one week's births may not be representative of those occuring at other times of the year.

Certainly, in some conditions it is known that there are statistically significant variations in prevalence according to the month of birth. Nevertheless, variations are never very profound, nor are the spring months usually those that are dramatically different from the rest.

The differences between opinions on the value of longitudinal studies generally lie in different expectations of the data. It should never be assumed that these surveys can replace the small in-depth studies of small homogenous groups of children, nor can they obviate the need for intervention studies or other more intensive methods of investigation. What they can do, with the relatively blunt tools at their disposal, is to sketch in the broad outlines of the various facets of childhood development. They can point out those factors which warrant further in depth study, and those for which study is not needed. They can and should be hypotheses generators. They should also be able to be used to cast doubt on traditionally-held beliefs, and if necessary knock the sacred cows of established thinking, whether in the medical, educational, sociological or psychological fields.

Further information may be obtained on:
(a) The 1946 cohort from Dr M. E. Wadsworth, Department of Community Medicine, University of Bristol.
(b) The 1958 cohort from Dr K. Fogelman, National Children's Bureau, 8 Wakley Street, Islington, London EC1V 7QE.
(c) The 1970 cohort from Professor N. R. Butler, Department of Child Health, University of Bristol.

REFERENCES

1948 Maternity in Great Britain. Oxford University Press, Oxford
Atkins E, Cherry N, Douglas J W B, Kiernan K E, Wadsworth M E J 1981 The 1946 British Birth Cohort: an account of the origins, progress, and results of the National Survey of Health and Development. In: Mednick S A, Baert A E, Bachman B P. Prospective Longitudinal Research: An Empirical Basis for the Primary Prevention of Psychosocial Disorders, pp. 25–30. Oxford University Press, Oxford
Butler N R, Bonham D G 1963 Perinatal Mortality: The first report of the 1958 British Perinatal Mortality Survey. E & S Livingstone, Edinburgh
Butler N R, Alberman E D 1969 Perinatal Problems: the Second Report of the 1958 British Perinatal Mortality Survey. E & S Livingstone, Edinburgh
Butler N R, Goldstein H 1973 Smoking in pregnancy and subsequent child development. British Medical Journal iv: 573–575
Butler N R, Golding J, Haslum M, Stewart-Brown S 1982 Recent findings of the 1970 Child Health and Education study: preliminary communication. Journal Royal Society of Medicine 75: 781–784
Calnan M, Peckham C S 1977 Incidence of insulin—dependent diabetics in the first 16 years of life. Lancet i: 589–590
Chamberlain R, Simpson N 1979 The Prevalence of Disease in Childhood. Pitman Medical Publishers, London.
Chamberlain R, Chamberlain G, Howlett B, Masters K 1975 British Births 1970, Vol. 1: The First Week of Life. Heinemann Medical Books, London
Chamberlain G, Philipp E, Howlett B, Claireaux A 1978 British Birth 1970: Vol. 2: Obstetric Care. Heinemann Medical Books, London
Davie R, Butler N, Goldstein H 1972 From Birth to Seven: A report of the National Child Development Study. Longmans, London
Douglas J W B 1960 The extent of breast feeding in Great Britain in 1946, with special reference to the health and survival of children. British Journal of Obstetrics and Gynaecology of the British Empire 57: 335–361
Douglas J W B 1951a Health and Survival of Infants in Different Social Classes: A National Survey. Lancet ii: 440–446

Douglas J W B 1951b Social Class Differences in Health and Survival during the First Two Years of Life: the Results of a National Survey. Population Studies 5: 35–58

Douglas J W B, Mogford C 1953 Health of Premature Children from Birth to Four Years. British Medical Journal i: 748–754

Douglas J W B 1975 Early hospital admission and later distrubances of behaviour and learning. Developmental Medicine and Child Neurology 17: 456–480

Douglas J W B, Blomfield J M 1958 Children under Five. George Allen and Unwin Ltd, London

Fedrick J. Alberman E D 1972 Reported influenza in pregnancy and subsequent cancer in the child. British Medical Journal ii: 485–488

Fedrick J. Adelstein P 1973 Influence of Pregnancy Spacing on outcome of pregnancy. British Medical Journal iv: 753–756

Fogelman K, Wedge P 1981 The National Child Development Study (1958 British Cohort).In: Mednick S A, Baert A E, Bachmann B P. (eds.) Prospective Longitudinal Research: An Empirical basis for the primary prevention of psychosocial disorders. Oxford University Press, Oxford

Golding J, Butler N R 1984 From Birth to Five: a study of the Health and Behaviour of a National Cohort. Clinics in Developmental Medicine

Herbst A L, Ulfelder H, Poskanzer D C 1971 Adenocarcinoma of the vagina: association of maternal stilboestrol therapy with tumour appearance in young women. New England Journal of Medicine. 284: 878–881

Kiernan K E, Colley J R T, Douglas J W B, Reid D D 1976 Chronic cough in young adults in relation to smoking habits, childhood environment and chest illness. Respiration 33: 236–244

MacCarthy D, Douglas J W B, Mogford C 1952 Circumcision in a National Sample of 4 year old Children. British Medical Journal iv: 755–756

Marmot M G, Page C M, Atkins E 1980 Effect of breast-feeding on plasma cholesterol and weight in young adults. Journal of Epidemiology and Community Health 34: 164–167

Miller D L, Ross E M, Alderslade R, Bellman M H, Rawson N S B 1981 Pertussis immunisation and serious acute neurological illness in children. British Medical Journal 282: 1595–1599

Palmer S, Butler N R, Golding J 1983 Long-term sequelae of Pertussis immunisation in children with contraindications.

Peters T, Golding J, Fryer J, Lawrence C, Butler N R, Chamberlain G 1983 Plus ça Change: a comparative analyses of predictors of birthweight. British Journal of Obstetrics and Gynaecology (in press)

Richardson K, Hutchison D, Peckham C S, Tibbenham A 1977 Audiometric Thresholds of a National Sample of British 16-year olds. A longitudinal study. Developmental Medicine and Child Neurology 19: 797–802

Rodgers B 1978 Feeding in infancy and later ability and attainment: a longitudinal study. Developmental Medicine and Child Neurology 20: 421–426

Rush D. 1982 Paper presented at the Colston Symposium, Bristol

Sheridan M D, Peckham C S 1978 Follow-up to 16 years of school children who had marked speech defects at 7 years. Child Care, Health, and Development 4: 145–157

Stewart-Brown S, Haslum M, Butler N R 1983 Evidence for an increasing prevalence of diabetes mellitus in childhood. British Medical Journal 286: 1855–1857

Taylor B, Golding J, Wadsworth J, Butler N R 1982 Breast feeding, bronchitis, and admissions for lower-respiratory illness and gastroenteritis during the first five years. Lancet i: 1227–1229

Taylor B, Wadsworth J, Butler N R 1983 Breast feeding and Intellectual Ability at 5. Developmental Medicine and Child Neurology (in press)

The community paediatric team—an approach to child health services in a deprived inner city area

INTRODUCTION

A deprived inner city area presents the Health Service with particular chal-
lenges in providing care for its children and their families. Similar demands
are also placed upon Education and Social Services. The problems are often
complex. Our influence on the 'cycle of disadvantage' may be minimal
(Rutter & Madge, 1976; Black Report, 1980; Blaxter, 1981). The Health
Services may 'mend', Social Services protect and aid, Education Services
teach, yet the true target which is virtually 'a change in culture' remains
beyond our reach. It will continue to be so as long as our services concentrate
upon superficial repairs. Our approach needs to be truly preventive and to
rest as much on teaching skills, self help and personal responsibility as on
direct fixing. Without this we encourage dependency and discourage personal
decision making; the families also lose confidence and self esteem.

Changes to Community Health Services in policy, training and health care
delivery have been widely advocated and hotly argued (Sheldon Report,
1967; Brotherston Report, 1973; Court Report, 1976; Preston Report, 1979;
Clarke Report, 1981; Royal College of General Practitioners, 1982; Forfar
Report, 1982; Anderson Report, 1982).The title of the Court Report (1976)
'Fit for the Future' summarises this new emphasis in paediatrics. In contrast
to the approach of this report, others who have looked at narrower
professional interests may fail to meet the overall needs. Progress must
involve doctors, community nurses and administrators advancing in step
with Education and Social Services, using common policies.

THE TEAM (Fig 16.1)

The community paediatric team is our attempt within an inner city area of
Nottingham to provide this close integration of services and to develop them
to meet the needs of the local community. The team grew from the appointment of one senior lecturer in Child Health with particular responsibility for
paediatric problems in the inner city area. A medical establishment with a
total sessional commitment of 20 sessions per week was provided using

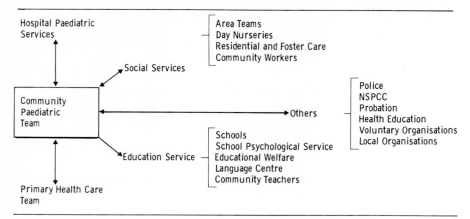

Fig. 16.1 The community paediatric team

existing health service resources for employment of child health doctors. There was therefore no increase in establishment, but rather a new statement of the clinical role of these doctors, breaking away from traditional patterns. A geographical area served by two main health centres was defined. Within this area the team provides the medical care into the schools, child health clinics and day nurseries. The community is small enough for the individual schools and clinics to be well known to the members of the team and for them to work closely with the community nursing staff. Regular meetings have allowed uniform policies to develop and have enabled us to provide support and advice at local level to community nurses, individual teachers and social workers. Informal contacts with general practitioners enable many paediatric problems, which might otherwise be referred to hospital, to be dealt with within the primary care setting. Some child health clinics are run by general practitioners and some by the community paediatric team. Whichever the arrangement, there is much discussion about problems. Some children are seen jointly, others are referred to our clinics, and others are discussed but not referred. School children are seen in the school clinic or at school. The school clinic is also used as a source of referral by general practitioners. In addition to the paediatric input, there is also a visiting ENT surgeon and a consultant opthalmologist. Both child health clinics and school clinics have facilities for investigation and treatment. Treatment and referral of patients is therefore a closely integrated activity. In the same way we work closely with the Area Social Services team and the Schools' Psychological Service. The team also relates to the University Hospital where there are shared clinical appointments between the hospital and community.

Introduction of change

The community team approach only works with individual motivation, goodwill, easy access for informal discussion, a sense of trust between the workers, combined with drive, flexibility and the willingness to take on personal responsibility.

Within the team the roles of individual workers are defined. In the past the overlap and repetition of work between health visitors, school nurses and doctors has been most wasteful and it has been to our advantage that the community nursing staff are increasingly taking on the role of primary screening. The doctors see all children when they attend clinic for the first time and follow up those at high risk, plus any which the parents or the community nursing staff request them to see. In school, other than for school entrants, routine examinations have been abandoned. Only children with previously identified problems or those requested by school nurses, teachers and parents are seen by the doctor. There is a comprehensive system for school nurse health appraisal (Latham, 1981) and a developing involvement of the doctor in the school health education programmes. Non-attenders whom the health visitors are concerned about are seen jointly in the home. Our present programme was shaped by much discussion and learning from one another, making a compromise between what is ideal and what is feasible within each individual professional's area. The expanded role of the community nurse in primary screening has, we believe, been achieved without any loss in terms of problems identified, but with gains in our ability to handle those problems. Table 16.1 demonstrates the success of this policy in one primary school, where the school nurse's assessment was checked by all children being seen by a doctor.

Two of the 'missed' conditions would have been detected by scrutiny of old notes and the remaining three had little functional significance.

Table 16.1 A community nurse's performance in primary screening in one school

Total number of pupils	124
Number of children with abnormalities	48
Predicted by school nurses	40
Predicted by teachers	15
Predicted by parents	10
Total predicted	43
Total selected	54
Conditions missed	5

The tasks of the Community Paediatric Team

We have defined the tasks that we wish to perform and have developed flexible programmes which provide consistency in their implementation and in the roles of the various workers within that framework. Tasks defined are:
   1. Prevention through:
      (a). health education
      (b). parent counselling
      (c). immunisation

2. Screening procedures leading to early diagnosis of:

(a). disorders of growth

(b). disorders of development (motor, intellectual, speech, vision and hearing)

(c). somatic disorders, e.g. scoliosis, congenital dislocation of the hip, undescended testes, hernia, heart disease

(d). emotional problems

(e). children experiencing emotional or physical deprivation or abuse

(f). children likely to have special educational needs

3. Management:

(a). parent counselling on training, behaviour and general child-care problems

(b). handicapped school and pre-school children with particular reference to their education needs

(c). problems related to groups of children such as schools or day nurseries

(d). management of paediatric medical problems in conjunction with their general practitioners or the hospital paediatric service

4. Advice to individual teachers, social workers and careers officers on children within the team's area

5. Evaluation of the health and other needs of children within the team area and the implementation of new programmes where current facilities seem lacking

6. Teaching medical students, doctors, community nursing staff

THE INNER CITY COMMUNITY

The County Deprivation Study (Nottinghamshire County Council, 1975) identified the inner city area as one of particular concern. The indices of child health shown in Table 16.2 were found to be far higher in the deprived areas.

The increase in post-neonatal mortality found by Madeley (1978) in the inner city area is no longer seen, but indices such as non-accidental injury continue to be identified as higher in our inner city area.

Table 16.2 Indices of child health in an inner city area as compared with the average for Nottingham

	Deprived areas	Average
Admitted to Neonatal Unit per 100 births	27.8	12.2
Admitted to hospital in 1st year of life per 100 births	55	27
On Child Abuse Register per 1000 children	4.5	1.5
Infant deaths 0–1 year per 1000 children	40	15.8

Our population consists of three main groups: Asians, West Indians and our local white population. Many of the latter have lived in the same locality for generations (whilst their more successful relatives have moved out). Within this small area there is however a high mobility and also a degree of circulation to and from other inner city areas such as Manchester and Liverpool. In some patches the Asians and West Indians are in the majority, forming up to 90% of the population in schools.

Primary care, by and large, is not zoned within the inner city area so that in one health centre we have to deal with children registered with 41 individual GP's (32 practices) and in the other with 57 GP's (43 practices) (Spencer & Power, 1977). The families tend to make heavy and often inappropriate demands on primary care. They also make extensive use of emergency services and the Children's Casualty Department at the University Hospital. Although quantitively they use more health services than their more priviledged neighbours, the well known result is not better health but worse health. An analysis of 399 consecutive admissions to the Children's Hospital by Wynne & Hull (1975) showed that social class V, although forming 8.1% of the population, accounted for 33.6% of the admissions. Over 20% were admitted primarily for social reasons. Perception of illness may be poor and compliance with treatment or keeping appointments even worse.

What underlies the particular vulnerability of our population? Many lack practical skills in areas such as literacy, budgeting, cooking and child care. Many parents have had disadvantaged childhoods and cannot give to their own children experiences they themselves have not received. Some seem to go straight from unsatisfactory childhood to unsatisfactory parenthood at 16 or 17 becoming immature 'adults' whose own needs are so great that they cannot set them aside for those of their children. Most important they lack confidence and self-esteem; they have not developed a sense of responsibility for their own lives (never mind those of their children) and see control of events as coming from outside themselves rather than from within. This is understandable in terms of their own histories in which authority in one form or another has intervened to make decisions for the family. Long-term unemployment, imprisonment, poverty and poor housing increase the sense of hopelessness, giving a lack of purpose and drive. They do not plan, even in the very short term, as the future might not seem to be within their control. The lack of planning extends to daily activities such as meals, shopping, cleaning clothes and activities for the children. This picture is obviously not true of all families but does provide a framework for understanding those with greatest difficulties.

Our Asian children are often first or second generation immigrants from the poorest parts of the Asian sub-continent. Many of the parents are illiterate and a large number of the mothers do not speak English. From one point of view it is remarkable how well many of the children do perform in school, but for some differences in culture and language, combined with over-crowding and lack of opportunities at home, place them at a disadvantage at school. Depression seems common among the parents (particularly the mothers) who have found adaptation to life in Britain difficult.

Many of the white and West Indian families are single parent families. Even with good skills it would be difficult to manage on low incomes with poor housing. Some of the housing consists of tower blocks, some of lower rise housing estates which at first view seem all concrete stairs and gangways, and others of old terraced houses privately rented.

The community contains excellent nursery school provision which is under-subscribed and four Social Service day nurseries with long waiting lists. The parents often do not understand the difference between the two types of facility.

Deprivation is associated with developmental delay, particularly in language development, social and cognitive skills and in general knowledge and awareness of the world about them (Wedge & Prosser, 1973). Remedial provision in school is too late for many children where the roots of their failure lie in restricted opportunities in the pre-school years. This poor start is compounded by the lack of interest and encouragement in education shown by many parents. Attendance records are often appalling.

The Area Social Services team carries a heavy load of problems such as non-accidental injury, neglect, requests for day care, reception into residential care, parents in need of support, marital and financial problems, violence, alcohol, teenage pregnancy, truancy and stealing by children. They are often only able to deal with the crises and theory must give way to the practicalities of handling an almost unlimited demand for help from one part of the population, and unlimited resistance to receiving help from others and a restricted amount of trained resource available. The built-in stress upon professionals in this situation is obvious.

This stress is also felt by the health workers who also have to meet demands with limited resources. The further resources are placed from the area of need, the less likely it is that they will be used. We have therefore developed a very local service. The inverse care law, described by Zinkin & Cox (1976) states that those families most in need of health care are those least likely to attend. This provides a challenge for the health service to make itself not only acceptable but accessible.

NEW DEVELOPMENTS

Immigrant families

Many families have a poor knowledge of English both written and spoken. This leads to difficulties in history taking and health teaching as well as in understanding labels on bottles, powdered milks and official forms. The first step was an ante-natal English class containing health teaching and English lessons. This is run by a midwife, an English teacher and an interpreter. The second step was an English class run within our own child health clinics with similar aims, involving a health visitor, an English teacher and an interpreter. A playgroup leader is available to look after older children.

Volunteers from the local Asian community have not only helped with translation in the home or clinic, but have also aided us as valuable consultants explaining much about culture, diet and attitudes towards health and disease.

Toy library

The child health clinic is seen not solely as a screening clinic, but as a place for health education, a place for social contact and for the children to play. The toy library fills an important need for the community. It is used by nursery schools and day nurseries as well as by mothers attending the clinic. Many homes have few or no appropriate toys for the children. Toys afford a means of bringing more stimulation into the homes and creating activities for parents and children to do together.

'For you and baby'—The Nottingham Baby Book

This is our approach toards a parent-held record of their child's development. It combines in a 36-page booklet, a record of the first year of life and simple written information. The reading age of 11.6 years brings it within the ability of most of our parents. It is heavily illustrated with the pictures carrying much of the information that is in print. Many of the pictures are intended to be amusing (Fig. 16.2) and we hope that the book will be fun to use. The content of the book is development (towards walking, towards talking, finding your hands), general care (feeding, sleeping, crying, play and safety), common illnesses, when to call the doctor and a record of clinic visits. The section on development is filled in by the parents and we hope will provide a basis for encouraging them to observe their own child. The book emphasises the essential partnership of parents and professionals in the care of children and the support of parents.

Children in day nurseries

Our sector of the inner city area of Nottingham contains four day nurseries. It was apparent that they contained a high concentration of social and developmental problems. Contacts with the parents of the children and with other agencies dealing with families could be poor. To some extent they seemed apart from the 'therapeutic' approach of other professionals, yet they had the care of the child for most of the day. The familiar custodial model seemed to operate, yet the staff were aware of this and dissatisfied with its limitations.

With the full help of the nurseries a series of programmes were set up, some initiated solely by the nursery staff and some as joint activities with the community paediatric team or other agencies. The nurseries themselves set

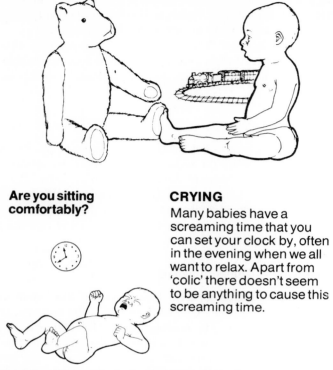

Are you sitting comfortably?

CRYING
Many babies have a screaming time that you can set your clock by, often in the evening when we all want to relax. Apart from 'colic' there doesn't seem to be anything to cause this screaming time.

Fig. 16.2 Examples of illustrations in the Nottingham Baby Book

up parents groups and a book lending service which formed a bridge between nursery activities and the home.

Language development was a major area of concern. Up to 50% of the children had a standard score of below −1.0 in the Reynell Scale, as shown by Bath (1981). Based on these assessments, she set up individual language programmes for children, carried out by herself or the nursery nurses. These programmes were most successful and brought other advantages. The nursery staff generalised their skills learned using the programmes to other children. They developed very impressive skills in observation, recording and understanding different aspects of the child's development. The findings of assessment and programmes were explained to parents.

Individual programmes have also been set up to tackle other types of developmental and behaviour problem.

Although many children in the nurseries are on observation registers, surveillance and immunisation in this group is often incomplete and indeed many clinic records are blank. A high incidence of conductive hearing losses is to be expected (up to 30%) and yet many children do not attend for hearing testing. The inverse care law is again at work. A research programme, using tympanometry, is running in all the city day nurseries—to date 70 children from among a nursery population of 700, (12 nurseries in all throughout Nottingham), have been found with significant but previously undetected conductive hearing losses.

A new surveillance programme

Only a small proportion of the work in the community is screening. The rest is responding to needs and demands as they arise. However, many districts have 'surveillance programmes' where they have not stated the conditions being screened for, the procedures to be adopted, accepted limits of normal and agreed action for those outside these limits. Moreover, confusion as to who should do this surveillance has resulted in wasteful duplication. The team decided to trim our original screening programme that consisted of the almost traditional complete examination at 6 weeks, 8 months, 1 year, 18 months, $2\frac{1}{2}$ to 3 years, $4\frac{1}{2}$ years. We decided to do less but to do it well. We also decided to be flexible, to leave aside the rigidity that demanded full developmental and physical assessment on each visit, and to structure our consultation depending on the history from the mother, the past medical history and to carrying out screening tests of established value such as those for dislocation of the hips or hearing tests. This discipline has to some extent been difficult to acquire, particularly by the author who enjoys serial developmental tests, even if their value is not established. After each examination, subsequent appointments are based on the needs established rather than any traditional scheme. These changes have enabled us to perform fewer, but far more meaningful examinations. We hope that our new records aid communication and form a simple system for recording and classification of problems.

The family centre

The family centre has emerged as our attempt to meet the almost insatiable needs of those families where there are the greatest deficiencies in parenting. The children are frequently in care or in hospital and the parents in trouble with the law. The centre was set up with the following aims:
  1. To promote practical parenting skills related to:
  (a) play and stimulation
  (b) day-to-day physical care
  (c) awareness and management of health problems
  2. To promote better home management, through a home economics programme
  3. To promote literacy
  4. To provide insight for parents into the needs of children and parents both in family life and in education
  5. To promote satisfaction for parents in parenting. To help parents to enjoy their children

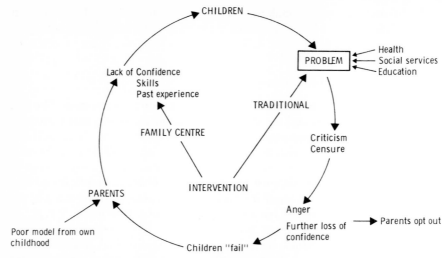

Fig. 16.3 The cycle of events in families with multiple problems

6. To reduce dependence on agencies for day-to-day care and acute problems.

The staff consists of a full-time social worker who is the co-ordinator of the project, a health visitor, a community teacher and a playgroup leader, plus a wide range of volunteers such as a nursery nurse, a hairdresser and a cook. Figure 16.3 illustrates the working of the centre and how we hope to interrupt the cycle shown.

The centre is open four mornings a week including lunchtime. On Monday and Tuesday programmes are run on topics such as health, family life, living with children, making decisions, boredom, and 'understanding my moods'. Wednesday is devoted to other activities such as jumble sales, outings, arts and crafts, adult literacy, cooking, hairdressing and family centre meetings. On Thursdays there is a contact group for new families and for those who have passed through the centre. The length of time any one family attends is usually 3 to 6 months.

The family centre is to many eyes an extended family, with the team losing some of their professional identity and the protection that this affords. The families learn to trust us, they share in the decision making and attend their own case conferences. The confidence that they require to do this has been acquired in the centre. They are anxious to show guests around the centre and enjoy the success of fund raising activities which were previously seen as activities that other people did.

Within the centre, the parents are responsible for their children and are encouraged to include them in activities such as cooking. We attempt to 'keep our hands off the children'. Where problems arise, parents are taught the skills and encouraged to solve them themselves.

The family centre is funded as a research project. An evaluation of this approach is planned in the next year (1983). Our subjective assessment is that the project has been successful. Perhaps in our previous professional contacts we have prejudged the families. This has caused us to concentrate on 'the problems'. We have discovered intelligence and confidence in these families. We have seen these emerge and have appreciated the difficulties that even small steps have presented them and the courage required to make those steps against a background of personal deprivation and past failure. Is this 'Pygmalian'?

THE PLACE OF THE COMMUNITY PAEDIATRIC TEAM IN THE REORGANISED HEALTH SERVICE

Our experience in the inner city area of Nottingham has demonstrated the feasibility of integrating hospital and community based services for children. The development of this concept would be a combined District Paediatric Service. This development would be in the best interests of the children. It would also provide a stable base, linked both to primary and secondary care that would both strengthen Community Child Health Services, and prevent the clinical isolation of those working within them. We feel that in providing services to our community we have looked critically at its needs, individual professional roles and the types of programme that they carry out.

Acknowledgements

I am grateful to Professor David Hull, and Dr Eleanor More (Specialist in Community Medicine, Child Health) for supporting the development of this programme and all the team members who have made it work.

REFERENCES

The Anderson Report 1982 Report of the working party on career structure and training of community health doctors. British Medical Journal 284: 359–362
Bath D 1981 Developing the speech therapy services in day nurseries: a progress report. British Journal of Disorders of Communication 163: 159–173
The Black Report 1980 Inequalities in health. Report of a research working group. Department of Health and Social Security.
Blaxter M 1981 Studies in Deprivation and Disadvantage. 3. The Health of the Children. Heinemann Educational Books, London
The Brotherston Report 1973 SHHD, towards an integrated child health service. Report of a working party on child health services, Edinburgh. Her Majesty's Stationery Office
The Clarke Report 1980 Report of the joint working party on community doctors. British Medical Journal 281: 955–955
The Court Report 1976 Fit for the future. Committee on child health services. Cmnd 6684, London, Her Majesty's Stationery Office
The Forfar Report 1982 Report of the joint working party on the training of clinical medical officers in child health. British Medical Journal 284: 637–640
Latham A 1981 Health appraisal/surveillance by school nurses. Health Visitor 54: 25–26

Madeley R 1978 Relating child health services to needs by the use of simple epidemiology. Public Health 92: 224–230

Nottinghamshire County Council 1975 The County Deprived Area Study

The Preston Report 1979 British Medical Association report of the working party on community health doctors. British Medical Journal i: 503–504

Royal College of General Practitioners 1982 Healthier Children—Thinking Prevention

Rutter M, Madge N 1976 Cycles of Disadvantage. A Review of Research. Heinemann, London

The Sheldon Report 1967 Standing Medical Advisory Committee, Child Welfare Centres. Her Majesty's Stationery Office, London

Spencer N J, Power F C 1977 Child health clinic survey. Prepared for North and South Nottingham District Health Care Planning Team (Child Health)

Wedge P, Prosser H 1973 Born to fail. Arrow Books in association with the National Children's Bureau

Wynne J, Hull D 1977 Why are children admitted to hospital? British Medical Journal ii: 1140–1142

Zinkin P M, Cox C A 1976 Child health clinics and inverse care laws: evidence from longitudinal study of 1978 pre-school children. British Medical Journal ii: 411–417

The functions of child health clinics

INTRODUCTION

Although the role of child health clinics has greatly changed since their introduction early this century, in many people's minds the clinic remains the traditional model providing subsidised infant foods, essential immunisations, and screening for such remedial abnormalities as dislocatable hips and undescended testes. However, parents nowadays bring their children to child health clinics for a wide variety of reasons: often it is for reassurance, but often too for specific and sometimes complex problems of illness and behaviour. The variety of medical problems which may present to a clinic doctor has been described by Illingworth (1979), which underlined the need for clinic doctors to have had adequate paediatric training.

Thus, the challenge of the community health services at the present time is to retain the best of the traditional model whilst evolving to meet the wider health needs of families with young children. With the decrease in emphasis on the physical pathology these needs are often to do with the behaviour of the child, which has not previously been considered a provenance in which traditional medicine was interested. Nevertheless, illness, behaviour and development are all inter-related and cannot now be viewed in isolation. Nor can they be separated from family or environmental factors, as we know that family stress, social conditions and maternal depression can adversely affect children's health (Haggerty, 1980).

In some areas services have adopted the problem orientated approach and with scarce resources are abandoning the attempt at total cover. However, it is still an important aim to provide cover for all children, not only to ensure high immunisation uptake but also because, even if one can identify a high risk population who will have an increased incidence of disease, it is still likely that the majority of disease will arise in the very much bigger group who are not at risk.

TRADITIONAL ROLES

Immunisation

Unfortunately, it tends to be forgotten that immunisation remains probably the best preventive health measure that the child health clinic, at present, provides. Maintaining a high immunisation rate amongst the child population therefore should remain a priority when considering the organisation and functions of child health clinics, especially as the National Child Development Study (Davie et al, 1972) found lower rates of immunisation uptake amongst children of lower social class parents (10% of children from social class IV and V were not immunised against polio, compared with 1% for social class I) as these very children are most likely to be at risk of higher morbidity from infectious diseases.

A current issue is whether immunisation sessions should be held separately from the normal child health clinic function as in some ways this is more efficient, especially if a nurse is available to give the injection whilst the health visitor and doctor concentrate on other aspects of child health. Ideally, the two sessions could run concurrently. At the present rates of pay a $2\frac{1}{2}$ hour session at which say 25 children are immunised would cost, in terms of the actual injection given, about £7 per session if a nurse was giving the injections, £22.10 if a clinical medical officer was giving the injection, and £67.50 if done by a general practitioner and charged to The Family Practitioner Committee. The disadvantage of having specific and separate sessions for immunisations is, of course, that parents frequently wish to discuss other problems at the same time. It seems likely that local areas have to decide for themselves what the most appropriate system of organisation between practice nurses, health visitors, GP's and clinical medical officers should be in regard to the immunisation policy.

Subsidised infant foods

In a recent survey in Oxfordshire (Macfarlane, personal communication) only 5.7% attending mothers considered subsidised foods to be a benefit of child health clinics. In many areas of England at the moment, not only can tokens be exchanged exclusively at child health clinics, but also child health clinics provide milk cheaper than those available over the counter in chemist shops. Many health visitors object to the role of acting as shop keepers in clinics and consideration needs to be given to the possibility of tokens being exchanged in chemist shops and ceasing to provide cheaper milk in child health clinics. Further, the exchange of tokens in child health clinics identifies certain parents within the social milieu of the clinic as being near poverty level.

Screening

The regular screening of children for certain abnormalities remains a contentious issue. It has classically been accepted that screening for visual abnormalities, hearing abnormalities, and language abnormalities, along with certain physical defects, such as undescended testes and dislocatable hip, fill the suggestion that screening tests should satisfy certain criteria. These criteria are: that the condition being screened for must have a significant morbidity or mortality and must be sufficiently prevalent to justify the cost of screening; the programme must cover the entire population, especially any individuals at particular risk of the condition; the condition, once picked up by screening must be treatable or controllable, and early treatment must have a significant advantage. Further, that adequate resources must be available for the definitive diagnosis and treatment of all individuals picked up by the screen; that the cost of the programme must be outweighed by the savings in human suffering and alternative expenditure that would occur if the condition was not diagnosed until the symptomatic stage. It should also be justified with respect to the false negative rate and in terms of the other ways in which such resources might be deployed. A false positive result in screening tests will also be costly in terms both of resources and of unnecessary anxiety to the parents. Beyond these, the test must be simple and convenient and the people who use it must believe that it is worthwhile. Within these terms recently even the value of early visual screening has been questioned (Hall et al, 1982) and it may well be that for certain conditions simply asking the parents whether they consider there is a problem may turn out to be equally or more effective than other forms of screening.

The issue of developmental screening is even more complex and a review of the evidence at present available in the literature suggests that the present methods for detecting neurodevelopmental abnormalities fall short of most of the above criteria. Standard tests are often used, such as The Denver Developmental Screening Test, based on small and non-representative samples and designed to measure delay, rather than abnormality. Furthermore, it does not differentiate between parental report and professional observation. There is limited evidence at present of any positive benefit from the management of delays detected by such methods. However, this is not to say that developmental testing techniques should not continue to be researched, but rather that all methods of screening, now and in the future, should be carefully researched using the above criteria.

Attendance

It is well known in many areas that attendance at child health clinics is disappointing. Patterson (1972) found in Westminster that 77% of babies attended for the 6-week examination but only 52% attended at 2 years and 44% at $4\frac{1}{2}$ years.

A similar pattern was found at one clinic in Camden before the start of the Thomas Coram study, described later in this chapter, with a drop-off in attendance after the age of 6 weeks (when it was 70%) to 58% at 1 year, 49% at 2 years and 47% at 3 years.

Attendance rates reported from child health clinics run by general practitioners vary hugely, from very high rates in one home counties practice (Curtin Jenkins et al, 1978) to rates of 59% overall attendance for developmental screening at a health centre in Glasgow (Bain, 1974). More recently Barber (1982) has reported greatly improved attendance rates at a Glasgow health centre with a significant detection of problems (discussed in more detail later).

A study of child health clinics in York (Graham, 1979) looked at attendance patterns within social class and reasons for the drop off in attendance. Initially, attendance rates were high for both middle and working class mothers, but by 5 months only 40% of working class mothers attended the clinic compared to 87% of social class I and II mothers. Also, considerably less working class mothers reported finding the advice of their health visitor helpful.

Graham stated 'the key question for the child health service is not why some mothers fail to attend the clinic, but why after an initial visit or two they fail to return.' Interviews with mothers suggested some reasons for this which related to an approach by the clinic staff which was felt to be critical, unsympathetic or judgemental. Hardly surprising then that the mothers failed to return—with the result that they were subsequently likely to be misjudged as being uninterested in their children's health.

A more positive picture emerges from other areas; for instance, a recent Oxfordshire study of parental views of child health clinics suggests that most parents do like going and that they feel the clinics fulfill a useful role (Macfarlane, personal communication).

Over a 12-month period, 103 child health clinics in Oxfordshire were visited, and 999 mothers interviewed. The great majority of mothers liked the clinics, and the main benefits mentioned were getting advice from the health visitor and gaining reassurance. Again, the social aspect of the clinic was mentioned by nearly a third of mothers. Complaints were few, although 12% of mothers did mention the long waiting time. Other complaints were of too infrequent clinics (1%), insufficient advice (1%), and inconvenient clinic times (1%), and five mothers were critical of staff attitudes.

The same study attempted to go some way towards looking at the reasons why certain parents did not attend child health clinics by asking the health visitors at all the clinics visited if they knew of parents within their area who regularly did not come. 150 families were identified in this way of whom 31 (21%) failed to visit because of transport difficulties, 54 (36%) did not attend either because they disliked the doctor or did not find the clinics useful, or did not want immunisation, and 23 (15%) did not attend either because they were too disorganised, or had diffuse social problems. Of the remainder, either the reason was not known or they were attending their GP at the surgery for developmental checks and immunisations.

THE BROADER FUNCTIONS OF CHILD HEALTH CLINICS

In this section I want to draw heavily on a recent study done at the Thomas Coram Research Unit in London, but first I will briefly review some of the other information available on child health screening programmes.

Glasgow

A pre-school developmental screening programme has been in operation by general practitioners and health visitors at the Woodside Health Centre in Glasgow since 1973. In the last 4 years, since amendments to the programme were made, the default rate has fallen to less than 10% at each age, and the results from one practice for this 4 year period have recently been published (Barber, 1982).

The minimum number of attendances requested was four (at 6 weeks, 7–10 months, 2 years and 4 years) with the health visitor completing the examination at home when children persistently failed to attend the clinic. At 7–10 months 8% of children had delayed or abnormal development, at 2 years 10% had developmental delay. Fifteen per cent of children (all ages) were found to have a previously undetected physical abnormality, and in total the percentage of children in whom a problem was detected requiring either intervention or follow up was 23%. The author made the point that 'it is of obvious importance to detect abnormal hearing before the age at which speech develops; it is equally important, but less obvious, that abnormal development in other social, manipulative, and interpersonal areas is also prevented by early detection and remedy.' From this study the pick-up rate of problems requiring action would certainly seem to justify the programme of developmental screening.

Three-year-olds in Westminster

A study examining a random sample of 132 3-year-old children in Kensington, Chelsea and Westminster found 54% of children with one or more problems requiring follow up or referral (Spies, 1979). Behaviour problems were about as common as developmental problems, and were found more often amongst children with language problems. A striking finding of this study (although unsurprising in view of the area policy on criteria for admission to day nursery) was that rates of most problems were twice as high in children attending day nurseries as in those who did not. Certainly, the data support the argument that one should ensure good paediatric cover for all day nurseries with adequate allocation of time.

Thomas Coram Research Unit Study

A recent study by the Thomas Coram Research Unit looked at the health needs and use of services of two populations of under-fives in North London in some detail. This study was inspired and launched by the late Professor Jack Tizard. One of the main aims of the study was to collect epidemiological data on the patterns of illness, development and behaviour problems in these young children.

The study took place in two geographical areas, each centred around a child health clinic and children's centre which provided both day nursery and nursery school facilities. The study areas had fairly typical inner urban characteristics, with nearly all the families living in flats.

In one area the social class was below the national average, and one-third of patients had been born outside the U.K. In the other, the parents' social class status was slightly higher than average, but the majority of families were bringing up their children in over-crowded conditions with inadequate access to play space.

Each area represented one health visitor's catchment, covering approximately 200 families. During the 5-year period of the study the two child health clinics were run by three doctors with considerable paediatric experience, and the children were seen at seven 'key' ages from birth to $4\frac{1}{2}$ years. Data were collected at these specific ages and the children were frequently seen at other times, whenever the parents wished to attend the clinic.

The service differed between the two areas, in that the children's centre in Paddington was in a new purpose built building incorporating the child health clinic on the first floor above the day nursery and nursery school. This centre also had a mothers' club, where parents could make tea or coffee, and an adjoining staffed play area for the children.

The centre became very much a focal point for many families of young children in the area and there were obvious advantages in having all facilities under one roof. Not least was the lack of complaints about waiting to see the doctor, as the time could be well spent along the other end of the corridor.

In the Camden area the clinic was a previously established local authority clinic in a fairly new building and adjoining a well-known children's hospital. The children's centre was approximately 250 yards away across a grassy square, and once children were attending there they were seen for medicals at the children's centre. There was a launderette at this centre, toy library and mother and toddler groups. The babies and young children were seen at the clinic which, on one afternoon a week, extended its hours until 6.30 pm to enable parents to come after work.

A yearly house-to-house enquiry ensured that all children living in the areas were known to the health visitor, who asked them to attend the clinic and followed up non-attendances with home visits. Children moving into the areas were included in the study, but we were unable to follow up those who moved out. In all, 900 children were seen over the 5 years with a total of over

3000 examinations. Some of the children were seen for all seven examinations between 6 weeks and 5 years, the remainder having a variable number of examinations before moving out of the areas.

During the study, attendance rates at the selected ages were over 96% at all ages. There was also a high attendance for non-routine visits between developmental checks, and these in fact represented two-thirds of all visits to the child health clinics. During the first year of life visits to the clinic averaged 13 (excluding developmental checks) at which there was always contact with the health visitor, and sometimes with the doctor. The clinics were run on a 'walk-in' basis as well as appointments for developmental checks, and attempted to be both friendly and flexible. Parents were encouraged to discuss any problems or worries they had related to their child and issues, such as housing difficulties, and marital problems were often brought up. There was no significant social class variation in the number of clinic visits in the first year, nor did we find social class differences between parents who were high attenders and those who were low attenders.

The findings

Data were available on the children's health, developmental and behavioural problems. At each age, around 20% of children were considered to have a problem requiring either intervention or follow up in one of these areas, and often the problems overlapped.

Developmental problems The most common of these was speech and language delay or abnormality; at 2 years 5% of children, and at 3 years 7% of children were considered to have a definite abnormality of speech and language, the assessment of the children's speech being validated by independent assessments by both a psychologist and speech therapist (Bax et al, 1980).

Other developmental problems were less common, and the rates of abnormal findings on motor development, vision and hearing are shown in Table 17.1 below. An assessment was made in each area of whether the child's development was normal, possibly abnormal, or definitely abnormal at each age. The rates given in the table are combined for the latter two.

Table 17.1 Percentage of abnormal developmental findings requiring intervention or follow-up

	Age				
	6 months (N = 335)	1 year (N = 273)	2 years (N = 295)	3 years (N = 328)	4½ years (N = 275)
Gross motor	2%	3%	2%	1%	3%
Fine motor	3%	2%	6%	10%	7%
Vision	4%	3%	1%	11%	8%
Hearing	12%	3%	3%	9%	7%

Table 17.2 Prevalence of behaviour problems

	6 months		1 year		2 years		3 years		4½ years	
	n	%	n	%	n	%	n	%	n	%
Parents worried about behaviour	11	3	23	8	34	11	45	15	35	13
Parents not worried	321	97	254	92	268	89	283	85	243	87
Total number	332		277		302		331		278	

Behaviour problems A questionnaire, based on that used by Richman et al (1975) was used to ask about various aspects of the child's behaviour at each age, and the parents were asked whether any aspect of their child's behaviour was a problem to them. A considerable number of children were reported to have problems, with the highest rates at 3 years, when 15% of parents were worried about their child's behaviour (Jenkins et al, 1980). The prevalence rates are shown in Table 17.2.

The most common problem in the younger children was night waking, which was strikingly more common than feeding problems, and often caused considerable distress and fatigue to parents. Waking on at least four nights a week was reported in 21% of babies at 1 year old, and 17% at 18 months, with an additional 6% and 9% waking two or three nights a week. Hence, 27% of parents of 1 year olds were suffering from very frequent disturbed nights.

In children over 2 years of age, parents commonly reported difficulty in managing certain behaviours. Night waking most nights was still reported in 15% of 2 year olds, and attention seeking and frequent temper tantrums were common. Twenty per cent of 2-year-olds were having tantrums at least once a day. Parents often sought advice as to how to manage these behaviours.

Although attendance rates at GP surgeries were high in this sample of children, behavioural and developmental problems were given as reasons for only 4% of GP consultations. The child health clinic was the venue where the large majority of parents sought professional help for these problems, usually in addition to advice sought from friends or relatives.

When asked what topic they had discussed at the clinic in a preceeding period, a fairly wide variety of topics was mentioned by mothers. They may, of course, mask a true reason for consultation, particularly where a mother is depressed. Behaviour, other than feeding, sleeping or toileting was discussed by 13% of mothers, similar to the proportion who remembered discussing worries about their child's speech or hearing, but considerably less than the rates for consultation for illness (Table 17.3).

Rates of illness Information about illnesses and accidents the children had suffered from, and attendance rates at GP surgeries and hospitals, were collected at regular intervals. The children had a physical examination on

Table 17.3 Topics discussed at clinic in previous 12 months

	Number of mothers*	%*
Feeding, sleeping or toileting	50	32
Other behaviour	20	13
Illness	49	31
Development	27	17
Speech or hearing	22	14
Pre-school provision	26	16
Housing	18	11
Mother's mental state	13	8
Total number	158	

* Some mothers discussed more than one topic

these occasions, hence data on the wide variety of health problems encountered in pre-school children was available, both from history and examination.

The proportion of children with one or more abnormal physical findings was 16–19% in children under 2, and 11–15% from 2–4½ years. In the under twos, the most common findings were umbilical hernias (4% at 1 year), undescended testis (4% of boys at 18 months), and squints (2% at 18 months). In the children over 2, upper respiratory tract abnormalities, skin conditions (e.g. eczema) and squint (4% at 3 years) were the most frequent findings.

In some cases the physical abnormalities were minor and often already noted by parents (e.g. umbilical hernias, haemangiomata), but in others parents were not always aware of the abnormality and referral was indicated (as for squint or undescended testis).

The rates of so-called 'minor' illness were high among children in this study, those being most commonly reported were recurrent colds or sore throats, ear infections, and bronchitis. Other illnesses were less common, but at each age around 20% of children had some significant illness.

The Inter-relationship of problems Not surprisingly, there was at all ages a strong association between recurrent upper respiratory infections and both bronchitis and ear infections. Of more interest was the strong inter-relationship found between illness and behaviour problems, and behaviour and developmental problems (Bax et al, 1983). Children who had recurrent colds, or ear infections, were significantly more likely to be night wakers, and to be difficult to manage. There were also strong relationships between ear infections and temper tantrums, particularly at 2 years, and between recurrent colds and feeding problems at 2 years. Of the developmental problems, the child with speech and language delay or abnormality was significantly more likely to have behaviour problems at 2 years and over.

Parents' views The parents' views of the two child health clinics in the Thomas Coram study were sought by interview and have been described previously (Hart et al, 1981). The majority of comments were favourable, with over 75% of mothers being satisfied with the advice and help given. The features which parents particularly liked, and mentioned, were the friendly welcoming atmosphere of the clinic, staff who had time for listening and explanations, the ability to walk in without an appointment, and the thorough examinations and explanations. Criticisms were about waiting times which were sometimes long, and the inability of clinics to prescribe.

The social aspect of the clinic was mentioned by many mothers. 'If it wasn't for the clinic I'd be a lonely person—it brought me out of my shell', and, 'it cheers you up—it's done wonders for me—even if you are quiet they encourage you to talk.'

GENERAL APPLICABILITY OF SUCH STUDIES

All the studies mentioned so far relate to inner urban areas, and the data reflect some of the particular problems of children and families in this type of environment. How best to provide appropriate primary care to families in Inner London has again been recently discussed both in the Acheson Report (DHSS, 1981), and the Royal College of General Practitioners Report (1981: The Jarman Report).

It is debatable how far results from studies in such areas apply to other areas where environmental factors are less adverse and there are likely to be less health and behavioural problems. However, certain general principles do apply, the main one being that one cannot separate the different aspects of child health, but must aim for a service which is both comprehensive and competent to diagnose and manage all the inter-related paediatric problems. The primary care service must have access to a paediatric consultant service relevant to the community and knowledgeable about its resources, and also access to a district handicap team.

The management of behaviour problems is not traditionally thought of as one of the roles of a child health clinic. However, unless problems are severe and reach the child psychiatry services, the clinic may be the only source of professional advice in the pre-school years. The findings from the Thomas Coram study are not unique, for instance, similar rates of night waking have been reported by Bernal (1974), Carey (1975), Ounsted & Simons (1978), and Blurton Jones et al (1978). The relationship between speech and language delay and behaviour problems was reported earlier by Stevenson & Richman (1976), in their large study of 3-year-olds. It is important to recognise this clinically, since the association between speech and language delay and behaviour problems can be demonstrated as young as 2 years.

Delayed speech is known to be correlated with later learning problems (Fundudis et al, 1979), and deviant behaviour in older children is more common in those with poor reading attainment (Rutter et al, 1970). The challenge is now to find intervention methods which will prove successful, although currently we do not know whether these should be aimed at the behaviour problem or the speech problem, or both. Children with speech and language delay, and/or behaviour problems represent around 10% of the population of 3-year-olds and one suspects that many of them remain undetected. Certainly, in most areas the intervention offered remains unmonitored as to its long-term effectiveness, and this is a field ripe for further research. Meantime, parents will continue to seek help for these and other problems, and the clinic should therefore be prepared to offer it.

A major criticism of child health clinics is that they have failed to adapt to the needs of their clients, and that they take a somewhat rigid approach to developmental screening. Both these criticisms are certainly, although not universally, true. With the devolvement of organisation to district level, the time is ripe for a critical look at individual clinics and more imaginative use of local resources and initiative. Attention should certainly be directed to the views of the clients—what sort of service do families want and need, are the clinics sited in convenient places, and are the hours appropriate?

It is well recognised that the attitude of health workers towards parents with young children is crucial in determining whether they will continue to use a clinic service. It is probably true also of the GP and hospital services although less so, since the circumstances provoking the consultation are somewhat different. Patronising or critical attitudes will put off many parents, particularly mothers whose confidence in their own role may already be undermined. Child health clinics can, and should, provide an opportunity for a mother to discuss her own health and feelings. Depression is extremely common among mothers of young children, as are minor health problems and marital problems, and often the health visitor is the first person to be aware of these. She can offer support and advice, and refer to the clinic doctor, GP, or other agencies when appropriate, for further help. This supportive role with families is an integral part of the function of a child health clinic, although one of the more difficult to evaluate.

The Clinic Doctor—GP or CMO?

Much debate has recently centred around the provision of primary care for children, and integration of the 'preventive' and 'therapeutic' services. The idea of a general practitioner paediatrician put forward in the Court Report remains an ideal for many, but he or she remains a mythical beast. The reality is that overall many GPs (between 10% and 20%) are already running their own child health clinics alongside normal surgeries, and that in certain districts, such as Oxfordshire, as many as 72% of all child health clinics are run by GPs. The recent working party report from the Royal College of General Practitioners (1982) suggests that this trend will escalate. The report makes a brief analysis of the present state of child health in the United Kingdom and makes a case for GPs undertaking the total care of children. It also acknowledges the deficiencies in child health care provided by many general practitioners.

Although some of the ideas and recommendations of the report are sound, there were certain naivities evident, not least in assessing the amount of time entailed in undertaking the extra work. It is assessed as approximately 10 minutes per child per year, which is a gross underestimate even for 'normal' children, but particularly if one assumes that 20% of children will have some problem requiring further evaluation and follow up.

The report is timely, and its conclusion that the separation of health surveillance from the rest of the medical care of children is totally inappropriate, is absolutely correct.

However, issues such as the workload and time required, adequate training for the doctors involved, and ensuring cover for all children (traditionally by the geographical 'patch') have yet to be fully worked out. Meantime, the evidence including that from the Thomas Coram study supports the need for continuing a preventive child health service, particularly in inner cities. Wherever possible this should be linked to primary care practices to facilitate communication, but the practical problems remain enormous, as exampled by the children attending one child health clinic in Camden who were between them registered with no less than 72 different general practitioners.

The health visitor

The health visitor is the lynch pin of the community paediatric service and has a unique role to play with young families. More recently her role has been extended to include developmental surveillance and it is obviously important that she be adequately trained in child development in order to be competent in this field.

Again, the time factor is of primary concern, and a note of caution should be sounded, for time spent on developmental screening will mean less time for other crucial activities, and priorities may need to be re-defined. It is obviously logical for health visitors to do some of the developmental screening, and exactly who does what should be worked out at a very local level. Certainly where there is concern about families who fail to attend clinics, the health visitor should be ready to do the surveillance at home. One hopes also that clinic doctors or GPs will back her up with home visits in these circumstances.

It is essential though to note that health visitors are already hard worked and in some areas have large case loads, and cannot always find time to support depressed mothers or visit frequently their 'at risk' families. Their case loads too include many elderly people, whose needs will also encroach on paediatric visiting time. It would be a pity if they got caught up in developmental screening to the detriment of valuable work in other areas. Ideally, the team of health visitors and doctor in any one clinic should work together to decide who does what, and this will depend on local priorities as well as individual skills.

CONCLUSIONS

In summary, child health clinics still have an important part to play in the health care of pre-school children. With local initiative, flexibility, and imagination they can go a long way towards providing the sort of service that is attractive and useful to parents.

This service needs to take a broad view of preventive health, to meet more of the needs of young families. We can convince ourserlves that detecting squints and undescended testes is a useful exercise, as the results are measurable. Data on the effectiveness of other aspects of clinic work, such as advising on behaviour problems or supporting a depressed mother, may be currently lacking, but it is time to view these issues as real and as affecting children's health. We need to continue to look at such problems, and develop tools to measure the interventions offered.

A good child health clinic should be flexible as to who mans the service, as to the ages at which children are seen for surveillance, and in the approach to families as well as clinic hours and the siting of the clinic. Meeting social needs as well as providing health education should be an aim, and activities such as language classes for immigrant mothers, keep-fit classes, single parent groups, and mother and toddler groups are to be encouraged.

Essentially, there should be continuity of health visitors and doctors, working closely together, avoiding giving conflicting advice, and deciding together who does which aspects of the work. The accent should be on assessment rather than screening. There continue to be many children in need of a competent community paediatric service. The challange of the eighties is to resist any weakening of that service, and to look critically at it and use its resources more imaginatively.

REFERENCES

Bax M, Hart H, Jenkins S 1980 Assessment of speech and language development in the young child. Pediatrics 66: 350–354
Bax M, Hart H, Jenkins S 1983 Behaviour, development and health of the young child—implications for care. British Medical Journal 286: 1793–1796
Bain D J G 1974 The results of developmental screening in general practice. Health Bulletin 32: 189–193
Barber J H 1982 Pre-school developmental screening—the results of a four year period. Health Bulletin 40: 170–178
Bernal J F 1973 Night waking in infants in the first 14 months. Developmental Medicine and Child Neurology, 15: 760–769
Blurton Jones N, Rossetti Ferreira M C, Farquar Brown M, Macdonald L 1978 The association between perinatal factors and later night waking. Developmental Medicine and Child Neurology, 20: 427–434
Carey W B 1975 Breast feeding and night waking. Journal of Paediatrics, 87: 327–328
Curtis Jenkins G., Collins C, Andren S 1978 Developmental surveillance in general practice. British Medical Journal, i: 1537–1540
Davie R, Butler N, Goldstein H 1972 From birth to seven: a report of the National Child Development Study. Longman, London

Department of Health and Social Security 1981 Primary Health Care in Inner London. The Acheson Report: London Health Planning Consortium

Fundudis T, Kolvin I, Garside R 1979 Speech retarded and deaf children: their psychological development. Academic Press, London

Graham H 1979 Women's attitudes to the child health service. Health Visitor, 52: 175–178

Haggerty R J 1980 Life stress, illness and social supports. Developmental Medicine and Child Neurology 22: 391–400

Hall, S, Pugh A, Hall D 1982 Vision screening in the under-5s. British Medical Journal 285, 1096–1098

Hart H, Bax M, Jenkins S 1981 The Use of the child health clinic. Archives of Disease in Childhood 56: 440–445

Illingworth R S 1979 Some experiences in an area health authority child health clinic. British Medical Journal i: 866–869

Jenkins S, Bax M, Hart H 1980 Behaviour problems in pre-school children. Journal of Child Psychology and Psychiatry 21: 5–17

Ounsted M K, Simons C D 1978 The first-born child: toddler problems. Developmental Medicine and Child Neurology 20: 710–719

Patterson M T 1972 Developmental screening of pre-school children. Community Medicine 128: 423–425

Richman N, Stevenson J, Graham P 1975 Prevalence of behaviour problems in 3 year old children: an epidemiological study in a London borough. Journal of Child Psychology & Psychiatry 16: 277–287

Royal College of General Practitioners 1981 A survey of primary care in London. Occasional paper 16

Royal College of General Practitioners 1982 Healthier children—thinking prevention. Report from General Practice 22

Rutter M,Tizard J, Whitmore K 1970 Education, Health and Behaviour. Longman, London

Stevenson J, Richman N 1976 The prevalence of language delay in a population of 3 year old children and its association with general retardation. Developmental Medicine and Child Neurology 18: 431–441

Spies J 1980 Child Health Surveillance Survey. Kensington Chelsea and Westminster Area Health Authority

The past, present and future of the health services for children in school

AN HISTORICAL PERSPECTIVE

The need for and the origins of the service

From its origin in 1908 the School Health Services was intended to help prevent the malnutrition, disease and disability that was then rife amongst school children. For this reason it was organised as a community health service, overseen by the local medical officer of health (MOH) who also became the principal school medical officer (PSMO). This preventive function was apparent from the importance attached to routine medical inspections. These were originally made statutory at three specific ages and their purpose and conduct was explicitly stated in terms which today still seem appropriate as objectives for the service as a whole: 'the early detection of unsuspected defects, checking incipient maladies at their onset', and 'furnishing the facts which will guide education authorities in relation to physical and mental development during school life' (Board of Education, 1907).

These inspections not only confirmed an unacceptable level of disease and disability in elementary schoolchildren (Table 18.1) but also revealed a need for treatment facilities that were not available at the time. Consequently, local education authorities (LEAs) were required to provide these facilities themselves under the Education Act 1918 and they did so mainly by setting up special school clinics, including minor ailment clinics.

With the opening of more and more special schools the service was from its onset concerned with handicapped children, school doctors being given responsibility for recommending special education particularly for those children with physical disabilities, visual defects, mental retardation and epilepsy.

The school nursing service was an integral part of the statutory medical services organised by the PSMO, and its responsibilities included cleanliness inspections and dealing with infestation. This role has gradually extended since 1945 when regulations required school nurses to be qualified health visitors.

For 60 years the basic features outlined above remained the principle func-

213

Table 18.1 Aspects of health in school children, 1915–1971: the changing prevalence of selected defects found to require treatment per 1000 pupils examined (England and Wales)

Defect	1915*	1931	1951	1971
Malnutrition	133	12	29†	3‡
Skin disease	18	12	11	16
Infestation	204	140	23	21
Heart disease	36	2	NA	2
Lung disease	36	NA	NA	6
Nose and throat disease	207	70	35	12
Ear disease	25	5	3	12
Hearing defect	111	4	3	10
Speech defect	13	10**	3	7
Vision defect	173	96	92	67
Dental disease	691	680	707	559

* 90 LEAs only.
** For year 1932.
† Physical state classified as 'poor' on 3-point scale ('good', 'fair', or 'poor').
‡ Physical state classified as 'unsatisfactory' on 2-point scale.

Table 18.2 Special clinics for school children (England and Wales, 1938–1980)

Type	1938	1951	1962	1973	1980†
Minor ailment	1279	1781	1896(1)*	1413	1105
Ophthalmic	774	589	982(420)	934	714
Orthoptic	—	33	137(73)	149	290
Orthopaedic	382	224	453(231)	291	161
Physiotherapy and remedial exercise	121	96	705(81)	455	588
ENT	57	113	228(110)	247	228
Audiometry	—	13	322(23)	412	511
Audiology	—	—	—	902	1378
Speech therapy	—	650	1339(9)	1610	2217
Child guidance	—	82	325	424	297
Paediatric	—	14	103(62)	55	253
Chiropody	—	29	182(2)	337	606
Enuresis	—	—	79(4)	292	510
Asthma	—	—	57(12)	72	118
Obesity	—	—	—	—	273
'School doctor'	—	—	—	1518	1832
Miscellaneous	31	240	1539(55)**	482	532

* Figures in brackets show the number of such clinics provided under arrangements with Regional Hospital Boards.
** This figure includes 1214 immunisation clinics.
† Figures for 1980 are for England only.

tions of school doctors and nurses. The service flourished with the medical staff level reaching an all time high in 1950 (one full time doctor for every 6250 pupils). As a result a higher proportion of children in each statutory age group received medical inspection than at any other time, 5 500 000 pupils: at the same time LEAs had increased not only the number but also the range of treatment facilities in school clinics (Table 18.2). This latter development was in response to a continuing change in the epidemiology of medical problems in school children (Table 18.1).

The part played at the time by the preventive health services, including the school health services, in the striking improvement in the health of pupils was difficult to gauge but arguably significant. For notwithstanding the imminent introduction of a national health service, the Education Act 1944 continued to require LEAs to maintain their school health services and statutory medical inspections, and to secure treatment for all pupils whatever their age. In applying the principle that all pupils should receive education according to their age, ability and aptitude LEAs were obliged under the Act to continue to rely on school doctors to advise them as to which children needed special educational treatment and which were ineducable.

The recent history of the service

In contrast, over the last 15 years the traditional methods of the service have been challenged, with some of its most cherished functions being criticised, its relevance to the current difficulties experienced by both pupils and teachers questioned, and its very existence as a separate service keenly scrutinised.

New regulations governing the school health service were issued in 1959. They withdrew the obligation for LEAs to organise medical inspections at pre-ordained ages and left their frequency to the discretion of PSMOs. The latter were encouraged to be more selective in the use of re-examinations by doctors as a method of health surveillance (Department of Education and Science, 1964) and to study ways in which these might be limited to children who showed at least some evidence of actually needing them. Ten years later only half the LEAs had experimented with selective examinations and several had reverted to age-based routine examinations. But a review of these arrangements concluded that neither periodic routine nor selective examinations were particularly efficient (DES, 1972) as a method of maintaining a check on the health and development of school children once they had been fully examined on school entry. In 1979 more than one-third of school doctors' examinations were still repetitive inspections of pupils aged 7 to 16 and the majority of school health services were using selective examinations.

The statutory nature of periodic medical inspections understandably resulted in their remaining a priority task for the services, requiring considerable administrative back up and organisation of doctors' and nurses' work programmes by office staff. This frequently lead to a rotary pattern of service in schools with a doctor and nurse being detailed to attend one school for as long as it took to carry out all outstanding statutory inspections at approximately 6–8 minute intervals and then another school and so on.

The emphasis at these examinations tended to be on finding the physical defects that doctors had been conventionally trained to detect, rather than looking for those disabilities affecting speech and language and development (learning) and behaviour, which were becoming equally important. Furthermore, due to the organisation of the system, continuity of care and rapport with teachers was difficult to achieve, with class teachers seldom receiving the support and advice they would have liked (Fitzherbert, 1982). The need for the introduction of school counsellors in secondary schools to help adolescents with their psycho-social and sexual problems is a classical example of the traditional support services, both medical and psychological, having failed to adapt to meet the needs of their customers.

Because of the use of formal ascertainment of handicapped pupils, i.e. ascertainment according to the letter of the law which required a medical certificate stating the nature and extent of a pupil's disability and the category of handicap children in which he should be placed, there was an increasing discomfort inside and outside the service at the pre-eminent role of doctors in decisions about the special education of handicapped children. The categories of handicap were legally defined in special education terms, and categorisation (by a school doctor) was tantamount to a transfer to a special school. The gradual use of more informal and multi-disciplinary assessment (DES, 1975) resulted in a rationalisation of the use of expertise, but in the process the role of the doctor appeared to many to have been eroded.

More recently the recommendations of the Warnock Committee (1978) concerning assessment (now embodied in the Education Act 1981) were singularly bureaucratic and unimaginative with regard to the medical contribution. Those relating to the special education of handicapped children in ordinary schools—hailed as an innovation but first advocated 25 years earlier (Ministry of Education, 1954)—have again not influenced practice and hence have not changed the responsibilities of most school doctors.

Whilst the Education Act 1944 re-affirmed the legal duty of LEAs to secure treatment for their pupils, the National Health Service Act 1946 also re-affirmed the roles of the GP and the hospital in providing respectively primary and specialist medical care. It was clearly the intention of the NHS Act that the GP with whom a child was registered should be the principal person for the prescription of free medical care. Not only was this administratively convenient but it reinforced the principle of investing primary health care with one doctor. Preventive health care was not at that time regarded as a form of care 'usually provided by' GPs and hence they were not specifically under contract to give it (although some had always done so). It was therefore expected that LEAs would meet their obligations to secure the treatment of pupils by referring them either to their GP or to a hospital: that minor ailment clinics and other school clinics would gradually close down, and that the school health service would at last be able to concentrate on the promotion of health and prevention of ill-health.

In the event, this proved to be too naive and casual an understanding of the need for services in schools, and what at first may have seemed a rational division of responsibility has been a recipe for a crisis in clinical practice. On the one hand, the number of school clinics more than doubled between 1951 and 1973 and most of the minor ailment clinics were still operating even in 1980 though chiefly in urban areas. In addition school doctors started more of their own clinics offering parents help with their management of obesity, enuresis and a wide range of problems in health and development.

There is a tendency to pretend that none of what school doctors do either in these clinics or in schools is therapy because they are not in a position to prescribe free medicine. This however is not how parents see it (Lucas, 1980) and the doctors know from experience that in many instances prevention and treatment are indivisible. Their inevitable involvement in therapy (sometimes even with the use of medicine) indicates that in many cases primary health doctors are failing to meet the therapeutic health care needs of school children. Yet community medicine—as the body responsible for the service—has refused to relinquish control of what it regards as its 'clinical arm', unmindful of the fact that its intransigence accentuates both the isolation of clinical medical officers within the NHS and the unrealistic dichotomy between preventive and therapeutic clinical practice. The Court Report (1976) condemned this situation in asserting that 'all trained doctors who are involved in the clinical care of children must be empowered to treat as well as to ascertain, diagnose and advise'; and more recently GPs have themselves re-affirmed 'the essential union of prevention with care and cure' (Royal College of General Practitioners, 1981).

On the other hand, as GPs have increased their participation in the preventive care of pre-school children, both directly and by the attachment of health visitors to group practices, the suggestion has been made (Royal College of General Practitioners, 1982; Ministry of Health, 1963) that they should likewise provide all the health care of children of school age. The need however for special health services in schools has been carefully considered and repeatedly confirmed (Porritt Report, 1962: DHSS, 1973: Court Report, 1976: Black Report, 1980: Children's Committee, 1981). The recommendations of the Court Committee for GPs (paediatricians), child health visitors, school nurses and consultant community paediatricians to staff the child health services would have gone a long way to meeting both these points of view but they proved unacceptable to the professions (DHSS, 1978) and since then there has been little progress in resolving the issues.

School doctors have never been obliged to undergo special training unless called upon formally to examine a child who might need special education as an educationally subnormal pupil (DHSS, 1980). This was a legacy of the decision to base the school health service within the public health services controlled by the MOH. Clinical work in the maternity and child health and school health services was part of the training of an assistant medical office for a diploma in public health and promotion to a post as deputy MOH. Alternatively, these services were offered as sessional work for any medical practitioner of almost any age and irrespective of his professional experience. This had a disastrous effect on the status of assistant medical officers as clinicians, already prejudiced by the way in which the child and school health services had grown up in isolation from other branches of medicine. Both the status and the isolation were made worse when the public health services remained with their local authorities outside the NHS when it was created in 1946. This situation was corrected when the NHS was reorganised in 1974, and it was acknowledged that clinical (assistant) medical officers were not in the same line of business as community physicians (DHSS, 1974) thus heralding a future for most of them as child health doctors. An appropriate training and career structure were subsequently promised (DHSS, 1978) but neither have yet materialised. These then were the principal theories and realities concerning the school health service when the study reported below was launched in 1978.

PRESENT PRACTICE

The North Paddington Primary School Health Project (NPPSHS)

This project was based on the premise that 'small is beautiful', and that improvement in the school health service is more likely to come from a more comprehensive, personal, self-critical service tailored to the needs of individual schools, than from modifications at district level. So the study was carried out by doctors and nurses actually serving a group of schools, with research assistance, and entailed an assessment of the health service needs of the pupils and their teachers, and of current practice and its effects, as well as a readiness to alter service methods according to the findings. No such project had previously been made and it was also unique in being a combined medical, nursing and psychological study.

The schools involved were the 15 inner city primary schools in North Paddington, London. Their size ranged from 82 to 360 pupils, with a total population that has been slowly declining. Six had a nursery class and five were high on the educational priority area (EPA) index then used by the Inner London Education Authority. The social class distribution of the school entrants in 1978, based on their father's employment status, showed that a disproportionate number came from the lower social classes: 21% were in single parent families. The mothers of half the entrants were born outside the United Kingdom.

A service has to be judged in relation to its function: it has to be both effective and efficient for those it serves, and enjoyable for those who provide it. Six main objectives were identified for the services in the project schools: the manner in which these were attained will only be summarised here (see Bax & Whitmore (1981) and Watt, (1982) for fuller reports).

Health cover. The standard programme of health surveillance initially adopted for all the schools in the study consisted of an entrant medical examination, a pure tone screening test of hearing, and an annual health interview including vision test and growth measurements.

In 1978, 99% of the 354 5-year old school entrants were examined: 90% of their parents attended. Ninety-four per cent had the hearing test and 77% the vision test and measurements of height and weight in 1979. The nurse's annual health interview was omitted for technical reasons. Ninety-nine per cent of the entrants still attending the schools in 1980 were re-examined, 92% of their parents supplying information about their health and development since the age of 5 and 68% attending the re-examination.

Health check. The entrant examination included a traditional physical examination, plus neurodevelopmental tests covering gross and fine motor skills, speech and language, hearing and visual perception, and general intelligence. The parent was interviewed by the nurse to obtain details of the child's birth and medical history, and information about early development and home background. For research purposes the parent completed a modified Rutter behaviour Scale A.

Fifty-six per cent of the entrants were normal in health and development, and the same proportion were normal 2 years later (71% of another group of 325 7–8 year-old children examined in 1978 in their first year in junior school were also normal). Only 72% of the entrants had received a booster immunisation against diphtheria, tetanus and poliomyelitis by the age of 7 although 90% of them had earlier completed a primary course.

Sixty per cent of the entrants had not been seen for health and development checks since the age of 2; half the entrants in whom problems were found (see below) had no record of pre-school surveillance and most of the problems that were found among those who had attended clinics had not been present at their last visit, usually at the age of 3.

Ninety-two per cent of the entrants passed their vision test in 1979 (6/6 in one eye and not worse than 6/9 in the other, using Sheridan's Test) and 88% passed their pure tone hearing test (not less than 20 decibels at four frequencies).

Health care. The prevalence of problems among entrants and juniors in 1978 is given in Table 18.3. The term 'problem' is used advisedly: some children had a condition to which a diagnosis could be put, others had patterns of development or behaviour that were deviant rather than pathological. Although some of these conditions and patterns were intrinsically serious, most of them were not in themselves severe though they could significantly interfere with educational progress, activities or adjustment in school. All of them called for some form of action—from observation to treatment or referral—and always for advice on management to parents and/or teachers.

Parents had previously sought advice from their family doctor for only 6% of the problems revealed at entrant examinations: 4% of parents did not follow the school doctor's advice to take their child to the GP or to make an appointment to see a specialist in hospital.

Half the problems among both entrants and first year juniors subsequently resolved in the next 12 to 18 months and another 20 to 30% had been reduced (Table 18.3).

Health education. For clinicians, health education can be personal or formal. Personal health education occurs when doctors and nurses talk to

Table 18.3 Problems and their outcome among infant school entrants and first year juniors (North Paddington Primary School Health Study, 1978–1980)

Problems	Among 351 entrants			Among 325 juniors		
	Number	%	% resolved in 12–18 months	Number	%	% resolved in 12–18 months
Physical	52	15	58	64	20	56
Visual	27	8	15	30	9	43
Hearing	26	7	35	4	1	33
Speech and language	28	8	56	4	1	75
Behaviour (incl. enuresis)	30	9	48	11	3	46
Cognitive	50	14	54	13	4	66
All problems	213	—	48	126	—	53
Children with problems	153	44	—	95	29	—

children and parents during the course of a clinical interview and is virtually impossible to quantify. Formal health education occurs when they talk to a class or group of pupils specifically on a health topic, or when they advise a teacher about the content of health education she plans to give her own class. Only one nurse in the NPPSHS had a group of girls for health education: the other nurses and doctors did not contribute to formal health education at all.

Help for teachers. Each head teacher and class teacher were interviewed for their opinions of the health and school psychology services. Head teachers were almost unanimously satisfied with the health service. Most of them found the psychologists helpful when they visited but these visits were infrequent and seldom allowed time for even brief discussion about problems other than serious behaviour disorders.

Class teachers saw both services differently. Many of them were unaware of the health service arrangements in their school. Three-quarters said they met the school doctor once a term or less and many complained of not receiving all the medical information they felt they needed about individual children. Feedback was 'haphazard' and 'difficult to get', and 10% did not think they should approach the doctor in person. They were even more critical of the psychology service: half had never met the psychologist and the majority regarded the service with indifference.

Help for parents. A sample of parents was also interviewed for their opinions of the health services. Four out of five were satisfied on the whole with the services in school, and this was the same proportion satisfied with their family doctor and hospital services. However, a quarter of them were not aware that the school nurse saw each child individually once a year and only 2% of the pupils seen by the school doctors during a sample (Autumn) term in 1979, were at the request of parents though when their child was invited for re-examination at the age of 7 20% they had a problem they would like to discuss with the school doctor.

The work of school doctors and nurses

The manner in which school doctors and nurses carry out their work obviously has an important influence on the efficiency and quality of the service. Information about this was obtained in the study from interviews, and from diaries and time/activity schedules kept by the staff over sample periods.

The nurses visited each of their schools two or three times a week, spending from $2\frac{1}{2}$ to nearly 4 hours (mean $3\frac{1}{4}$ hours) per week on educational nursing for every 100 pupils. Seventy per cent of this time was spent on clinical work, including liaison, 20% on clerical work and the rest on sundry activities including travelling. In spite of mostly (sometimes highly) unsatisfactory medical rooms they had a high degree of job satisfaction but they felt there was insufficient liaison with other professional staff except health visitors based on the same clinic.

The doctors were also aware of the limited time spent talking to class teachers and the poor liaison they had with speech therapists and educational psychologists in the schools, and with GPs and child psychiatrists outside. They visited their schools either weekly or fortnightly for a total time of 7 to 16 hours (mean 10 hours) per 100 pupils per term. Eighty-five per cent of this time was spent on clinical work, the remainder on administrative work.

Some general findings of the study

The NPPSHS confirmed that there is still, in an urban area, a high prevalence of problems among infant school children including physical disorders but those associated with hearing, speech and language, and learning and behaviour, predominate.

It has also shown how health services in schools are essentially caring services because care is an important method of prevention. The doctors were instrumental in resolving two-thirds of the problems identified in the pupils, partly through referral to other services (one-third of referrals were to opthalmologists) but equally through their own management of obesity, skin conditions, hearing loss, enuresis, sleep and feeding problems, psychosomatic symptoms and various other behaviour difficulties. The study showed that this was not a reduplication of what the family doctors were doing. The study has also shown how health services in these schools can be effective without resource to rotary staffing and routine periodic medical examinations, though every so often the methods employed need to be reviewed. For instance, the standard programme of health surveillance adopted initially reached virtually all the children entering the infant schools and provided continuity of cover for a high proportion as they moved through to junior schools. The entrant examination used proved effective in eliciting problems in health and development for which the doctors and nurses could provide help. In particular, the neurodevelopmental tests have been shown to correlate highly with a battery of standardised psychological tests administered by an educational psychologist and they have proved at least as efficient in identifying children who subsequently encounter learning and behaviour difficulties at seven years of age. All children entering school in 1978 who had transferred to a special school by the age of nine had failed the neurodevelopmental tests at five. The pick-up rate for difficulties in hearing using the pure tone screening test at the age of 6 was nine children per 100 tested, and that for visual defect using Snellen's Test was two to three per 100 tested.

Rates of booster immunisations were not high and the contribution of health staff to formal health education was unsatisfactory. Equally disappointing was the number of teachers and parents who knew little about the health service, and the fact that so many class teachers reaped no benefit from either the health or psychological services.

Once recognised many of these service deficiencies can be tackled. For example, discussions with teachers in each school resulted in a more systematic arrangement for doctors and class teachers to meet, which varied according to the circumstances and inclinations of the staff in different schools. When interviewed again 18 months later the proportion of teachers who were getting sufficient medical information had increased from a half to two-thirds. The experimental service provided by the research psychologist led many teachers to appreciate psychological advice, especially when this was offered on a sessional basis in the classroom. And parents have been helped by receiving a pamphlet describing the services available through the school doctor and nurse, and the use of a standard enquiry when the children reach seven as to their health and development since entry to school and the offer of an appointment to talk to the doctor if they were concerned about these.

The NPPSH demonstrated all too clearly how school doctors and nurses are still working largely in isolation from their colleagues in primary and secondary care service. This is one of a number of more general issues brought out by the study and although the latter was confined to primary schools in an inner city area the following conclusions are also relevant for services in schools in other urban and perhaps even rural areas.

HEALTH SERVICES IN SCHOOLS IN THE FUTURE

The time has gone when the school health service should be regarded as a separate entity. We should be talking about, and organising and financing, health services for children in school.

A wide range of problems arise in the health and development of children seen in school and doctors and nurses must be able to deal with them as they are found. Integrated services offering treatment as well as prevention must not only be readily available but also easy to use. If the needs of patients really are to come first (and this is far from being the case at present) health services in schools as in other community settings must be organised as supplementary rather than complementary, overlapping rather than merely adjacent to family doctor services.

Special clinics for dealing with the problems outlined above are still required but they should cease to be nominally for school children. Instead they should be supplementary specialist clinics for all children organised in association with the appropriate hospital department but usually sited in community health premises. When a school doctor works in such a clinic he should do so in the capacity of suitably qualified member of the paediatric department.

Administration

Health services in schools need to be decentralised and administered from community health services clinics. Every school should have its appointed doctor and nurse, based on the clinic, and they should provide the programme of health surveillance they think each school requires. Health surveillance is a clinical responsibility and it is not the function of district health authorities to determine clinical policies: senior clinical medical officers should resist the temptation to standardise health services in schools under the pretext of monitoring them. Decentralisation is necessary in order that trained school doctors and nurses can assume a personal responsibility for the service they provide—as befits professional staff—and give a more personal service to children, teachers and parents, and create and maintain the essential link at practitioner level between health services in school and family doctor services. Besides agreeing a health programme they should organise their own visiting times with head teachers, and arrange locums as necessary. They should together maintain a single health record for each pupil, which should be locked up in the school where it may be needed without notice. All letters to parents and other professionals should be sent under their own signatures, not that of the district medical officer, and teachers should know that in the first instance it is to them that any enquiry concerning health matters should be made. They should accept the additional function, with help from community physicians, of gathering epidemiological data about their schools' populations, an important factor in tailoring services to needs.

Staffing levels

The NPPSHS concluded that the medical time required in an inner city primary school was not less than 1 hour per term per 10 children; for the nurse it was 20 minutes per week. This medical time is equivalent to one full time doctor during school terms for 3500 children; the comparable national figure was one for 6750 pupils in 1980 though prior to 1974 it was nearer 5625. The nursing time is equivalent to one full time nurse for 900 children, the comparable national figure in 1978 being 1950.

The fact that the NPPSHS staffing levels appear to be nearly twice as generous as existing levels for the country as a whole underlines the need for flexibility in the provision of health services in schools; the national figure makes no allowance for differences between schools in rural and urban areas, nor between primary and secondary schools. It also raises the issue of limited resources for health services in schools and in facing this health authorities will need to decide their priorities.

Positive discrimination in the provision of health services in school

The principle of equality in the provision of services has long been applied through basic and supplementary grants to local authorities but the concept of positive discrimination is relatively new. The idea is that extra resources should be made available for services in areas in which they are most needed (if necessary at the expense of areas where they are needed less) in an attempt to alleviate the consequences of social disadvantage. This policy was pioneered in the education service after the Plowden Committee (reporting on children in primary schools) (Plowden, 1966) demanded that schools and the children in them in deprived areas should be given 'priority in many respects' and asked LEAs to identify 'educational priority schools and areas' (EPAs) which needed special help to raise standards above the national average and to provide educational environments which sought to compensate the children for the effects of their socially depressed surroundings.

Positive discrimination by health services in favour of disadvantaged children is already official policy (Ennals, 1978) but there is little information about its application at district level either in general or specifically in health services in schools. The inequalities in health that still occur among children—and school children are no exception and the disparities in the health services provided for them are such that a strong case can be made for positive discrimination in health services in schools. At present this operates only in so far as most private schools do not have health services provided by district health authorities but it should be extended to maintained schools. This would mean first that those schools in which there was a high intake of disadvantaged children with high rates of problems in health and development would need to be identified; initially this could be done by adopting existing EPA classifications of areas and schools but eventually it could be refined with epidemiological data gathered in each school. Then it would mean maintaining a full service in these schools at all times as a matter of priority, even if other schools had an inadequate service or none at all in the event of resources becoming severely restricted.

Positive discrimination might also need to be applied to clinical practice. Not all children in EPA schools have problems in health and development and disadvantaged children are found to some extent in schools in both urban and rural areas not designated EPA. It might be necessary for school doctors and nurses to identify which children in any school needed preferential health care. Discrimination in the selection of individual children for whom health care should be provided, to the possible exclusion of some, is alien to many clinicians but it could be an inevitable consequence of health authorities having limited resources.

Before this point is reached health authorities, and school doctors and nurses themselves, need to be sure that doctors are used in a uniquely medical role and nurses are used to their full effect, and that neither waste their time on tasks of doubtful value.

The responsibilities of nurses

With the abandonment of statutory and more recently routine periodic medical examinations the nurse has become the key health worker in schools, and rightly so because of her closer contact with children, teachers and parents. The role of the doctor is now that of consultant in educational medicine in support of the nurse. The extent to which she seeks this support depends on her training and experience and the expectations of her employers and the doctors with whom she works. But there is much to be said for extending her training from 3 to 12 months to equip her for a more responsible role as a school nurse practitioner (Hilmar & McAtee, 1973). For this to be a practical proposition in this country there would first need to be a significant change in the heirarchical relationship between nurse management and school nurses. This is already creating difficulties as school doctors increasingly work with clinical autonomy (Tyrrell, 1981) but it is frankly incompatible with the level of clinical responsibility envisaged for school nurse practitioners.

The contribution of the school doctor

The introduction of school nurse practitioners would reduce, but certainly not dispense with, a medical input to health services in schools for there will always be some children needing a medical examination followed by discussion in school between doctor and teacher. Requests for this arise in all schools because of problems that require a diagnosis, and often medical management.

In addition, in secondary schools students must have direct access to a doctor. The medical time that can be saved by nurses undertaking health interviews rather than doctors carrying out re-examinations urgently needs diverting to an adolescent consultation service available to pupils on their own initiative or following referral by teachers or parents.

In primary schools, theoretically the entrant examination might be shortened or dropped or used with more discretion. The examination in the NPPSHS took 15 minutes because it was not so much a screening as a clinical assessment requiring judgement as to the need for intervention. Intervention was however necessary in half the children and took another 5 to 10 minutes. One of the features of paediatric work in the community is the time that is spent on unhurried consultation with parents and teachers. The nature of the children's problems requires this and rarely a spot diagnosis and prescription, and health education cannot be dispensed in seconds. GPs are prepared to schedule 10 minutes for a school entrant examination in their surgery (Royal College of General Practitioners, 1982) but this would be resorting to a pattern that has long been discredited.

It may be argued that neurodevelopmental assessment of entrants is unnecessary if pre-school surveillance is regular and when so many LEAs have their own screening programme in infant schools. But to do so would be to confuse screening with assessment, to under-rate the importance of early and comprehensive assessment, and to overlook the potential of the entrant examination for preventive health care. The need for review of health and development on entry to inner city infant schools is very apparent from the NPPSHS data on pre-school clinic attendance and the scale of problems at 5 not reaching GPs.

A better case can be made out for reducing the number of school entrants examined than for diminishing the content and quality of the examination. At the best of times it is sensible to use medical examinations with discretion. In populations outside cities there may well be many children whose preschool checks have been regular and satisfactory, and who need no more on starting school than screening tests of growth, vision and hearing by the school nurse.

Training for school doctors

It is essential that doctors who practice educational medicine should first have had a special training. Based on paediatrics, learned in hospital and in the community, it must include experience in audiology as well as ENT work, and especially in paediatric neurology and psychiatry. An apprenticeship is essential for gaining practical experience in educational medicine under tutorial supervision and also an understanding of the roles of speech therapists and educational psychologists, the work of education and social services, and the function of departments of community medicine in organising and monitoring services. This training needs to be combined with that for the health care of pre-school children and would require a period of 2 years to complete.

There are at present no facilities for any kind of training in community child health care but it has been suggested that an appropriate programme could be devised that would at the same time satisfy the conditions for

vocational training for general practice. This would make any doctor satisfactorily completing such a 3-year training eligible to be either a principal
in general practice or a child health doctor in the community, or to pursue
higher specialist training in paediatrics. This proposal is first and foremost
an expediency for achieving an ultimate objective of general practice
becoming the only source of every aspect of primary care, in the home and
in the school. It does not adequately safeguard standards of practice in child
health care, including educational medicine (nor for that matter in general
practice). It would be possible for a doctor to receive a certificate of
prescribed experience whether he had completed 2 years training in paediatrics and child health or none at all, but the certificate would not show this.
The onus would then rest on health authorities to employ in their health
services in school only those doctors with suitable experience in educational
medicine, with no regulations or even guidelines as to what would be suitable; past experience is far from reassuring in this respect.

CONCLUSION

The school health service was conceived in idealistic terms as a preventive
service but it had its roots in the harsh realities within schools and quickly
assumed a therapeutic function as well. These two facts ensured that in its
early years its work was always relevant and contributed in a very special
way to the health and education of pupils.

Just when the physical health of school children was seen to have vividly
improved, the isolation of the service was exacerbated by its exclusion from
the newly-formed NHS, its therapeutic role was rudely interrupted, its
organisation and methods became needlessly stereotyped, and it began to
lose touch with the changing needs of pupils and teachers.

The potentialities of the service have never been denied and the study
quoted in this chapter shows how some of them can be realised by doctors
and nurses jointly in modern times. The possibility of the withdrawal of
health services from schools seems remote but there is a very real danger of
the medical input being minimised. This could happen as a result of the
legitimate extension of the nurse's contribution; the failure to recognise the
need for competence and discrimination in the delivery of health services in
school; and the misguided concept that general practice can now provide the
kind of integrated medical care that is currently required in school.

Health authorities should settle their priorities for health services in school
with due regard for differences in need that may exist in general between
primary and secondary schools, and rural and urban schools. The doctors
and nurses who provide the services in schools should organise these themselves with administrative back-up, allowing for differing needs between the
schools for which they are responsible. As general practice still shows little
interest in the learning and behaviour problems of school children and
resolutely refuses to countenance specialisation within primary care, notwith-

standing the dictum that there should be one service which covers the child from the early pre-school years through school and adolescence (Court Report, 1976), medical services in schools along with special clinics for children should now be ranked as specialist services and organised as part of a district paediatric service staffed by suitably qualified doctors (Whitmore et al, 1979).

REFERENCES

Bax M C O, Whitmore K 1981 The health service needs of children in primary schools: Report to the Kensington, Chelsea and Westminster AHA(T). London.

Black D 1980 Inequalities in Health: Report of a Research Working Group to DHSS. HMSO, London

Board of Education 1907 Circular 576: Memorandum on Medical Inspection of Children in Public Elementary Schools. HMSO, London

Children's Committee 1981 The School Health Service: A Position Paper. National Children's Bureau, London

Court S D M 1976 Fit for the Future: Report of the Committee on Child Health Services. HMSO, London

Department of Education and Science 1964 Report of the Chief Medical Officer, 1962 & 1963. HMSO, London

Department of Education and Science 1972 Report of Chief Medical Officer, 1969 & 1970. HMSO, London

Department of Education and Science 1975 Circular 2/75: The Discovery of Children Requiring Special Education and the Assessment of their Needs. HMSO, London

Department of Health and Social Security 1973 Report from the Working Party on Collaboration between the NHS and Local Government on its Activities to the End of 1972. HMSO, London

Department of Health and Social Security 1974 Health Service Circular (Interim Series) No. 13: Community Medicine in the Reorganised Health Service. HMSO, London

Department of Health and Social Security 1978 Health Circular (78)5: Health Services Development, Court Report on Child Health Services. HMSO, London

Department of Health and Social Security 1980 DDL(80)1 (revised): Ascertainment of Children Requiring Special Education: Courses Approved for the Purpose of the NHS (medical examinations—educationally subnormal children) Regulations. HMSO, London

Ennals D 1978 Eleanor Rathbone Memorial Lecture. Health Circular (78)5 HMSO, London

Fitzherbert K 1982 Communications with teachers in the health surveillance of school children. Maternal and Child Health, March: 100–103

Hilmar N A, McAtee P A 1973 The school nurse practitioner and her practice. Journal of School Health XLIII, 7: 431–441

Lucas S 1980 Some aspects of child health care: contacts between children, general practitioners and school doctors. Community Medicine 2: 209–218

Ministry of Education 1954 Circular 276: Provision of Special Schools. HMSO, London

Ministry of Health 1963 The Field of Work of the Family Doctor: Report of the Sub-Committee of the Standing Medical Advisory Committee. HMSO, London

Plowden, B 1966 Children and their Primary Schools; a Report of the Central Advisory Council for Education (England). Vol. 1. HMSO, London.

Porritt A 1962 Review of the Medical Services in Great Britain: Report of the Medical Services Review Committee. Social Assay, London

Royal College of General Practitioners 1981 Health and Prevention in Primary Care: Report from General Practice No. 18. RCPG, London

Royal College of General Practitioners 1982 Healthier Children—Thinking Prevention: Report from General Practice No. 22. RCGP, London

Tyrrell S 1981 Confusion over accountability of clinical medical officers. British Medical Association News Review, December

nised by the parents and their children, who seldom actually use the metal foot supports so generously prescribed (Köhler, 1973a).

Furthermore orthopaedic screening is not carried out until school age, when all children are examined for structural scoliosis, usually by doctors, nurses or teachers, using the 'forward-bending' test. A recent screening of 17 000 school children in Southern Sweden (Willner & Udén, 1982) revealed that 3.2% of the girls and 0.5% of the boys had a scoliosis of at least 10° the lower limit generally recommended when using forward-bending test as the screening method.

Otherwise, systematic screening programmes for children have been used as a routine in testing vision, hearing, speech, general development and examination of blood and urine. There is also a standardised growth and development chart from birth to the age of 18 where the individual child's performance is compared with statistical means and ranges. All results from the examinations are collected in a health record that follows the child from birth into school (Fig. 19.1). This includes a report from the maternity ward concerning the pregnancy and the neonatal period. In this way there is a useful line of health information about the child, from conception to school, forming an accurate, although maybe blunt instrument of judging the child's physical, mental and social development.

Evaluation studies

Although evaluation has seldom, if ever, been built into the routine preventive programmes, there are some research studies that could serve as models and point out the more useful examinations and screening methods.

Dental health

The most pronounced health problem for the preschool children in the 60's was dental decay: 74% of the children had caries, and 20% were recorded as emergency cases in need of pulpotomy or extraction of two or more molars in combination with 15 or more decayed surfaces. A very active, local programme for dental health was instigated in schools, pre schools and Child Health Centres, and public knowledge of reasons for dental decay and their prevention was greatly increased. As a result, another cohort of 4-year-old children 10 years later was caries-free in 70% and the number of emergency cases was reduced to a small number of individual cases (Holst & Köhler, 1973).

Auditory screening

Early detection of deafness is of course vital for the child and much research is going on to develop techniques for testing newborns. This, however, is at the moment only done on newborns at risk, e.g. pre-term children.

At about 8 months of age, a simple test of hearing, the so-called BOEL test is widely used in Swedish babies. BOEL is formed from the initial letters of the Swedish sentence 'Gaze orients after sound' and is constructed to provide the infant's response to sound—the distinct turning of the head in the direction of the sound source (small calibrated silver bells) hidden in the examiner's clutched fist and brought up behind the infant's ear. In a study of 10 000 infants in a county (Lindsjö, 1980) 1.4% were referred after failing the test. When examined by an audiologist, half of them were normal and sensorineural hearing impairment was diagnosed in seven children. Including those detected earlier, the total prevalence of severe hearing impairment in children 0–3.5 years of age was 0.08%. The test was very good at detecting these serious hearing defects, but was not so useful as a tool for disclosing developmental or motor delay (something it had been argued it would be useful for (Barr et al, 1978)).

Later, at 4 years of age, another hearing test with pure tone audiometry is performed. At this time, as expected, very few severe or progressive cases of hearing impairments are found, but about 3% of the children have a hearing loss due to not properly resolved middle ear infections (Köhler & Holst, 1972). When the screening is repeated at 7 and 10 years of age, the same frequency of abnormal hearing due to infections is found, one-third having the same problem at each examination (Köhler, 1977; Kornfält & Köhler, 1978, Kornfält, 1981).

Vision screening

All children at 4 years of age are now routinely examined for visual defects by a monocular screening of distant visual acuity using linear E:s at 5 metres, accepting 5/5 as normal. This simple method is shown to be highly efficient in detecting those who need treatment—mainly children with hypermetropia and strabismus. Other methods tested—cover-test at a distance of 0.5 metres, observing the eye movements and examination of the binocular vision with the Wirt Fly Stereo test—are found to be unreliable; they can possibly be used if you have very high ambitions, but should never be used as the only test (very low sensitivity, but high specificity) (Köhler &Stigmar, 1973). Retesting the children with a linear E-chart at a distance of 5 metres when they come to school at 7 years of age confirms the usefulness of the earlier screening: very few eye disorders were missed during the pre school age and the risk of finding a new significant eye disorder in a 7-year-old child was more than six times greater for a child who was not examined in his pre school years. The risk of finding an amblyopic child was more than 10 times greater (Köhler & Stigmar, 1978). The results of treatment were better among those who were detected early.

Since myopia develops rather fast in school children, distant vision screening is usually repeated every year. At 12 years of age, the colour vision is tested to be able to advise colour-blind children against certain occupations. The value of this colour test has never been assessed.

Child Health Services

Birth-day

Name

Address

GIRL   Adopted
Foster child

| Mother's birth-day | Nationality | New addresses | phone | date |

Name

Profession

Family situation
married   co-hab.   alone   other family sit.

| Father's birth-day | Nationality |

Name

Profession

Siblings

Pre-school, day care   phone   date

| Born year | mth. | day | sex | Name |

Vaccinations

Diseases

BCG / PPD	Diptheria Tetanus	Polio	Measles Mumps Rubella		Whooping cough	year	allergic dis.
					Measles		Diabetes
					Parotitis		
					Chicken pox		Visual dysf.
					Rubella		Hearing dysf.
							Other chronic dis.

Neonatal period OK

Diag. from hosp./special.

| In, date | Out, date | Clinic | Diagnosis |

date   date

Handicap register   Register for mentally retarded

healthy

LIC BHV-1   Flicka 1981-11 (SOSB 36380)

Fig. 19.1 The health record card completed for every child in Sweden from birth to school age.

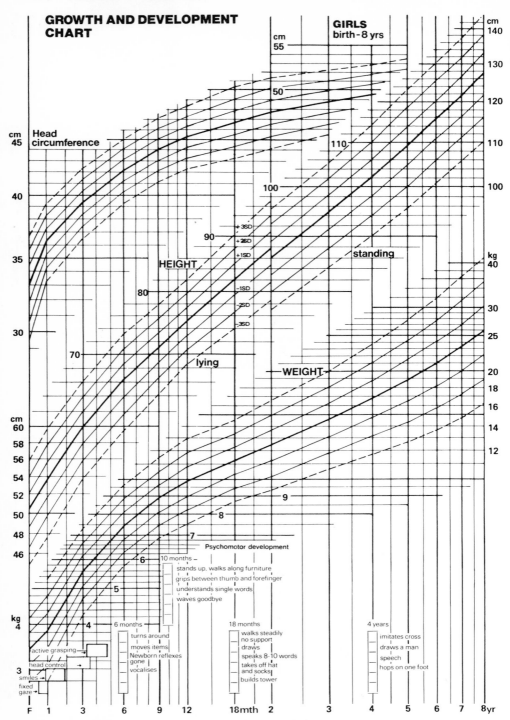

GROWTH AND DEVELOPMENT CHART

GIRLS birth-8 yrs

Head circumference

HEIGHT

standing

lying

WEIGHT

+3SD
+2SD
+1SD
-1SD
-2SD
-3SD

Psychomotor development

10 months
stands up, walks along furniture
grips between thumb and forefinger
understands single words
waves goodbye

6 months
turns around
moves items
Newborn reflexes gone
vocalises

active grasping
head control
smiles
fixed gaze

18 months
walks steadily
no support
draws
speaks 8-10 words
takes off hat and socks
builds tower

4 years
imitates cross
draws a man
speech
hops on one foot

Fig. 19.1 Cont'd

Karlberg, P. – Engström, I. – Klackenberg, G. – Klackenberg – Larsson, I.
Lichtenstein, H. – Svennberg, I. – Taranger, J. 1972, copyright

	Birth date																
AGE	MONTHS												YEARS					
	0	1	2	3	4	5	6	8	10	12	18	2	2,5	3	4	5,5	7
DATE,																	
Living quarters																	
Outer environment (traffic, air)																	
Inner environment (diseases, abuse)																	
Behaviour (feeding, sleep)																	
DISEASES																	
ACCIDENTS																	
FEEDING																	
Breast milk																	
Cow's milk																	
Normal diet																	
Special diet																	
Vit. AD																	
STATUS	Sign																
General																	
Skin																	
Motor dev.																	
Gross motor																	
Fine motor																	
Tonus reflexes																	
Lungs																	
Heart																	
Femoral pulses																	
Stomach																	
Genitals																	
Hips																	
Head																	
Back, legs																	
Mouth																	
Hearing																	
Speech																	
Eyes																	
Vision																	
TEETH																	
Malocclusion																	
Decay																	
Fluor. in drinking water																	
HEALTH EDUCATION (group, individual folder, verbal)																	
Food and physical exercise																	
Development OK																	
Play and stimulus																	
Accidents																	
Smoking, alcohol																	
	0	1	2	3	4	5	6	8	10	12	18	2	2,5	3	4	5,5	7
	MONTHS												YEARS					
Psycho-social environment																	

Fig. 19.1 Cont'd

Weight as newborn		Height as newborn		Head as newborn		Type of contact	contact by		
						home visit clinic	Physician Nurse	hearing ass. soc. worker	dental hygienist dentist
con- tact	date	age	weight	height	head	phone pre-school			dental nurse

Fig. 19.1 Cont'd.

Pilot studies of testing for hypermetropia by adding 'plus' lenses, indicate that the method is inaccurate and can quite safely be omitted (Köhler &Stigmar, 1981).

Health examination of 4-year-old children

Some 10 years ago a special health examination was introduced in Sweden when it was realised that the attendance rate to the Child Health Centres rapidly decreased as the children grew older: almost 100% of infants attended, some 90% of 1–2-year-olds, 50% of 4–5-year-olds, and only 20% of 6-year-olds. A low attendance rate could of course mean that some children with handicaps were not detected and treated prior to the school entry at the age of 7. The age of 4 was chosen as a compromise between the wish to detect the handicaps early, and the wish to use reliable and simple methods. The programme was designed to cover the child's physical, mental and social health and comprised physical examination by a physician, dental examination by a dentist, screening of vision, hearing, blood and urine, assessment of mental development and social adaption by a psychologist, and a questionnaire and an interview of the parents regarding previous paediatric and developmental history.

In a few counties, the examination has been properly evaluated and the immediate results show that the offer was well accepted by the parents, resulting in the attendance rate rising to about 97%. Gross disabilities and handicaps had usually already been detected at an earlier age. Newly detected, functionally important health problems were only found with any frequency in fields not fully covered by the existing routines at the Child Health Centres, e.g. vision and hearing disturbances, dental decay, and emotional problems. As a result, from several of these studies, it could be concluded that about 25% of the children had a health problem that was likely to have a significant and prolonged impact or to hamper the full exploitation of the environment, either immediately or in the future (Köhler, 1973b; Sundelin et al, 1982) (see Table 19.1).

Table 19.1 Percentage of 4-year-old children with health problems considered to be of functional significance (Köhler, 1973b)

Health problem	Per cent
Vision	8.9
Hearing	1.7
Neurological	2.8
Heart	0.6
Surgical	1.1
Orthopaedic	0.4
Other physical	0.7
Dental caries	7.9
Emotional disturbances	5.0

Long-term follow-up studies of this programme for 4-year-olds are now emerging from several research centres (Köhler, 1977; Kornfält & Köhler, 1978; Kornfält, 1981; Sundelin et al, 1982). The results are difficult to measure, the methods are crude and incomplete, but they probably reflect existing limitations on evaluation methods. The general conclusion is that the measurable, direct impact of the screening on the health of the children is marginal. The programme seems to have contributed very little to the prevention of most problems, with the possible exception of visual screening and the dental programme.

The symptoms of behaviour problems found at the age of 4 years have very little prognostic value for problems prevailing at 10 years of age (Sundelin et al, 1982). Some individual children and families are, of course, offered immediate help and assistance, and do indeed profit by it. This is, however, no guarantee for their future health.

The best prognostic value seems to be found, not in the individual, but in the family environment. Perhaps the best method to detect early problems with the children is to study the family and to listen carefully to the needs and complaints of the parents.

Screening of anaemia and bacteriuria have been abandoned, because anaemia is practically non-existent in Sweden and because asymptomatic bacteriuria is no longer considered to be the hidden threat to health that it was some 10 years ago (Köhler et al, 1979; Lindberg et al, 1978).

CONCLUSION

After careful evaluation in admittedly limited areas and on selected populations, it is safe to conclude that only a few of the screening methods have been shown to fulfil the criteria of a proper screening test, i.e. with high sensitivity and specificity, detecting a decent number of cases where effective and efficient treatment is available. These tests usually belong to the area of physical health. The value of formal screening for mental, behavioural, linguistic or social development in small children has still not been convincingly proved and, therefore, tests have not generally been introduced. It is not reasonable or probable that the complicated biological and social background of developmental retardation should be easily revealed by simple questionnaires or tests. Nor is it realistic to expect that the findings at a very early age will predict with certainty problems later in childhood and adulthood, because this disregards the complex interplay between inherited tendencies and environmental influences and underestimates the adaptive capacity of the growing mind and body. However, pilot research studies in this field are being and should be undertaken.

An information system for children's health

The first prerequisite for a successful screening programme is to reach the target group—in this case children and their parents. Practically all Swedish children visit the Child Health Centre regularly. Therefore it is important that the screening tests are incorporated in the general health surveillance programme and that the tests are performed by the ordinary staff, usually the nurses, rather than research specialists. For people used to dealing with children, the techniques of screening are easy to learn and are part of their continuing education.

However, if you want to get a full picture of children's health in order to register development and changes, to spot health hazards, to note differences between groups and areas, then these cross-sectional medical examinations and screening programmes are insufficient. What is needed is a continuous and systematic surveillance of all children's physical and mental health, taking into account objective and subjective health concepts and placing them in a social context.

At present no such system exists. What is available is reliable mortality figures, scattered data on hospital care, a few studies on children's primary care, a growing number of studies on preventive care and, of course, an enormous amount of information hidden in various medical social, and educational registers. However, there has been no attempt to compile and coordinate these sources and there is a lot of information missing as well. Unlike adults, children are not the target for continuous 'welfare studies' that try to assess their state of well-being in the population.

The politicians in Sweden have realised that there is a lack of knowledge in this field and the government has recently appointed a committee to produce a new national information system on children's health and well-being. Thus, this committee will look into what cross-sectional studies of children's health situation we need and at what ages, so as to be able to observe changes in health and disease panorama over time. Further, it will examine what longitudinal surveys we need so that we may answer questions about the impact of early health deficiencies on later health problems and well-being. The committee will also discuss what research resources are needed to compile, analyse and coordinate all this information from studies, surveys and registers in such a way that it can serve as a comprehensive information system.

Such a system, together with research resources will form the necessary background for the planning of medical and social services for children and, in the long run, for an active and rational family policy.

REFERENCES

Alm J, Larsson A, Zetterström R 1981 Congenital hypothyroidism in Sweden. Acta Paediatrica Scandinavica 70: 907–912

Barr B, Stensland-Junker K, Svärd M 1978 Early discovery of hearing impairment: a critical evaluation of the BOEL test. Audiology 17: 62–67

Holst K, Köhler L 1973 Preventing dental caries in children. Report of a Swedish programme. Developmental Medicine and Child Neurology 17: 6026–6040

Kornfält R, Köhler L 1978 Physical health of ten-year-old children. An epidemiological study of school children and followup of previous health care. Acta Paediatrica Scandinavica 67: 481–489

242   PROGRESS IN CHILD HEALTH

Köhler L 1973a Physical examination of four-year-old children. Acta Paediatrica Scandinavica 62: 181–192

Köhler L 1973b Health control of four-year-old children, An epidemiological study of child health. Acta Paediatrica Scandinavica Supplement 235

Köhler L 1977 Physical health of 7-year-old children. An epidemiological study of school entrants and a comparison with preschool health. Acta Paediatrica Scandinavica 66: 297

Köhler L, Holst H-E 1972 Auditory screening of four-year-old children. Acta Paediatrica Scandinavica 61: 555

Köhler L, Stigmar G 1978 Visual disorders in 7-year-old children with and without previous vision screening. Acta Paediatrica Scandinavica 67: 373–377

Köhler L; Stigmar G: 1981 Testing for hypermetropia in the school vision screening programme. Acta Ophtalmologica 59: 369–377

Köhler L Svenningsen N; Lindquist B 1979 Early detection of preschool health problems— role of perinatal risk factors. Acta Paediatrica Scandinavica 68: 229–237

Lindberg U, Claesson I, Hansson L-A, Jodal U 1978 Asymptomatic bacteriuria in school girls. VIII. The clinical course during a 3 year follow-up. Journal of Pediatrics 92: 194

Lindsjö A 1980 BOEL hörselscreening med utvecklingsdiagnostiska fördelar. Läkartidningen 77: 4556–4559

Sundelin C, Mellbin T, Vuille J-C 1982 From four to ten: An overall evaluation of the general health screening of four-year-olds. In: Anastasinov NJ, Frankenburg W K, Fandal A W (eds.) Identifying the Developmentally Delayed Child. University Park Press, Baltimore

Thomas T L 1983 Treatment of congenital dislocation of the hip. Developmental Medicine and Child Neurology 25: 97–99

Willner S, Udén A 1982 A prospective prevalence study of scoliosis in Southern Sweden. Acta Orthopaedica Scandinavica 53: 233–237

Is screening worthwhile?

INTRODUCTION

Screening is a term used to cover different kinds of investigation with different ends in view. Medical screening is directed towards the detection of occult disease or defect by the application of tests, examinations and other procedures which can be applied rapidly. Its aim is to sort out apparently well persons who may have a disease from those who do not have a disease. In this respect its function is to distinguish those individuals who would benefit from further clinical investigation from those who need no further examination. The economical application of medical screening procedures to large unselected groups of apparently well persons is known as mass screening. In a discussion of the development of screening principles in medical practice Hart (1975) has emphasised the need for distinguishing between monophasic and multiphasic screening programmes. In monophasic screening the intention is to identify the presence or absence of a specific individual disease, whereas in multiphasic screening the assessment of normality is set against the detection of a number of different diseases. Of necessity, multiphasic screening involves the use of a test battery, although monophasic screening could rely upon single or multiple test data. Until 40 years ago the health screening of a community was regarded as somewhat of a luxury. Emphasis was placed on selective monophasic screening of those people thought to be at special risk. In Britain, the introduction of the National Health Service in 1948 brought an increased awareness of health standards with a rapid trend towards multiphasic screening programmes. In medical practice today, there is a place both for selective monophasic and mass multiple screening programmes. The principal common aim is that the results of the screening procedure should eventually benefit the individual in the subsequent advice or action taken. The principal common problem which faces the user of a screening programme is to decide whether it is all worthwhile. The answer to this question will, of course, depend upon many factors and in this chapter we describe how this may be achieved for any screening problem by the application of decision analysis.

All screening procedures are undertaken to produce evidence of some kind. This might be in the form of signs, symptoms, or data from laboratory investigations of the results of some administered test. With this in mind it is important at the outset to emphasise that no data, evidence, information or its interpretation is free of error. Even when evidence results from sources which involve precise and reliable techniques of measurement there is always, to a greater or lesser degree, an associated error rate in the measurement and in the inferences we draw from it. The corollary of this is that uncertainty is present in much of human judgement and consequently the drawing of inferences or choosing actions under risk or uncertainty is an appropriate description of clinical decisions (Lusted, 1967). Within this context we can describe the screening problem as a procedure requiring two choices:

1. The selection of a test (or battery of tests).
2. The making of a judgement on the basis of evidence provided by the test.

In making these choices we would normally consider many factors which fall under two broad headings.

Firstly, there is the information to be gained by testing. Does the test discriminate between the populations of interest, e.g. between those who could benefit from treatment and those who do not need treatment? Furthermore, how much better off are we at the end of the screening procedure in making the kind of judgement we wish to make? We shall use the language of probabilities to express our states of knowledge before and after testing and as a measure of information gained by testing.

Secondly, there is the value and priority we ascribe to the information provided by screening, and to the success or lack of success of our resulting decisions. Here we must consider the benefits and cost of testing (where cost includes many dimensions such as financial, time of testing, discomfort to patient, etc), in terms of the relative weight or importance we give to alternative outcomes of the testing procedure. Included in this is the problem of the selection of test criteria which helps us to relate our judgement to test performance. We shall use the concept of utility to represent the worth or value we attach to the consequence of our actions.

THE SCREENING PROBLEM

The simplest screening problem can be illustrated by a 2 × 2 table relating the presence or absence of a disease to the outcome of a screening test which gives positive or negative results. The idealised screening test is shown in Fig. 20.1a. Here there is a perfect agreement between the test result and the presence or absence of the disease. Such a situation is also represented in Fig. 20.1b where we imagine a group of patients screened by an ideal test. In this state of certainty the decision problem before us is relatively trivial.

The practical screening situation is shown in Fig. 20.2a. By contrast with the idealised screening test result, the uncertainty in this problem is due to

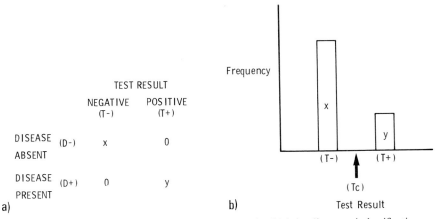

		TEST RESULT	
		NEGATIVE (T-)	POSITIVE (T+)
DISEASE ABSENT	(D-)	x	0
DISEASE PRESENT	(D+)	0	y

a)

b)

Figs. 20.1 (a) and (b) The idealised screening test result which implies no misclassifications from test performance.

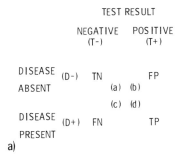

		TEST RESULT	
		NEGATIVE (T-)	POSITIVE (T+)
DISEASE ABSENT	(D-)	TN (a)	FP (b)
		(c)	(d)
DISEASE PRESENT	(D+)	FN	TP

a)

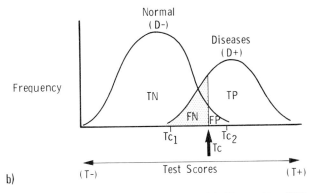

b)

Figs. 20.2 (a) and (b) The practical screening situation with false positive (FP) and false negative (FN) misclassifications. In the contingency table above the values (a), (b), (c) and (d) represent the number of individuals found in each category giving respectively a true negative (TN), false positive (FP), false negative (FN) and true positive (TP) result.

the presence of a small but significant number of misclassifications denoted as false-positive (FP) and false-negative (FN). The remaining two cells contain true-negative (TN) and true-positive (TP) results. From Fig. 20.2a we can define two measures of test performance:

$$\text{The sensitivity of the test} \; = \frac{TP}{FN + TP}$$

$$\text{The specificity of the test} \; = \frac{TN}{TN + FP}$$

Both these measures are conditional probabilities.

> Test sensitivity = $P(T+/D+)$ is the conditional probability of a positive test result (T+) given that the patient has the disease (D+).
> Test specificity = $P(T-/D-)$ is the conditional probability of a negative test result (T−) given that the patient does not have the disease (D−).

Clearly a good screening test is one where both sensitivity and specificity are high. The same problem is shown in Fig. 20.2b. Assuming test scores are measured on a continuous scale, the frequency distributions of test scores from the two populations of normals and diseased will overlap. The problem is to choose a test criterion score (Tc) such that test scores (T+) which are greater than (Tc) result in a decision for disease present (D+), while test scores (T−) which are less than (Tc) result in a decision for disease absent (D−). For any given single test criterion score (Tc), error rates of FP and FN will occur as shown. If we move the test criterion score (Tc) to the left (i.e. to a lower test score) we decrease one of the error terms FN but at the expense of increasing the other error term FP. Similarly by selecting a higher test score as criterion (Tc) we will reduce the error term FP but will simultaneously increase the error term FN. In other words, by varying the criterion score Tc we vary the trade-off between test sensitivity and specificity and also between the relative costs associated with screening errors of false-positive or false-negative classifications. If the purpose of screening is to identify the normal, we are likely to make FN very small and as a consequence accept a large number of FP among the population requiring further investigation. There is, of course, a further option available which is to choose several criteria on a test. For example, it is possible to ensure small ratios of error rates FP and FN by selecting two criteria in the decision problem. As shown in Fig. 20.2b, test scores less than C_1 could result in a decision for (D−); test scores greater than C_2 result in a decision for (D+) while those test scores falling between C_1 and C_2 would be indeterminate decisions requiring further evidence from other sources.

In the past, the criterion cut-off point for clinical decisions has been chosen on the basis of clinical impressions or expert clinical opinion. An alternative to this has been to choose arbitrary points on statistical distribution curves to justify selection. More recently, both these former methods have been replaced by a rational process which makes use of ideas of probability, utility and decision analysis.

Receiver operator characteristics

A useful diagrammatic way of representing the problem for defining an appropriate criterion cut-off point in a screening test is the Receiver Operator Characteristics (ROC) curve—a term developed in the electronic engineering field and widely used in psychology as a means of representing the detection of signal against a noisy background. An ROC curve is simply a plot of test sensitivity $p(T+/D+)$ against test specificity $P(T-/D-)$. Specificity is either plotted on a reverse scale or the derivative $(1-$ specificity) is plotted in the usual manner on the abscissae. A typical form of ROC curve is shown in Fig. 20.3a. Here are shown the decision curves for two tests A and B. Points along any curve (e.g. Tc_1, Tc_2) represent different test score values which can be used in the test as criteria or cut-off points (e.g. for T+ and T−). The broken line represents the curve for a test which could *NOT* discriminate at all between two populations (e.g. normal and diseased). On the other hand the closer the curve approaches the upper left hand corner of the graph the better is the test at discriminating between the two populations. Test B is therefore a better screening test than test A.

The ROC curve is therefore a means of providing two separate measures for a detection or discrimination problem—one an index of the power of the test to discriminate between the two populations (d_A, d_B) and the other the decision point selected as criterion score $(Tc_1$ or $Tc_2)$, (see Figs. 20.3b and 20.3c).

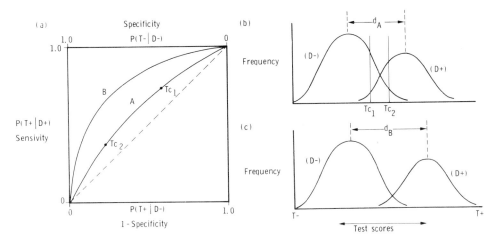

Fig. 20.3 (a) Receiver operator characteristics (ROC) curves showing two levels of discrimination (A, B) and two values of the test criterion score (Tc_1, Tc_2). (b) and (c) Relationships between levels of discrimination d_A, d_B and test criterion scores Tc_1, Tc_2 for the ROC curves of (a).

Derived measures form ROC curves

We have gone some way to answering the original question concerning a basis for comparing and so choosing between alternative screening tests. We can also derive further measures of diagnostic quality. These will influence the choice of an optimum cut-off criterion and also the average net benefit derived from performing the screening.

Optimum criterion

Once the ROC curve for a screening test is known we must choose some test criterion or cut-off value. In deciding this criterion we must consider all the factors associated with the outcome of Fig. 20.2a (i.e. the costs and benefits of the test). These might be:

(i) Benefits   TN —relief of patient anxiety
               TP —a function of the efficacy of treatment
(ii) Costs   FP —unnecessary detailed clinical investigation, medical treatment or surgery, including hazards of side effects of treatment, anxiety to patient or relatives
               FN —a function of the seriousness of the disease and loss of pride for the clinician

These factors can be arranged to determine the slope β of the tangent to the ROC curve at the optimal criterion point. This may be expressed as:

$$\beta = \frac{P(D-)}{P(D+)} \frac{(\text{Benefit TN} + \text{Cost FP})}{(\text{Benefit TP} + \text{Cost FN})}$$

where $P(D+)$ and $P(D-)$ are the probabilities of the disease being present and absent respectively in the population studied. β is also equal to the ratio of the ordinate of the $(D+)$ distribution to the ordinate of the $(D-)$ distribution for specific test scores (see Fig. 20.2b). If $\beta = 1$, which corresponds to the point on the ROC curve farthest from the diagonal indecision line, then the optimum criterion value is at the point where the two frequency distribution curves for $(D+)$ and $(D-)$ cross. On the other hand, if the costs and benefits of FP and TN balance those of FN and TP then the optimum criterion value becomes the point on the ROC curve where the slope of the curve is equal to the ratio of the probabilities of $(D-)$ to $(D+)$. Methods by which costs and benefits can be quantified as utilities are illustrated in the example described on page 255.

Average net benefit

Lusted (1976) has proposed the following formula for assessing the net benefit (NB) of screening. This can be thought of as the reduction in cost resulting from the screening or diagnostic study and may be determined as follows:

$$NB = (C_{FN} - C_{TP}) \cdot P(D+) \cdot P(T+/D+) - (C_{FP} - C_{TN}) \cdot P(D-) \cdot P(T+/D-) - \bar{c}$$

where C_{FN} = cost of false-negative
C_{TN} = cost of true-negative
C_{FP} = cost of false-positive
C_{TP} = cost of true-positive
$P(T+/D+)$ = sensitivity
$P(T+/D-)$ = 1 – specificity
and where $\bar{c}$ is the cost of not performing the study (i.e. no treatment or a negative decision by default) and is given by:
$$\bar{c} = C_{FN} \cdot P(D+) + C_{TN} \cdot P(D-)$$

BAYES' THEOREM

As suggested in the Introduction, screening and diagnosis can be distinguished; diagnosis being a second stage procedure aimed at establishing the most probable hypothesis (disease) among the set of possible hypotheses (diseases). The number of diagnostic hypotheses entertained at any one time seems, due to the limited capacity of short term memory, to be at most five (Kozielecki, 1982). Clinicians will use different problem solving strategies in eliminating most hypotheses and in generating the few considered most probable. Both the screening and diagnostic phases can be illuminated by Bayes' theorem of conditional probability.

The Bayesian approach is based on the realisation that screening tests are always given against a background where some states (e.g. diseases) are more probable than others. Only by considering both the context in which the screening or diagnosis is to be done and the test evidence, can a real assessment be made of the value of the test information in differentiating between alternative states, be they normal and abnormal or disease X and disease Y.

For instance, consider the screening situation in Fig. 20.2a. It follows from Bayes' theorem that the probability of the disease being present given a positive test result may be expressed as:

$$P(D+/T+) = \frac{P(D+) \cdot P(T+/D+)}{P(D+) \cdot P(T+/D+) + P(D-) \cdot P(T+/D-)}$$

i.e.
$$= \frac{P(D) \left[\dfrac{d}{(c+d)}\right]}{P(D+) \left[\dfrac{d}{(c+d)}\right] + P(D-) \left[\dfrac{b}{(a+b)}\right]}$$

Similarly, the probability of no disease given a negative test would be:

$$P(D-/T-) = \frac{P(D-) \cdot P(T-/D-)}{P(D-) \cdot P(T-/D-) + P(D+) \cdot P(T-/D+)}$$

i.e.

$$= \frac{P(D-) \left[\frac{a}{(a+b)}\right]}{P(D-) \left[\frac{a}{(a+b)}\right] + P(D+) \left[\frac{c}{(c+d)}\right]}$$

The other two conditional probabilities of interest are the complements of these:

i.e. $P(D-/T+) = 1 - P(D+/T+)$

and $P(D+/T-) = 1 - P(D-/T-)$

The implications of Bayes' theorem surprise many clinicians, particularly when the disease incidence $P(D+)$ is low. Consider for example, the use of an excellent screening test with 99% sensitivity and 99% specificity in the detection of a disease which occurs in 0.5% of the population. We find from Bayes' theorem that the probability of the patient having the disease given a positive result on the test is only 0.33. In other words, two out of three patients with positive test results do not have the disease, and the best conclusion is 'disease absent' following positive test results. On the other hand, the probability of the patient not having the disease given the test result is negative, in this example, is 0.9999. Such a test is therefore very good indeed at detecting the normals but not so good at detecting the diseased. This result gives support to the view that screening separates normal from those awaiting further investigation who, as Hart (1975) says, '*may* have a disease'.

Screening populations where the disease incidence is low is the rule rather than the exception. The above example shows that positive test evidence from a good screening test may not overturn the overwhelming prior evidence in favour of a decision for clinical normality. It is necessary, therefore, that those who use clinical screening procedures are aware both of the efficiency of the screening test and also the incidence of the clinical condition for which screening is being conducted. Furthermore, it is important to realise that both these factors may be a function of change. For example, the efficiency of a screening test may not only be different for different population groups as the manifestation of the clinical abnormality is more or less evident, but if it involves the application of clinical skills it will also depend on the expertise of the examiner.

The influence of both these factors may be illustrated in the detection of congenital dislocation of the hip. It is a matter of common experience that paediatricians have considerable difficulty in diagnosing cryptic deformities in a newborn child. Detection is frequently poor not only because of low test sensitivity as a consequence of the difficulties associated with the clinical examination itself, but also because of the greater likelihood that no deformity is present. The diagnosis of congenital dislocation of the hip is in fact difficult to make with clinical certainty at birth, but after the first 3 months its detection rate improves (i.e. test sensitivity improves) as it becomes easier to recognise from clinical examination due to progressive limitation of hip movement. In other words the sensitivity of the screening procedure increases with the age of the child. But against this variable detection rate is the clinical knowledge that the earlier the detection, the greater is the likelihood of avoiding lasting deformity. In deciding on what age within the first year of life to conduct this screening test, a decision has to be made to find an acceptable balance between the opposing constraints of test sensitivity and successful clinical management. Too many false-positives from early screening soon after birth may involve costly additional after care management in addition to unnecessary parental anxiety.

The prior incidence of the clinical abnormality is also a changing value in the condition of congenital hip dislocation. In 1970, for example, the incidence in Western Europe and North America was 0.1% of births. But as the survival rate of live births has improved over the last decade, especially in those instances involving breach births or marked uterine compression, the incidence of congenital hip dislocation has now more than doubled to give a priority probability of 0.5% of births. Doctors and nurses should therefore be vigilant of the changing incidence values in congenital deformities since this will clearly influence detection rates.

Multiple test data

Bayes' theorem generalises to several items of evidence and several diagnoses. The general form of Bayes' for two or more tests is:

$$P(D_1/x_1x_2 \ldots x_n) = \frac{P(D_1)P(x_1/D_1) \ldots P(x_n/D_1)}{\sum_{\text{all } k} \{P(D_k)P(x_1/D_k) \ldots P(x_n/D_k)\}}$$

The set of diseases $D_1 \ldots D_k$ should be mutually exclusive and the set of tests mutually independent. However, on the latter point Bayesian performance may be maximised by using a few of the most diagnostic of the available variables even if they are highly redundant, (Fryback, 1974; Jacquez & Norusis, 1976). If independence between tests is desired where there is clear evidence of high correlations between them, the data from tests can be combined. For example, suppose screening is required to distinguish between 'normal' and 'doubtful' from evidence of 'pass' or 'fail' on two tests. A 2 × 2 table for 'normals' can be constructed with rows: pass test 1, fail test 1; and columns: pass test 2, fail test 2. A similar 2 × 2 table can be constructed for 'doubtfuls'. The Bayesian expression is used with test performance probabilities selected from one of the four headings: pass test 1, pass test 2; pass test 1, fail test 2; fail test 1, pass test 2; fail test 1, fail test 2, depending on the test scores from the patient.

The Bayesian view

When probabilites defined as relative frequences of occurrence are available, the above use of Bayes' theorem is non-controversial, being a logical consequence of the laws of probability. However, the Bayesian view is more radical in holding that probability can be subjectively interpretated as 'degrees of belief' for which an ideally rational person conforms to the mathematical principles of probability. For example, if my degree of belief that a patient has a disease is p then my degree of belief that the patient does not have the disease should be (1-p). For a Bayesian, prior opinion expressed in the form of subjective probabilities should be incorporated into the formal procedures so that judgement can be publicly displayed. In the absence of further evidence, the initial subjective probabilities might well conform to the incidence probabilities. However, this need not be the case as the probabilities stand for opinions held by the clinician. Thus beliefs (prior probabilities) are modified by evidence to yield new beliefs (posterior probabilities) which then become in turn prior probabilities for subsequent new evidence. A scientist or clinician should quantify his opinions as probabilities either by calculation or more practically in the case of a clinician, by subjective estimation before collecting data, then proceed to collect the data and subsequently use Bayes' theorem formally to revise those opinions. Ideally therefore, for a Bayesian, learning should go by these revised probability values.

A high posterior probability associated with a hypothesis does not guarantee its truth but only indicates it is the most likely among those considered. So by this cyclical or iterative process data is collected which bears on the relative truth of alternative hypotheses (or diagnoses). The Bayesian argues that the traditional null hypothesis is rarely of interest and represents only one of several alternative hypotheses. Moreover, in assessing the null-hypothesis one relies on fairly arbitrary conventions whose Bayesian equivalents would be to conclude in favour of a hypothesis when you are 95% or 99% certain.

DECISION ANALYSIS

In decision analysis all possible outcomes or consequences of an action must be stated, must be assigned a probability estimate and must be assigned a value of importance. The Bayesian approach to decision making requires that a rational person pursues a course of action which makes the best consequences most probable. A maximum is sought for the expected value (EV) of a consequence where:

$$EV = \sum_{i=1}^{m} P_i v_i$$

in which P_i denotes the probability of event i and v_i denotes its value. Bother variables can be assessed either objectively or subjectively as probability and value, or as subjective probability and utility respectively. In the Bayesian framework where both variables are subjectively assessed we seek to maximise subjective expected utility (SEU).

Measuring belief as subjective probability

In many situations, definitive clinical data is not available and the clinician must rely on his own past experience. In such circumstances it is beneficial to make clinical estimates explicit by means of subjective probabilities. Of several alternative methods the 'equivalent urn' is perhaps the simplest.

Suppose we wish to assess a clinician's belief about the success or failure of a particular treatment. We may present him with the following two lotteries:

Lottery 1 Win £100 if the treatment succeeds, win £0 if the treatment fails.

Lottery 2 Win £100 if a black ball is drawn from the urn, win £0 if a white ball is drawn.

(Imagine an opaque urn containing 100 balls, p of which are black and (100 – p) of which are white). The task is to find the value of p for which both lotteries are equivalent to the decision maker. This value of p is the subjective probability representing the individual's personal belief about treatment success.

For example, if when there were 50 black and 50 white balls in the urn, lottery 1 was preferred to lottery 2 then we assume that the subjective probability of the treatment's success is >0.5. If on the other hand with 90 black and 10 white balls in the urn, lottery 2 was preferred to lottery 1 then the subjective probability of the treatment's success must be <0.9. The normal method of limits can be used to home-in on the threshold point where the individual is indifferent between the two lotteries. If this occurred when there were 75 black and 25 white balls in the urn we conclude the subjective probability of the treatment's success is 0.75. The concept of a matching range or a range of equivalence can be used as an indicator of the variance of the measurement with the mid-point of the range the best index of uncertainty.

This method of paired comparision between lotteries can be extended to the case of three or more discrete variables. If the three uncertainty options were: patient gets worse (prob. P_1); patient stays the same (prob. P_2); patient gets better (prob. P_3); then the first decision could be 'patient gets worse' (P_1) against its complement 'patient does not get worse' ($1–P_1$) or ($P_2 + P_3$). Once this probability has been assessed a second decision could be made on the alternative 'patient stays the same' (P_2) against 'patient gets better' (P_3).

Finally the ratios between the values must be preserved so that all three values add up to unity.

Measuring value as utility

Utility measurement is concerned with the assignment of subjective values of consequences or outcomes. The utility ascribed to the consequence of an action is always contingent upon the particular conditions, and the method of assessing utilites takes this relative feature into account.

The assessment begins by assigning a utility of 1 to the outcome which is considered the best of those available and a utility of 0 to the outcome which is considered the worst of those available. Paired lotteries are then presented to the decision maker to determine the utilities of intermediate outcomes. For example, in assessing the utility of the intermediate outcome I_1 the decision maker is presented with two options:

Lottery 1 Receive I_1 for certain

Lottery 2 Receive the best outcome with probability p and the worst outcome with probability $(1-P)$.

The value of P for which the decision maker finds the two lotteries equivalent represents the utility outcome I_1. The procedure is then re-presented for a new intermediate outcome I_2. Only a small number of intermediate outcomes is needed to generate a utility function from which other utilities can be interpolated. The shape of the utility function reflects the risk taking behaviour of the decision maker, (see Fig. 20.4).

Many decision problems require utility functions of more than one variable. For example, in the dislocation of the hip problem we considered parental anxiety, cost of after care management, and state of health. One of the simplest practical ways of dealing with this problem is to use a weighted additive utility model:

$$u_x = \sum_{i=1}^{k} b_i x_i$$

where x_i denotes the value of dimension i while b_i denotes its weight. Weights can be assigned to dimensions by simply letting numbers reflect the relative importance of the dimension. (For further details of all measurement procedures see Kaufman & Thomas, 1977; Kozieleki, 1982; Aspinall & Hill, 1983). It is advisable to precede such strategies of compensation by a threshold strategy which eliminates from consideration those outcomes which do not reach an acceptable level on any dimension.

THE MODEL

In designing a screening programme according to the foregoing principles the following five stages should be observed:

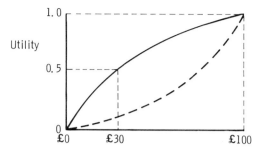

Fig. 20.4 Utility function expressed in monetary terms for a risk avoider (————) and a risk seeker (----).

Stage 1. The screening or decision problem is clarified by drawing a simple decision tree to represent actions and events in the sequence in which they occur. Here the decision maker must specify the realistic alternatives open to him and the areas of risk and uncertainty involved.

Stage 2. The probabilities and utilities must be attached to all appropriate branches of the decision tree.

Stage 3. The subjective expected utility (SEU) (assuming probability and value are subjectively assessed) is calculated for each node of the decision tree working from right to left (i.e. the reverse order in which the events occur in time).

Stage 4. The action with the greatest SEU is the chosen one.

Stage 5. The sensitivity is checked by adjusting the judgemental inputs to reflect their variance, e.g. pessimistic values which are 'almost certain to be exceeded' can be used as input. This has the effect not only of checking the stability of the decision tree but also of highlighting the crucial factors in the decision problem.

A simple example

Consider the question of whether to introduce a new screening test into a clinic. Let us assume there are three consequences of the decision involving: State of health(H), cost of screening(C), discomfort to the patient(D).

Assume H has three levels $H_1 H_2 H_3$ where H_1 is most preferred. The intermediate outcome H_2 is assessed at a utility of 0.7. Utilities for $H_1 H_2 H_3$ are therefore 1, 0.7, 0 respectively.

Assume C has two levels C_1 = no cost, C_2 = cost of screening test including time and capital outlay. Utilities for C_1 and C_2 are therefore 1 and 0 respectively.

Assume D has two levels D_1 = no discomfort, D_2 = discomfort to the patient arising from the application of the screening test. Utilities for D_1 and D_2 are therefore 1 and 0 respectively. (For simplicity, we will ignore consequences of not detecting the condition at an early stage with subsequent later costs, discomforts and altered probabilities of recovery).

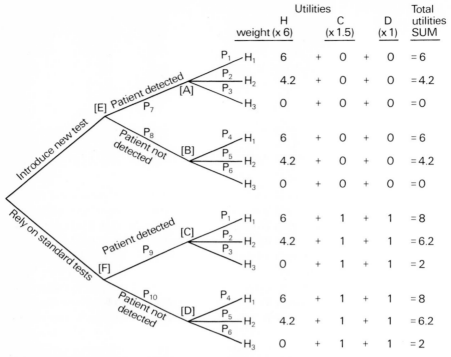

Fig. 20.5 Decision tree for a screening problem with uncertainties assessed as subjective probabilities and values assessed as utilities for the estimated states of health (H), cost of screening (C) and discomfort to the patient (D).

Suppose the decision maker considers H four times as important as C which is half again as important as D. Weights for dimensions H, C and D are therefore 6, 1.5, 1 respectively.

The problem is illustrated in Fig. 20.5 in which utilities have been calculated for clarity, but probabilities specified as P_1 to P_{10}.

For junction A

$$SEU = 6P_1 + 4.2P_2 + 0P_3 = U_A$$

For junction B

$$SEU = 6P_4 + 4.2P_5 + 0P_6 = U_B$$

For junction C

$$SEU = 8P_1 + 6.2P_2 + 2P_3 = U_C$$

For junction D

$$SEU = 8P_4 + 6.2P_5 + 2P_6 = U_D$$

For junction E

$$SEU = U_A P_7 + U_B P_8 = U_E$$

For junction F

$$SEU = U_C P_9 + U_D P_{10} = U_F$$

If $U_E > U_F$ then the best decision would be to introduce the new screening test. If $U_F > U_E$ the clinic should continue to rely on existing standard tests.

SOME PRACTICAL PROBLEMS

It will be realised that it is only possible to determine the sensitivity and specificity of a clinical test where there is an accepted validating criterion against which the performance of that test can be compaired. Consequently, if a test is quoted as having a sensitivity of 0.9, this implies that another test procedure must exist for which the sensitivity is defined and accepted as being 100%. Such a test procedure is known as the validating criterion. In screening, the validating criterion is generally taken to be the result of full clinical examination. The theoretical assumption here, of course, is that there are no misclassification errors associated with decisions based upon the clinically determined information. Occasions do arise, however, when new tests are developed for the earlier detection of a disease or clinical condition in babies for which existing testing procedures have proved inadequate. In such instances, the evaluation of the new test should be based on the results of a prospective study. Performance on the new test may then be assessed against the currently accepted validating criterion of a full clinical investigation when the child is old enough to be examined reliably.

Nevertheless, some new tests are introduced into clinical practice where validation is either not available or perhaps not even possible. The new test therefore becomes its own reference datum. An example of such a test in child health is the recent introduction of the Auditory Response Cradle which has been designed for the detection of hearing impairment in neonates. It is claimed that this test will function on babies as young as 1 day old, whereas currently accepted procedures of hearing assessment require the child to be $2\frac{1}{2}$ to 3 years of age before reliable results are obtained. The value of the new test, it is argued, is that although nothing can be done surgically or medically in most instances of neonatal hearing impairment, it is possible to amplify the sound level to permit for an improvement in normal language development. Since the incidence of babies at risk from hearing impairment is of the order of 0.1%, it will be appreciated from Bayesian inference that even if the new test is found to have a sensitivity and specificity of 0.999 (and very few tests are as good as this), the probability that hearing impairment is present in the light of evidence from the test is no better than chance at $P = 0.5$. It is clear, therefore, that paediatricians whose patient management would be influenced by results from an Auditory Response Cradle must interpret the test data in one of two ways. Either they ascribe subjective probabilities of $P = 1.0$ to the test outcomes for the presence or absence of hearing impairment requiring treatment or management (i.e. the test is seen as the defining criterion for the presence or absence of the condition), or they implicitly assign far greater importance or utlity to not providing hearing assistance in an undetected defective child (i.e. false-negative) than to the inappropriate treatment or management of a child with normal hearing (i.e. false-positive). This example serves to illustrate the difficulties associated with the introduction of a new test in the absence of a comparable validating criterion and emphasises to the user of such a test the need for quantifying the emphasis which is being placed on decisions associated both with misclassifications and correct test outcomes. We have shown how Bayesian principles of decision analysis may be used for this purpose.

In the practice of screening it is self-evident that a screening test designed to detect a specific clinical condition will be of little or no value in screening for other conditions. Consequently, most mass screening programmes are multiphasic involving tests on a variety of functions. It is important there-fore, to distinguish between multiphasic test batteries and specific test batteries. The former involves independent screening for several unrelated clinical conditions, while the latter involves using independent tests as a means of improving specificity and/or sensitivity in the detection of a single clinical condition. (For the use of test batteries in colour vision screening see Chapter 5).

One of the problems associated with screening for specific conditions is that by concentrating our attention on looking for a single sign or set of signs, it is possible to overlook other signs which would indicate the presence of a different pathology. This becomes a particularly important problem if the screening procedures involve clinical judgement. What is not generally appreciated in these circumstances (such as in the screening examination for congenital hip dislocation), is that we approach the patient with preconceived ideas of what to expect and what not to expect. An effect of this attitudinal or perceptual bias is such that we interpret the information received from the screening examination in terms of our past experience and expectations. There are numerous examples of this sort of problem in radiological screening procedures where frequently inter and intra observer variation in reading radiographs is surprisingly high. We therefore need to be aware of the fact that where clinical judgements are involved most of these will be influenced by unconscious factors involving both past experience and what we believe to be true. According to Abercrombie (1969), we may learn to make better judgements if we become aware of the factors that influence their formation. Clearly, the less dependent a screening test is on clinical experi-ence for collection of the information about an individual, the less likely it is to be influenced by personal perceptual factors.

CONCLUSION

In this discussion of screening we have adopted the functional definition that it is a procedure designed to distinguish between those individuals who would benefit and those who are not likely to benefit from further clinical investigation. In doing so, it is necessary to invoke the concept of differentiating between clinical normality and disease. Because health and disease know no sharp boundaries we accept there are considerable difficulties attached to the concept of what is normal. The user of a screening programme, therefore, should be aware of the limitations associated with defining the condition for which the test is a predictor. A misleading but frequently prevalent attitude in screening is to look upon those individuals who pass a test as being free from the condition which the screening programme is designed to detect. As we have shown, this assumption cannot be made unreservedly because of the possibility of false-negative misclassifications. Consequently, in practice, the emphasis in screening is usually to reduce the number of false-negatives to an acceptable size and thereby aim towards a high test specificity. Where a single cut-off criterion is used, it will be realised that this is always achieved at the expense of test sensitivity.

In assessing the appropriateness of a cut-off criterion on a screening test it will be evident that the user needs to draw on many sources of information, but difficulties frequently arise because hard evidence is not always available. In these instances it is important that procedures are adopted for making explicit clinical impressions about the likelihoods and utilities associated with the various test outcomes. Earlier approaches to the economics of screening assumed that such procedures were not available for quantifying the benefits in relation to costs (see Teeling-Smith, 1975). We have shown, however, that the application of a Bayesian approach to decision analysis provides a framework within which all relevant factors may be considered quantitatively. By this means the designer or user of any screening programme has a rational model and procedure for evaluating its efficiency and utility. Whatever the purpose for which a screening test is to be used it is therefore possible to provide an informed and reasoned answer to the question 'Is screening worthwhile?'

REFERENCES

Abercrombie M L J 1969 The Anatomy of Judgement. Penguin Books, Harmondsworth
Aspinall P A, Hill A R 1983 Clinical inferences and decisions. Ophthalmic and Physiological Optics, 3 (3), in press
Fryback D 1974 Bayes' theorem and non-independence of data in a medical diagnosis task. University of Michigan, MMPP, pp 74–77
Hart C R 1975 Screening in General Practice. Churchill Livingstone, Edinburgh
Jacquez J, Norusis M 1976 The importance of symptom non-independence in diagnosis. In: F T de Dombal, F Gremy (ed) Decision Making in Medical Care. North Holland, Amsterdam
Kaufman G, Thomas H 1977 Modern Decision Analysis. Penguin Books, Harmondsworth
Kozielecki J 1982 Psychological Decision Theory. D Reidl, London
Lusted L B 1967 Medical decision making. Digest 7th Int. Conf. on Medical and Biological Engineering, Stockholm
Lusted L B 1976 Clinical decision making. In: F T de Dombal, F Gremy (ed) Decision Making and Medical Care. North Holland, Amsterdam
Teeling-Smith G 1975 The economics of screening. In: C R Hart (ed) Screening in General Practice. Churchill Livingstone, Edinburgh

Index